T0211344

TREATING OUT OF CONTROL SEXUAL BEHAVIOR

Douglas Braun-Harvey, LMFT, CGP, CST, is a sexual health author, trainer, and psychotherapist who bridges sexual and mental health and facilitates organizational change. In 2013, Doug Braun-Harvey cofounded The Harvey Institute, an international education, training, consulting, and supervision service for improving health care through integration of sexual health. He teaches and trains nationally and internationally, linking sexual health principles with drug and alcohol treatment, group psychotherapy, HIV prevention and treatment, and child maltreatment. Since 1993, he has been developing and implementing a sexual health-based treatment approach for men with out of control sexual behavior (OCSB). Previous publications include *Sexual Health in Recovery: Professional Counselor's Manual* (2011) and *Sexual Health in Drug and Alcohol Treatment: Group Facilitator's Manual* (2009). He has earned several distinctions, including the 2013 Carne's Award from the Society for the Advancement of Sexual Health, a 2011 Sexual Intelligence Award, the 2011 President's Award from the National Association of Lesbian and Gay Addiction Professionals, and the 2011 Society for the Scientific Study of Sexuality Western Region Public Service Award for promoting sexual health awareness and providing the intellectual framework for integrating sexology and chemical dependency. Mr. Braun-Harvey is a licensed marriage and family therapist (MFT), certified group psychotherapist (CGP), and certified sex therapist (AASECT Certified). He is on the web at www.DBHnow.com and in private practice in San Diego, California.

Michael A. Vigorito, LMFT, LCPC, CGP, is a sexual health consultant, author, and psychotherapist. As a consultant, Mr. Vigorito trains behavioral health providers to integrate sexual health into their systems of care through routine sexual health screenings, sexual risk reduction counseling, and culturally competent interventions. As a clinician, Mr. Vigorito developed, supervised, and conducted therapy in integrative behavioral health programs that worked with substance addiction, mental illness, and HIV/AIDS. In his Washington, DC, private practice, Mr. Vigorito provides individual, couple, and group psychotherapy specializing in sexual health, including out of control sexual experiences, sexual dysfunctions, sex/drug-linked behaviors, and sexual dissatisfaction. He is licensed as a marriage and family therapist (MFT), licensed clinical professional counselor, and is a certified group psychotherapist. Mr. Vigorito is also a member of the American Group Psychotherapy Association; the Society for the Scientific Study of Sexuality; and the American Association of Sex Educators, Counselors, and Therapists. More about Mr. Vigorito can be found at www.iCounselingServices.com.

TREATING OUT OF CONTROL SEXUAL BEHAVIOR

RETHINKING SEX ADDICTION

Douglas Braun-Harvey, LMFT, CGP, CST
Michael A. Vigorito, LMFT, LCPC, CGP

SPRINGER PUBLISHING COMPANY
NEW YORK

Springer Publishing Company, LLC
11 West 42nd Street
New York, NY 10036
www.springerpub.com

Acquisitions Editor: Nancy S. Hale
Production Editor: Pamela Lankas
Composition: MPS Ltd, India

ISBN: 978-0-8261-9675-0
e-book ISBN: 978-0-8261-9676-7

15 16 17 18 19 / 5 4 3 2 1

Library of Congress Cataloging-in-Publication Data

Braun-Harvey, Douglas, author.
    Treating out of control sexual behavior : rethinking sex addiction /
Douglas Braun-Harvey, Michael A. Vigorito.
        p. ; cm.
    Includes bibliographical references and index.
    ISBN 978-0-8261-9675-0—ISBN 978-0-8261-9676-7 (ebook)
    I. Vigorito, Michael A., author. II. Title.
    [DNLM: 1. Sexual Behavior—psychology.   2. Sexual Dysfunctions, Psychological—therapy.
    3. Behavior, Addictive—therapy.   WM 611]
    RC560.S43
    616.85'83306—dc23
                                                                        2015023372

Printed in the United States of America by McNaughton & Gunn.

To the hundreds of men who entrusted us with their sexual health care.

Contents

FOREWORD

Over 100 years ago, Freud discussed his theories about sexuality, describing how repression and the cultural mores of Victorian society, as well as the unchained instinctual search for pleasure, significantly disrupted child development and the behaviors of adults. He would be totally amazed and confused by the lack of repression and the flaunting of sexuality in every aspect of modern Western life. He might assume that the release of repression and the advances in our understanding of sexuality would bring enlightenment, intelligent and open conversations about sexuality, and a clear perspective on the role of healthy sexuality in human development and behavior. Unfortunately, such is not the case. Sexual assault, rape, pedophilia and other nonconsensual sexual behaviors, as well as a host of other consensual or solitary sexual activities and sexual risk-taking behaviors abound in our society. Freedom often becomes license. Sexual behaviors, which are inherently reinforced and evolutionarily important, spiral out of control for individuals, for our institutions—like college campuses and the military—and for our society as a whole.

Human sexuality is an integral part of being human and the foundation of intimate relationships and a healthy society. It is not a necessary evil or something that should be shrouded in secrecy and shame. Pathologizing, stigmatizing, labeling, and criminalizing deviations from what are considered "acceptable" sexual behavior have not helped individuals and, more important, societal leaders and healers to understand sexual health or to adequately address sexual behaviors that feel out of control. As with all appetitive human behaviors, the goal is to manage and self-regulate so that the behavior is in the zone of what I call "self-regulated behaviors" that are under self-control and are upregulated or downregulated as needed based on internal and external feedback about the behavior. However, all appetitive behaviors can spiral out of control— seeking satisfaction without responsibility, engaging in repetitive patterns that are harmful—bringing serious consequences and becoming less and less pleasurable as they become more and more automatic and excessive. Such are the out of control sexual behaviors described in this book.

However, the focus should not be solely on loss of control or problematic sexual behaviors. As described in the World Health Organization's (WHO; 2006, p. 6) definition of sexual health, the focus should be on "physical, emotional, mental and social well-being in relation to sexuality." Yet, sexual health involves an even larger conversation, and should be focused on "pleasurable and safe sexual experiences, free of coercion, discrimination and violence" (WHO, 2006, p. 6).

Doug Braun-Harvey and Michael Vigorito have entered the field of human sexual behavior with a clear perspective on the discipline's extensive history of confusing and conflicting conversations and research about excessive and harmful sexual behaviors. Their focus on out of control sexual behaviors and the deeply humanistic and respectful manner in which they address these behaviors is not only refreshing but offers all providers an exciting new view and innovative way of addressing these behaviors in an effective, compassionate, and client-centered manner. In this volume, they help providers to begin to confront the often hidden prejudices and superficial knowledge about sexuality that they bring to conversations with clients. Offhand remarks, embarrassed silence, stigmatizing comments, or complete uncritical acceptance are not the foundation for the types of conversations that individuals engaging in out of control sexual behaviors need. The process of change must begin with an understanding, open, caring, and collaborative conversation with any client considering whether, how, and what to change.

Although focused on out of control sexual behavior (OCSB), this volume offers a wealth of information about sexual health and how conversations about sex must move beyond sexually transmitted disease and pathology. We must shift the focus from "using condoms and protecting against pregnancy" to how to appreciate and understand our bodies and engage in behaviors that enable us to be physically, mentally, and sexually healthy and happy. Sex in the shadows, survivor sex, shame and stigma, as well as adverse early sexual experiences and poor education lead to the silence and secrecy that undermine sexual health. The wealth of information and the assessment and intervention strategies highlighted in this book can enable therapists and providers of all types to effectively bring the sensitive topic of sex into the daylight and open air of constructive conversations. Braun-Harvey and Vigorito offer a comprehensive and clear discussion and framework for addressing sexual health and out of control sexual behaviors in a collaborative and motivationally enhancing manner.

The process of change is a journey, and clients need empathy, support, accurate information, feedback, guidance, and the skills to make the change. These are needed so clients can successfully negotiate the multiple tasks of the journey to successful and sustained change. This book offers the authors' wisdom, accumulated through many years of experience helping people change, both in individual counseling and in groups focused on sexual health. Their experience makes the case vignettes and the many interactions highlighted in the text real and relevant. The principles and practices outlined here are very well described and come alive with the many and varied vignettes describing interactions between clients and counselor. Even more interesting, they describe some conversations between Doug and Michael as they colead groups and do not always agree on the best way to ask a question or make an intervention. This dialogue offers a way for the reader to explore different approaches and to understand that approaches to intervening with a client on any specific topic involving a choice should reflect thoughtful and sensitive listening to the client; empathy; and sound, critical self-assessment.

I am currently completing a collaborative project funded by the Substance Abuse and Mental Health Services Administration, titled "No Wrong Door," that is attempting to ensure that individuals entering primary care, mental health, and substance abuse portals seeking treatment will be assessed and offered treatment for all their concerns. More important, when needed, these individuals will be offered counseling not only for sexual risk reduction but also for sexual health. As we attempt to undertake this challenge, we need well-trained counselors who are able to address the sexual health needs of clients. One hopes this volume will empower generations of counselors to be more proactive and effective in meeting the needs of individuals with "out of control sexual behaviors" that often lead to significant interpersonal, social, and personal consequences, with the goal of helping them to achieve and maintain sexual health.

CARLO C. DICLEMENTE, PhD, ABPP

REFERENCE

World Health Organization. (2006). *Defining sexual health: Report of a technical consultation on sexual health 28–31 January 2002*. Geneva, Switzerland: Author.

Acknowledgments

Sexual health conversations matter. This book is an outgrowth of countless professional exchanges, research, and years of clinical application integrating a broad range of scholarship. Beyond the learning afforded us by the publications cited throughout this book are the discussions with trusted friends and colleagues that have guided, critiqued, and supported us as we organized our thoughts and experience into this clinical model for treating out of control sexual behavior.

We have relied upon numerous colleagues' critical feedback and generosity long before we imagined writing this book. A gracious thank you to Michael Berry, Vena Blanchard, Eli Coleman, Rebecca Cutter, Marcus Earle, Ralph Earle, Thomas Ellis, Marc Gilmartin, Irwin Goldstein, Bill Herring, Sheri Kirshenbaum, Marty Klein, Joe Kort, Chris Kraft, Jack Morin, Rory Reid, Esther Perel, Anna Randall, Edita Ruzgyte, Larry Siegel, Ricky Siegel, Tony Stiker, Charles Samenow, and the men of Doug's San Diego consultation group. We are so deeply grateful for your encouragement and willingness to honestly share your thoughts and to promote our ideas for out of control sexual behavior treatment.

We refined and developed our model over many years of professional dialogue and networking at conferences and professional forums. We have been privileged to present our emerging OCSB assessment and treatment model to the American Association of Sexuality Educators, Counselors and Therapists (AASECT); American Group Psychotherapy Association (AGPA); California Association of Marriage & Family Therapists (CAMFT); Guttman & Pearl Associates in Washington, DC; The Intimacy Institute in Boulder, CO; Professional Counseling Services in Phoenix, AZ; Psychotherapy Networker Symposium in Washington, DC; San Diego Sexual Medicine; Sex Therapy, Education and Medicine (STEM) in San Diego, CA; the Society for the Advancement of Sexual Health (SASH); and the Society for the Scientific Study of Sexuality (SSSS).

For over 20 years the San Diego psychotherapy community has been fertile ground for clinical wisdom and collaborative relationships. Treating out of control sexual behavior is a collaborative process that relies on a community-based treatment team to address the multiple factors contributing to men's sexual behavior problems. We thank Steve Alper, Garet Bedrosian, Dan Bjierke, Shannon Chavez, Clark Clipson, David Garmon, Randy Hicks, Jeff Jones, Peter McDade, Michael McDaniel, Katie O'Brasky, Dan Offner, James Reavis, Jennifer Rehor, G. Michael Scott, Davey Smith, Trish Stanley, Gloria Shurman, Paul Sussman, Jim Weinrich, and David Wexler. They have offered their collaborative spirit and tremendous talent to form a local treatment network for meeting our clients' diverse needs.

We invited colleagues from the San Diego treatment community to attend an external review process to further shape our assessment and treatment model. Thank you to Kathleen Burns, Anne Clarkin, John DeMiranda, David Garmon, Sue Goldstein, Diana Guest, Rose Hartzell-Cushanick, Tom Hollander, Al Killen-Harvey, Tom Horvath, Gregory Koch, Jim Lair, L. C. Miccio-Fonseca, Terri Martin, Bob McClure, Julieanne Myers, Charlie Nelson, Dan Offner, Diane Pendragon, Yaron Pruginin, Peter Roussos, Carrie Sakai, Joseph Severino, Peter Wayson, and Mary Wheeler. Their informative feedback and observations strengthened our early book outline.

After his relocation to the District of Columbia, Michael feels particularly grateful for the opportunity to collaborate and establish a local community network that made his transition both rewarding and enjoyable. Thank you to Peter Chirinos, Michael Giordano, Krystal Ginzl, Catherine Grothus, Gail Guttman, Chris Kraft, Sean LeSane, David McCall, Gwen Pearl, Tamara Pincus, Charles Samenow, and Chris Straley.

We are grateful for the generosity of time and critical thinking of trusted colleagues and content experts who commented on early chapter drafts: Stacy Bubhe, Neil Cannon, Clark Clipson, Eli Coleman, David Delmonico, John Giugliano, Elizabeth Griffin, Bill Herring, L. C. Miccio-Fonseca, and Julieanne Myers. Thank you.

Shamaine Cardoza, Michael Giancola and Joseph Severino participated in a professional Advanced Training Program with Doug in which they co-led groups and provided OCSB screening, assessment, and treatment under his supervision. Mentoring, supervising and educating these fine professionals was vital to developing the transferable knowledge and clinical application of the OCSB model well beyond the minds of its originators.

Since its inception, our editor, Nancy S. Hale, has believed in the value of this book. She understood the need for sexual health texts for clinicians and psychotherapists. Her flexibility and ongoing support were essential in each stage of development and publication. We are deeply grateful to Jesse Richards who created the visual representations of the OCSB Clinical Pathway that elucidate and enliven the OCSB model.

As in life, books also need good editors. In addition to the editing from our publisher, John Hammond, Peter Wayson, and Al Killen-Harvey contributed their editing skills and keen critical minds to the first two sections of the book. Their eye for clarity, composition, and maintaining reader interest were vital in shaping the final manuscript.

Lastly, our friends and family have been patiently waiting for our return from the two years spent composing this manuscript. Time usually spent nurturing these relationships was shortchanged by writing. We appreciate their patience and encouragement over the last two years and now delight in returning to the joy of these relationships.

A personal note from Doug to his husband and life partner of 28 years. Al, how do I express my appreciation and love for your attending to our home, friendships, family, and professional work? The seeds for this book germinated in your observation that I am happiest when I am writing and you were ready for me to write another book. Thank you for your generosity in making space for me to write on weekends and holidays, which too often meant not spending time with you.

These are important times for sexual health. Every sexual health conversation with our colleagues, friends, and family is reflected in these pages. *Treating Out of Control Sexual Behavior: Rethinking Sexual Addiction* is a true representation of how much we value collaboration and our investment in providing compassionate, respectful, and informed care to clients seeking help with their sexual health.

INTRODUCTION

Compulsive sexual behavior and sexual addiction treatment models were introduced over 30 years ago and sparked a debate that has yet to be resolved. Is sexual behavior dysregulation a disease rooted in a process addiction or a disorder stemming from a psychosexual pathology? With hundreds of sexuality, addiction, neuroscience, and psychological studies and thousands of psychotherapists providing specialized clinical interventions, there is still no consensus regarding etiological or best treatment practices for out of control sexual behavior (OCSB). However, the lack of scientific and clinical consensus has not discouraged men and women from seeking help for what they experience as sexual dysregulation. During these same three decades, the World Health Organization, the U.S. surgeon general, and other distinguished bodies began defining the concept of sexual health. Since the mid-1970s, notions of sexual health moved beyond the absence of sexually transmitted diseases and unintended pregnancies to encompass issues of human rights, consent, nonexploitation, pleasure, and access to sexuality education. Just as definitions of sexual health moved beyond the focus of disease prevention and treatment, could current discourse benefit from shifting the focus toward a sexual health approach for understanding and treating sexual behavioral problems?

Treating Out of Control Sexual Behavior: Rethinking Sex Addiction is our sexual health approach for the assessment and treatment of cisgender men motivated to change consensual sexual behavior that feels out of their control. In the following chapters, we introduce our conceptualization of OCSB and our assessment and treatment pathway, which grew from many years of providing individual and group psychotherapy to men of all sexual orientations motivated to improve their sexual health.

We began this project by delving into the literature on sex addiction, impulsive/compulsive sexual behavior, and hypersexual behavior. We were dispirited by the emphasis to establish and defend a singular pathological pathway or clinical disorder that did not reflect the symptom complexity found among our clients. It was common to read studies that merged consensual and nonconsensual sexual behaviors in their population samples or clinical approaches. Further, emerging substance addiction neuroimaging research was often overgeneralized and too eagerly cited as support for sexual addiction etiology. This resulted in sociocultural sex negativity being camouflaged within medical or mental health language while premature conclusions advanced diagnostic labels despite the lack of randomized clinical trails, evidence-based practices, or scientific consensus. Diagnostic labels were proposed as psychiatric disorders only to be rejected for lack of scientific agreement.

Absent a theoretical and clinical consensus among mental health professionals, our research expanded to human behavior and wellness literature. This led to articles and models that shed light on problems of decision making, self-regulation, and behavior. We studied positive psychology, sexology, attachment theory, mindfulness, and behavioral economics. We became increasingly interested in resolving men's sexual behavior problems by *moving them toward sexual health* rather than limiting treatment to what seemed an increasingly moribund goal of diagnosis and amelioration of a contentiously debated pathological state.

Our primary task was to synthesize and apply this diverse literature to OCSB treatment. It was not until we read the work of integrative psychotherapists that we fully appreciated what we had undertaken. Integrative psychotherapy explains human behavior by integrating physiological, affective, cognitive, behavioral, and systemic approaches understood within stages of human development and the wide range of human functioning (Erskine & Moursund, 2011). Integrative psychotherapy principles construct frameworks for understanding the multivariate factors that contribute to complex behavioral problems. The integrative psychotherapy mission, to join components of effective therapy that cut across theoretical approaches and client populations, affirms our investment in psychotherapy best practices as a foundation for OCSB assessment and treatment.

Our purpose for writing *Treating Out of Control Sexual Behavior: Rethinking Sex Addiction* is to provide clinicians a resource for establishing an individual and/or group psychotherapy relationship with men wanting to change and to improve their sexual health. Numerous books have been written that prescribe generalized counseling techniques for anyone in sexual addiction treatment. Absent from much of the materials was how to be a sexual addiction therapist in relationship with clients.

In his recent article, "What Should We Expect From Psychotherapy?" Stony Brook University psychologist Marvin Goldfried (2013) summarized five common change principles in effective psychotherapy:

1. Fostering the expectation that therapy can help
2. Forming an optimal therapeutic alliance
3. Raising client awareness about the factors contributing to their problems (in themselves, others, and their environment)
4. Facilitating corrective experiences
5. Ongoing reality testing

He additionally cites client motivation to change (Prochaska & DiClemente, 2005) along with interventions that enhance motivation (Miller & Rollnick, 2013) as significant components for effective therapy. The therapeutic alliance, however, is viewed as "most essential to the change process," which includes the therapeutic bond and the agreement on goals and methods by client and therapist (Goldfried, 2013, p. 867).

Our emphasis on the collaborative therapeutic relationship and creating a unique vision of each man's sexual health vision distinguishes OCSB treatment from most current addiction and psychosexual disorder models. Rather than proscribe a series of tasks for the client to complete under the direction of a trained certified therapist, this book guides clinicians on how to be a therapist in relationship with men seeking to build and define a personal vision of sexual health.

We were inspired by Goldried's "change principles" when structuring the three sections of *Treating Out of Control Sexual Behavior: Rethinking Sex Addiction*. Section 1 establishes the foundation for a sexual health approach to addressing out of control sexual behavior. In it, we review how our sexual health framework supports essential relationship skills to prepare client and therapist to enjoin in a collaborative process of change. Further, we introduce a dual-process model of human behavior to contextualize the internal and external factors that contribute to a client's out of control sexual behavior. Section 2 outlines the OCSB screening procedure and assessment plan. We describe the dual purpose of identifying vulnerability factors and competing motivations that contribute to sexual behavior problems and the psychotherapy techniques research suggests enhance client motivation for behavior change. Section 3 builds on the previous two sections by discussing combined individual and group therapy principles and practices designed to facilitate corrective emotional experiences and support men moving toward their personal vision of sexual health.

We begin the book by introducing you to composite client stories compiled from over 250 men treated since 1993. The book ends with treatment highlights from four of these cases. Sprinkled throughout the book are sample client dialogues that provide examples of individual and group psychotherapy to illustrate a particular aspect of the OCSB Model.

PROTOCOL DESIGN METHODS

We also want to be transparent about our motivations for applying the research and literature presented in the book. Evidence-based practices guided the development of our OCSB treatment model. However, the OCSB Clinical Pathway is also an outgrowth of integrating these studies with actual client symptoms and narratives. As so many clinicians know, the realities of practice require consistent decision making, flexibility, and reevaluation that are not always mirrored in social science experiments. Each OCSB protocol component balances the scientific literature with our clinical experience.

We first presented the early musings for our model at the 2008 Society for the Scientific Study of Sexuality, Western Region (SSSSWR) conference. In the ensuing 7 years, we have presented adaptations and refinements of what is now this book. We want to thank SSSSWR as well as the American Association of Sex Educators, Counselors and Therapists (AASECT), Society for the Advancement of Sexual Health (SASH), American Group Psychotherapy Association (AGPA), California Association of Marriage & Family Therapists (CAMFT), and the national meeting for the Society for the Scientific Study of Sexuality (SSSS) for providing opportunities for much needed dialogue and critical thinking in the development of our treatment method. In 2012, we conducted several external review sessions in San Diego to ascertain feedback from invited therapists, researchers, addiction treatment professionals, and sexologists. We are immensely grateful for the many esteemed colleagues from psychotherapy, sex research, sex therapy, and forensic psychology who agreed to preview and critique early chapter drafts.

PROTOCOL DESIGN INFLUENCES

Vetting the OCSB protocol did not remove our personal values from the protocol design. We began to see the influence of our personal experiences when we were formulating ethical principles for OCSB treatment.

Our emphasis on establishing an ethical foundation could not be separated from living as gay men in the 35-year shadow of the AIDS pandemic. A seminal historical narrative for us was remembering when providers were caught up in the sexual panic of the early stages of the AIDS crisis before the countervailing forces of public health research and patient-rights advocacy reshaped health care delivery. As a consequence of this legacy, we were skeptical of psychotherapeutic techniques designed to treat clients with sexual behaviors considered socially unacceptable and treated in the absence of rigorous scientific research. As a result, we grounded the OCSB Model in ethical standards of care to promote a psychotherapy space free of the similar sexual stigma that often contaminated the relationships between patient and provider during the AIDS crisis.

We regard the therapeutic alliance as the highest priority when conducting OCSB treatment. To best establish this relationship, it is incumbent upon providers to conduct a thorough self-evaluation to address any personal discomfort with sexual diversity that may interfere with their ability to empathize and join with their clients whose sexual behaviors are often deemed disgusting, perverted, dangerous, excessive, sinful, and unhealthy by mainstream society. We suggest you read this book with both your professional mind as well as a personal process for self-reflection. How do your life experience and sexual values influence your work? How do you resolve personal and professional discomfort with detailed sexual health conversations? What checks and balances do you use to suspend your judgments that, left unchecked, will inevitably disrupt the therapeutic alliance?

A SEXUAL HEALTH ALTERNATIVE

Without existing scientific or psychiatric consensus to establish a sexual regulation disorder, we built our model on the assumption that OCSB is a behavioral problem. We are open to a sexual disorder that differentiates a subgroup of consensual out of control sexual behaviors, but only after compelling evidence delineates a specific sexual pathology from a scientific process free of sexual judgments and cultural disapproval. We define OCSB as a sexual problem of consensual sexual urges, thoughts, or behaviors that feel out of control for the individual. We contextualize OCSB within a theory of human behavior on which clinicians organize the client's sexual health problems within principles of sexual health and focus change in the direction of each man's personal sexual health goals. We assess vulnerability factors and competing motivations that research suggests contribute to negative and dysregulated sexual experiences. The assessment process produces a Unique Clinical Picture to guide OCSB treatment. The combined individual and group treatment interventions are designed to address each man's vulnerability factors and competing motivations that impede his ability to achieve his vision of sexual health. The OCSB Clinical Pathway outlines a sequence for screening, assessment, and treatment of out of control sexual behavior.

We do not propose an essential method that "should" be universally applied by treatment professionals to treat OCSB. We offer a protocol for a sexual health dialogue in which clients define and realize their personal vision of sexual health. Sexual health conversations remain a rare and privileged exchange and are essential for treating OCSB. Ultimately, our hope is that by sharing our thoughts with you, the reader, we provide a clinical pathway to integrate within your current clinical practices, help foster curiosity with your clients, and expand your clinical approach in treating problematic and out of control sexual behavior in whatever professional context you work.

REFERENCES

Erskine, R. G., & Moursund, J. (2011). *Integrative psychotherapy in action*. London, UK: Karnac Books.

Goldfried, M. R. (2013). What should we expect from psychotherapy? *Clinical Psychology Review, 33*(7), 862–869.

Miller, W. R., & Rollnick, S. (2013). *Motivational interviewing: Helping people change*. New York, NY: Guilford Press.

Prochaska, J. O., & DiClemente, C. C. (2005). The transtheoretical approach. In J. C. Norcross & M. R. Goldfried (Eds.), *Handbook of psychotherapy integration* (2nd ed., pp. 147–171). Oxford, UK: Oxford University Press.

A SEXUAL HEALTH FOUNDATION

CHAPTER ONE

THE STATE OF THE FIELD

DAVID

It was my sixth appointment with Veronique and Jay. Married 8 years, they were in couple therapy for communication problems and overall relationship dissatisfaction. Sitting on the far side of the waiting room with her arms folded, Veronique stared straight ahead. Jay, with his head buried into his hands, was unaware that I entered the room. "David's here," Veronique said curtly as she stood up and walked past me to my office. Jay slowly followed.

I was barely in my chair before Veronique looked at me and asked, "Are you ready to hear a new one?" Her eyes were tearing. "I found it all" she said, louder and angrier. "He's been lying the whole time. I looked at his e-mail and found a secret account he's been hiding from me. Apparently he goes online and looks at porn and talks to women. He has files of pictures. It made me sick!"

Jay looked at me and said, "I got rid of it all, I don't want to do this anymore."

Veronique barely let him finish before yelling, "I can't believe a word you say! You'll say anything right now!" Jay looked at me silently.

CHARMAINE

As part of my graduate school internship, I co-led a weekly adult outpatient drug and alcohol treatment group with my supervisor. Susan was a highly respected and experienced certified drug and alcohol counselor. Each year, Susan welcomed a new intern to train with her as a coleader in her treatment groups. In the 3 months that I had been working with Susan, the group's membership increased from five men and women to nine. Around this time, one night's group began with Hector saying he had something to talk about. He was hesitant, choosing his words carefully.

Hector said, "I know we hardly ever discuss this, but I need to be honest about something that happened this week. I went to a clinic, an STD [sexually transmitted disease] clinic, because I was worried I might have something. Well, it turns out I did. I tested positive for gonorrhea. They gave me some meds and everything will clear up soon. But, I had to tell Phil, my partner. He was *so* mad. He said that he was done. That he was tired of my lying and drinking. I have been staying at my sponsor's house. I haven't used, but I am afraid and don't know what to do next."

I sat very still, staring at Susan for guidance.

BETH

As a psychiatrist in an outpatient medical group, I provide mostly diagnostic assessments and medication. My first appointment this afternoon was with Frank. I have been treating Frank's generalized anxiety disorder since it was first diagnosed 5 months ago. Frank has reported steady symptom reduction, so I anticipated an uneventful appointment. I noticed Frank's poor eye contact when he entered my office. He seemed distressed. After we were seated, I asked, "How are you?"

"I'm doing OK, except ... I have something I have to talk about," he replied.

Frank paused, his body motionless.

"You seem nervous about something," I said.

After several deep sighs, he murmured, "I need to talk about what happened at work. My boss called me into his office last week. They found out that I was downloading porn at my desk. I'd been doing this for years. My boss told me it had to stop or I'll be fired ... I can't lose my job! I couldn't believe I got caught. I'm so stupid!"

LYNN

When I scheduled my first appointment with Peter, he mentioned that he was married with three children and was troubled about something that was affecting his relationship. Within the first minutes of this session, he recounted a recent conversation with his minister.

"I talked with him about what I've been doing and he suggested that I see someone. You were the closest therapist who took my insurance, so I'm hoping you can help me. Raising three kids, I don't have much time or money to spend on therapy. But this is important."

"I'm glad you were able to make it in," I said. "You mentioned that your minister recommended therapy. What was the reason for the suggestion?"

"I've been cheating on my wife since we've been married. Every couple of weeks I watch porn on the computer. I know I shouldn't. I should only feel that way toward my wife, but sometimes I can't help it. When I told that to my minister, he said that I might be addicted to porn and that if I wanted to honor the vows of my marriage, I needed to stop. Is that something you can help me with? To only have sex with my wife?"

DANNY

Will tested HIV positive a couple of weeks ago. I usually see clients who have been living with HIV for several years, but, working as a psychologist at an HIV mental health clinic, newly diagnosed clients are occasionally scheduled. When he came in for his first appointment, he was outwardly upset.

"I have no one to blame but myself," Will exclaimed. "I've been out long enough to know better. But, I was careless. And the person who gave me my results drove that point home. The lady said I was a sex addict and should get treatment"

"What do you mean?" I asked.

"On her form, she needed to know how many sex partners I had over the past year. ... I'm not completely sure, so I said 10 guys, but it's probably more like 20. I didn't think 10 was that many compared to some of my friends, but she suggested that I try to reduce the amount of partners I have. Then, as if to confirm my carelessness, she tells me I'm positive and to get help for my sex addiction."

AMY

As a hospital social worker, I'm frequently asked to intervene when patients exhibit behavioral problems on the unit. Last month, I was working with Anthony, a single, 29-year-old man recovering from injuries related to a car accident. He was a sweet man who was handling his misfortune well. At least, that was my initial impression until I heard from one of the nurses that she walked in on him masturbating. That is not terribly uncommon, but it was the second time it happened with this patient and I overheard a nurse refer to him as a pervert. So, I thought I should check in to get a better understanding of what was happening.

At first, he denied that he was masturbating, which was curious, because that was not the issue. I was attempting to tell him how to masturbate appropriately, such as in the adjoining bathroom. But, the more defensive he became, the more suspicious I became. And then I realized— my assumption that he was accidentally discovered was incorrect.

"The nurse mentioned that there's been a couple incidents where they've walked in on you ..." I began.

Interrupting, Anthony said, "Look, I'm sorry. I didn't mean to upset anyone. I feel really bad. But, honestly, I'm not sure why I did it. I promise that I won't do it again."

MOMENT OF DISCLOSURE

David was faced with an intensely emotional moment involving a sexual dispute between intimate partners. Charmaine, like so many newly trained professionals, withdrew when presented with a detailed sexual disclosure and looked to her coleader/supervisor for guidance. Beth and Lynn were presented with clients in distress about their solo sexual behaviors, Danny's client was dealing with the consequences of his multiple-partnered sex, and Amy was faced with managing a sexual boundary violation.

Consider your response to these scenarios. What did you notice about yourself? How did you imagine yourself feeling? How would you have responded? Although these vignettes contain brief interactions, they are glimpses into clinical moments during which sociocultural conflicts about sexual dysregulation live and breathe among clinicians. Your reactions to these case examples (or response to real-life client sexual disclosures) provide insights into how the past 30 years of theoretical debate over sexual behavior problems have influenced your work. Despite the many tensions that currently exist in sociocultural, sexological, and psychological debates surrounding sexual behavior problems, therapists are still expected to assess and intervene when presented with these clinical situations. Like members in a quarreling family, our actions and reactions are affected by the tensions of the greater systems in which we reside.

We begin this book with clinical situations inspired by either Doug or Michael's clients or professional case consultations. More information about the clients Jay, Hector, Frank, Peter, Will, and Anthony unfold throughout the book. We follow these clients from the moment of disclosure to treatment completion as we introduce the assessment and treatment components of a process we call the Out of Control Sexual Behavior (OCSB) Clinical Pathway. Before delving into the OCSB treatment protocol or discussing clinical applications for problematic or OCSB, we focus on the therapist providing the service.

THERAPIST PREPARATION

Research suggests that the therapeutic alliance is essential for effective psychotherapy (Goldfried, 2013). The relationship between clinician and patient is more closely correlated with positive outcomes and is more often correlated with effective treatment than is the therapist's theoretical approach or matching of his or her clinical theory with a specific client population. The importance of this therapist and client partnership requires the interpersonal relationship to mature within each clinical relationship and sustain over the course of psychotherapy. Miller and Rollnick's third edition of *Motivational Interviewing* (2013) elevates the importance of the relational process by identifying it as the "spirit of Motivational Interviewing" (MI; p. 14), without which MI might be misconstrued as a set of tricks to influence clients to do what the therapist wants a client to do. To prepare for the complexities of facilitating sexual health conversations, we place a similar emphasis on the relationship components Miller and Rollnick identify as comprising the spirit of motivational interviewing: partnership, evocation, acceptance, and compassion.

Throughout this book, you will notice the prominence we place on client motivation for change. Central to OCSB treatment is a process for therapists to use to raise client awareness regarding their sexual behaviors with the goal of uncovering and *evoking* each man's motivation for change. Client motivation shapes OCSB clinical questions and the direction for OCSB treatment. The substance of therapist OCSB interventions stem from what the client wants to achieve for his sexual health rather than the sexual-disorder symptoms he should overcome or what the therapist thinks is sexually appropriate. OCSB treatment is ultimately a process for men to better understand the motivations behind their sexual behaviors and use this wisdom to improve their sexual health. The therapist and client relationship collaborate to clarify and maintain each client's personal vision of sexual health. In concordance with Miller and Rollick's (2013) strength-based approach to change, we designed our treatment protocol to optimize therapist and client curiosity about the client's behavior. It is this curious stance that provides a process for men to understand their OCSB as an attempt to fulfill honorable needs with problematic solutions.

The aspects of *acceptance* Miller and Rollick (2013) highlight stem from the work of Carl Rogers (1980): accurate empathy, absolute worth, autonomy, support, and affirmation. The concept of acceptance has particular significance in the treatment of sexual behavior problems because the various actions presented in treatment are often socially inappropriate, harmful to themselves and others, or criminal. People who engage in high-frequency sex, commit acts of infidelity, or become infected with sexually transmitted infections (STI) are often portrayed in the media as immoral, promiscuous, and unsympathetic. People with sexual problems or unconventional sexual interests are often deemed unworthy or undeserving of empathy. An acceptance stance is less likely among clinicians lacking adequate sexual health conversation skills and who implicitly or explicitly react disapprovingly to their clients' sexual behaviors. Unexamined personal sexual values and attitudes hinder therapist efforts to earnestly maintain an actively curious interest in the internal worlds of their clients. Consider whether the psychiatrist Beth would be able to remain empathetic with Frank after he disclosed his history of watching sex videos if she strongly believes porn exploits women. Or Charmaine, who during group therapy has a passing thought that Hector invited these consequences on himself. Or whether Amy felt repulsed by Anthony exposing his erect penis to the nursing staff. Prizing "the inherent worth and potential" (Miller & Rollnick, 2013, p. 17) of clients regardless of the sexual acts they have committed is a radical notion that is not fully realized in general psychotherapy training and practice.

The promotion of another's sexual health also depends on the therapist providing *compassionate* care. "Who is entitled to compassion?" is a common struggle that occurs when sexual problems arise in relationships. A client may arrive at the office as the "identified patient" because he did not honor his commitment with his romantic partner. Clients may assume that the therapist will withhold empathy for their situation until they have corrected the problematic sexual behavior. It is important for therapists to be prepared for this client assumption and avoid preconditions for forming the therapy relationship. This can be seen in men attending OCSB sessions as a condition of remaining married. In this circumstance, therapy risks becoming primarily a vehicle for the injured spouse's need for healing and security. Therapists will need to quickly differentiate the newly forming therapeutic relationship from the injured spouse's perceptions that compassionate therapy is an endorsement of client's exploitive and dishonest sexual behavior. OCSB treatment prioritizes establishing a therapy relationship conducive to the process of change, even when the client or his significant other might not believe he deserves it.

A variety of factors impede the therapist's attempts to establish an optimal relationship and apply the spirit of MI when sexual behavior problems are the presenting problem. We emphasize therapist preparation for conducting OCSB assessment and treatment because it is vital for therapists to stay attuned and connected when sexuality is the topic of psychotherapy. Two areas of preparation we highlight are therapist's knowledge and comfort with facilitating sexual health conversations.

Therapist Knowledge

The U.S. health care system has shown a lack of integration of sexual health knowledge. There is an even deeper void when men and women in this country present with sexual behavior problems. As surprising as this may sound, the vast majority of medical and mental health providers in the United States are under-trained, and personally uncomfortable with talking about sex. Sexologist Peggy Kleinplatz links health care training and confidence deficit with a general reluctance among health care professionals to initiate sexual health conversation with their patients (Kleinplatz, 2012). Although basic coursework in human sexuality is required at some institutions that offer training in these professions, a sexual health domain is rarely integrated into physician, nursing, psychology, social work, marriage and family therapy, addiction counseling or professional counselor curriculums, or postgraduate training (Maurice, 1999). In graduate and postgraduate training, most mental health professionals only learn introductory knowledge about sexual disorders. But, training that covers the enormous diversity of child, adolescent, and adult sexuality (Kleinplatz, 2012), and how to facilitate effective, person-centered sexual health conversations is limited. A recent forum to address gaps in medical school sexuality education found "little instruction on sexual health in medical schools and little consensus around the type of material medical students should learn. To address and manage sexual health issues, medical students need improved education and training" (Coleman et al., 2013, p. 924).

Postgraduate training for mental health professionals interested in treating sexual behavior problems is also limited. For example, sexual addiction certificate training programs lack a curriculum to develop therapist sexual health knowledge or sex therapy skills. The International Institute for Trauma and Addiction Professionals (IITAP), a limited liability company (LLC) that trains mental health professionals in sexual addiction treatment, has a well-defined process for sex addiction (SA) treatment certification (certified sex addiction therapist or CSAT), but requires no advanced training in human sexuality or sexual health. There is no comparable organization that provides a certification process for impulsive–compulsive sexual behavior (ICSB) or hypersexual disorder (HD) treatment. Some workbooks on sexual compulsivity, sexual addiction, and cybersex integrate sexual health concepts (Edwards, 2011; Edwards, Delmonico, & Griffin, 2011). However, these books are patient resources and do not address specific sexual health training or skills for professionals, nor do they advise their readers to evaluate their therapist's level of postgraduate sexual health and sex therapy education (e.g., Carnes, 2010; P. Hall, 2013; Magness, 2013).

The American Association of Sexuality Educators, Counselors and Therapists (AASECT) offers a process to become a certified sex therapist (CST). The AASECT certification process emphasizes treating sexual disorders and dysfunction. This focus reflects the origins of sex therapy to improve the psychological treatment of sexual functioning and satisfaction (Giugliano, 2004). Because OCSB is currently not recognized as a disorder or dysfunction, the AASECT certification process implicitly disregards OCSB education and skill development as an expected core treatment skill among CSTs. Unfortunately, a clinician may obtain a sex therapy certification without any education or supervised clinical experience in treating OCSB.

We believe medical and mental health sexuality education deficits leave providers, certified or otherwise, unprepared for the complexities of sexual health conversations and OCSB treatment. As a result, providers too often rely on limited sexological or sexual health knowledge. These knowledge gaps can inhibit clinical inquiry about client's sexuality (Harris & Hays, 2008), undermine treatment planning for sexual behavior problems, and contribute to therapist discomfort with sexual health conversations.

Therapist Comfort

Harris and Hays's (2008) survey of marriage and family therapists found a correlation between therapist discomfort with sexual topics and their unwillingness to initiate sexuality-focused interventions. Therapist knowledge, in and of itself, was insufficient for the survey respondents to reliably initiate or feel comfortable with clinical discussions about sex. Instead, the more discomfort the therapist felt about discussing sexual topics, the more therapists avoided initiating sexual conversations with their clients. An avoidant therapist risks not seeing the biases and treatment responses that deter the client from continuing to discuss sex. Therefore, we first address common emotional entanglements of avoidant therapists that contribute to their inability to address client sexual behavior problems before we turn our attention to our OCSB conceptualization and treatment protocol.

When therapists avoid sexual health conversations, it replicates the client's similar avoidance of uncomfortable affect states. There are not many topics in life that can generate discomfort like sex. What prevents sexual openness in the therapists will hinder them from initiating or addressing sexual health matters in session (Schnarch, 1991). Many health care professionals find themselves unprepared to manage their emotional activation in tandem with the clients' sexual presenting problem. The therapist's emotional activation may override his or her capacity for critical thinking and adversely influence his or her clinical responses with clients. The source of therapist activation could be anything. It may relate to personal discomfort about the details of his or her sexual behaviors or turn-ons. Therapists may have a historical or recent sexual violation that still hurts. They may be in the midst of resolving an intense regret over a recent sexual choice in their own lives. Without self-reflection regarding sexual discomfort, even the most experienced psychotherapists will lose their well-honed confidence and clinical acumen when a client reveals a sexual behavior problem.

Therapist defenses look different for each therapist. One way to understand therapist defenses in response to a client's talking about sex is to group them as an under response or an active, but judgmental response. V. W. Hilton (1997) observed that the most common failure of therapists is to avoid sexual issues altogether. These are the under-responders. This pattern was observed in Harris and Hays's (2008) research, which found a correlation between therapist anxiety regarding sexuality-related topics and low frequency of therapist initiation of sexual-related conversations with their clients. All too often, therapists rely on the client to initiate a discussion regarding an aspect of their sexual behavior that is dissatisfying. In this scenario, the therapist's avoidant defenses collude with client's avoidant defenses. General questions about client's satisfaction with his or her sexual behavior, function, and pleasure, as well as a discussion of sexual problems or sexual health are absent from treatment. A therapist's avoidance of sexual topics creates unnecessary burden and disincentive for clients who feel uncomfortable talking about sex to initiate a sexual health conversation. Faced with their therapist's avoidant defenses, clients might observe nonverbal facial cues, changes in therapist rate of speech, or interventions that steer the discussion away from sexual health. Clients may choose short-term relief from their own discomfort and follow the therapist's lead to a less anxiety-provoking topic. Clients are left with the choice to either tolerate the negative consequences associated with their sexual problems or push through their discomfort with talking about sex to address their sexual problem. It is a high price to pay for access to sexual health care.

Clients who link a specific negative consequence with their sexual behavior will often initiate talking about their sexual behavior with their existing therapist or find a therapist to help them with their sexual concerns. If therapists are not ready to facilitate an open discussion about a client's emerging self-discrepancy with his or her sexual behavior, they may simply move the focus toward a psychotherapy model, notion, or concept in which the therapist feels comfortable and professionally literate. For example, on hearing Hector disclose his gonorrhea infection and his relationship crisis, Charmaine and Susan might have moved the group discussion to the relapse risk linked with Hector's emotions resulting from this severe relationship crisis. They might quickly affirm Hector's clear determination to stay sober. They might even suggest he look into going to a 12-step program for sexual addiction. All of these responses could be motivated by one or both of the group therapists' anxiety and discomfort with discussing the specific sexual behavior details that resulted in Hector contracting an STI.

The active but judgmental therapist defense contributes to values-laden clinical interventions that negatively influence treatment. When therapists lack a sexological knowledge base acquired through medically accurate and scientifically informed sexuality education, they unfortunately rely on their personal experience, values, and attitudes to clinically respond to their client's sexual concerns. For example, Ford and Hendrick (2003) found therapists with a conservative sexological worldview tended to view their clients with multiple sexual encounters as having more pathology than the monogamous clients, who reflected their own values and sexual ethics. Hertlein (2004) studied psychotherapist conceptualizations of Internet infidelity. The therapists in this study attributed a significantly higher degree of SA to male clients and considered their female clients who viewed online pornography as atypical. Interestingly, men's online sexual activity was not considered unusual by the therapists in this study when the men engaged in the same frequency or kind of online sexual behavior as their female clients. This is consistent with the findings of Seem and Johnson (1998), who studied therapist responses to client gender-atypical behavior. In this study, therapists were more likely to respond negatively toward clients who did not act in a gender-stereotypical manner than toward their clients who acted in a manner consistent with expected gender norms. In addition, Hertlein

(2004) found correlations between therapists labeling client online sexual behavior as a sexual addiction and the therapist's level of religiosity. The clinicians who self-identified as more religious among the study participants were more likely to rate married clients' online viewing of sexually explicit material or Internet sex-chatting as a serious problem or as a sexual addiction.

These studies suggest a troubling circumstance in psychotherapy that arises when a therapist's lack of knowledge, discomfort with talking about sex, and lack of preparation for sexual health conversation aligns with a client's defenses against talking about his sexual activities and behavior. Perhaps assigning a sexual addiction or compulsive sexual behavior label unwittingly allows both client and therapist to each avoid uncomfortable emotions when talking about the intricate details of sex. Could it be that many psychotherapists and their clients prematurely move toward diagnosing sexual behavior as an addiction or compulsion to defensively avoid the painstaking intricacies of assessing each man's specific circumstances? This encourages clients to quickly experience the relief felt when accepting a therapist's diagnostic label as a support to their motivation to "get on" with treatment and to prevent whatever dire consequence is at hand (e.g., ending their marriage, job, or child custody). When therapists avoid uncomfortable sexual topics or fill their knowledge gaps with sociocultural judgments, they sacrifice developing an informed clinical picture.

We hope the screening, assessment, and treatment protocol described here helps therapists remain grounded in person-centered principles of psychotherapy by offering a map to facilitate a sexual health conversation with clients concerned about problematic sexual behaviors and OCSB. This book can also be part of a preparatory step toward increasing your sexual knowledge and comfort to facilitate client sexual health conversations. But, as we just discussed, knowledge alone is not enough to safely and effectively conduct sexual health conversation. It is imperative that therapists develop an ongoing self-awareness process to identify and resolve their discomfort and knowledge gaps when talking about sex.

A BRIEF HISTORY OF THE DEBATE

We move from the internal focus of therapist comfort and ability to talk about sex to a review of the various external factors that influence a psychotherapist assessment and treatment for OCSB. We review our perspectives of how the sociopolitical history surrounding diagnosis and treatment for sexual behavior problems led us to a sexual health model for OCSB. We also highlight sexual science research that informs the debate among various models for sexual behavior problems. We believe it is important to understand both the science and the cultural influences that intersect and contribute to the current controversy surrounding basic ideas and clinical approaches for OCSB treatment. Some readers may be very familiar with the historical markers that inform the existing circumstances. For others, our review of the competing models of sexual behavior dysregulation may be an important historical context to better understand our motivation and intent for proposing a sexual health approach to OCSB treatment.

Sexual Behavior Clinical Disorders

Simon Andre Tissot's *Treatise on the Diseases Produced by Onanism* (1832) has had an enormous influence on European and American medicine. Prior to germ theory, body fluids were a significant focus of medical theory and treatment. According to Tissot, semen was an essential fluid that drained vitality and degenerated the mind and body when expelled. Wasting semen was seen to disable organs, cause maladies such as syphilis and gonorrhea (then called social diseases), and be directly responsible for "degenerate promiscuity" and "whoring" (Money & Lamacz, 1989). Tissot fused the social vices of recreational sex, multiple sex partners, sex work, and sex outside of marriage with "the secret vice"—self-abuse (aka masturbation; p. 19). He linked perceived immoral partnered sexual practices with masturbation as the reason why some people degenerated into "whoring" and disease. Without the knowledge of germ theory, he proposed that semen loss from sexual dreams and masturbation, driven by lustful feelings, caused STIs and sexual degeneracy. Most important, Tissot believed lust could be spread to others through coarse, crude, and offensive indecent sexual behavior (lust as a contagion?). Not only were these social diseases believed to be the reason why certain people progressed into states of increasing sexual depravity, they were the etiological explanation for mental illness and sexual disorders. "Degeneracy theory became applied to the explanation specifically of psychiatric and sexological disorders during the middle of the 19th century" (Money & Lamacz, 1989, p. 20).

When nonmarital and nonprocreative sex can lead to psychosis or perversion, it does not take too long for procreative sex within marriage to become the only sexual activity safe from social and medical condemnation. The emerging field of psychiatry identified masturbation, unconventional sexual turn-ons, and recreational sex as symptoms of lustful wantonness that devolved into perverted sexual behaviors. Degeneracy found new life in the words of Freud and his contemporaries. Their medical theory shifted degeneracy caused by immoral wanton lustful fantasies to psychopathological regression (which was a step toward compassionate care). Degeneracy was now imbedded in a mental illness manifested by either an arrested development or a regression to an earlier stage of psychosexual maturation. Intrapsychic fixation from an unachieved psychosexual developmental task became the medical explanation for behaviors judged as sexual psychopathology. Sexual degeneracy theory was woven into the fabric of early psychiatric thought, merging mental illness with sociocultural values, and reflected publicly scorned, criminal, religiously condemned sexual desires or behaviors (Money & Lamacz, 1989). We benefit from the findings of modern scientific research that plainly dispute these historical notions of morbidity. These proposals are perfect examples of how sociocultural sexual values are expressed in notions about health and wellness in the absence of empirical evidence. Although we can now easily dismiss the idea that lust causes venereal diseases and organ failure as illogical and incorrect, the concept that sexuality degrenerates into a state of moral depravity and physical disability continues to find a home in sexual dysregulation constructs.

The primary focus of our review examines the current professional debate stemming from the sexual addiction framework popularized in the 1980s. Since the inception of the SA framework in *The Sexual Addict* by Patrick Carnes (1983), differences about etiology and diagnostic criteria for sexual dysregulation remain central to the mental health field and consumer literature. The embedded hypothesis within this framework threads through centuries of conflicting and overlapping approaches (Ley, 2012); although a comprehensive history of the sexual addiction concept is beyond the scope of this book, see Giugliano (2009), Ley (2012), Reay, Attwood, and Gooder (2015a) for a review. Other models to emerge alongside "sex addiction" (SA) include "compulsive sexual behavior" first postulated by Michael Quadland (1985) and further developed by Eli Coleman (1990). In 1987, "sexual impulsivity" was introduced by Barth and Kinder and "hypersexuality" by Martin Kafka (1997), then "dysregulated sexuality" by Winters, Christoff, and Gorzalka (2010), and finally "impulsive/compulsive sexual behavior" (ICSB) an updated revision of Coleman's compulsive sexual behavior (Coleman, 2011). Despite the emergence of competing models, SA captured the attention of the general public and mental health field. SA became the prevalent model in the consumer literature and, in the late 1980s, a guild of mental health care professionals was formed to promote a new area of therapy specializing in treating SA. Therapists using the SA model established diagnostic criteria as well as a clinical model of sexual addiction treatment.

Yet, SA specialists did not represent the entire provider community treating sexual behavior problems. Sex therapists, behavioral specialists, sex offender treatment providers, and psychiatrists were also treating clients concerned about sexual dysregulation. These disparate practitioners brought their own competing ideas, conceptualizations, and perspectives to their clinical work and research questions about problematic sexual behavior. Many were neither trained in the addiction field, nor believed that treatment methods linked with addiction were the best course of treatment for these issues. Although everyone was interested in helping clients address their sexual behavior concerns, disagreements about etiology and treatment methods merged with provincial conflicts between professional identities: sex therapist and sex addiction therapist. Thus, affiliation with a professional organization also identified the model of treatment with which these disparate professionals practiced. Sex therapists, addiction treatment professionals, Christian therapists, and generalists gravitated toward the professional organizations that aligned with their models of treatment. Increasingly heated conflicts among these diverse treatment professionals led to a split in the field.

Not only was *sexual addiction* a term used to label sexual behavior and around which a community of practitioners formed, the movement advocated for the inclusion of "SA" as an officially recognized psychiatric disorder in the *Diagnostic and Statistical Manual* (*DSM*; American Psychiatric Association [APA], 1952). It would not be the first time that disorders of sexual excess or dysregulation were listed in the *DSM*. The first edition (APA, 1952) included "nymphomania" as a diagnosis. It was removed in the second edition (APA, 1968) only to be re-added in the third edition along with "Don Juanism" (APA, 1980). References to nonparaphilic SA were made in the *DSM-III-R* (1987), but all references to sexual excess or dysregulation were removed in the *DSM-IV* and only alluded to in the definition for "Sexual Disorder, Not Otherwise Specified (NOS)" (APA, 2000). Seeming to confirm the expression "everything old is new again," "Sexual Disorder NOS" was removed and "HD" (Kafka, 2010) was proposed and rejected from the most recent edition of the *DSM* (5th ed.; APA, 2013). HD was not included because of "insufficient peer-reviewed evidence to establish the diagnostic criteria and course descriptions needed to identify these behaviors as mental disorders" (APA, 2013, p. 481). Thirty years of theory development that attempted to anchor problematic sexual behaviors to a specific psychiatric disorder, diagnosis, or treatment paradigm has led us to no clear accepted terminology or approach (Joannides, 2012; Kaplan & Krueger, 2010).

Areas Needing Clarity

In this section, we review three predominate models that advance excessive and dysregulated sexual behavior as a specific and distinct psychiatric disorder. Although a discussion about the emerging conceptualizations and diagnostic categories for out of control sexual experiences provides excellent material for professional debate, that is not our intention. Our objective is twofold:

1. To illustrate the limitations of the prominent models that motivated the development of our treatment protocol
2. To provide a clinical guide for therapy interventions in an era when therapists are faced with complex sexual problems and the psychotherapy field is deeply divided about whether to even call this issue a disorder

Sexual Addiction

Probably the most popular label used by the general public and the term that sparks the most contention among physicians, psychotherapists, sex therapists, and sex researchers is *sexual addiction*. In *The Sexual Addict* (republished as *Out of the Shadows* in 1994), Carnes defines *addiction* as "a pathological relationship with mood altering experience" (Carnes, 1983b, p. 4) and links sex to the experience that alters mood. He suggests using the SAFE formula to discern addictive from nonaddictive sexual behaviors. Sexual behavior is addictive if it is (S) secretive, (A) abusive to self or others, (F) used to avoid painful feelings, and (E) empty of a caring or committed relationship. He later adds 10 signs that indicate SA and 10 behavioral types (Carnes, 1991). Other researchers and theorists have amended or expanded the definition of *sexual addiction*. Schneider and Irons (2001) indicate three elements can be used to create an operational definition for any behavioral or chemical addiction: (1) compulsivity, (2) continuation despite harmful consequences, and (3) obsession or preoccupation with the activity. Weiss (2013) describes *sexual addiction* as "a dysfunctional preoccupation with sexual urges, fantasy, and behavior, often involving the obsessive pursuit of non-intimate sex, pornography, compulsive masturbation, romantic obsession, and objectified partner sex" (p. 1). Magness (2013) defines *sexual addiction* as a "progressive intimacy disorder" of patterned destructive sexual thoughts or behaviors the person is unable to stop. Other theorists and researchers apply problematic sexual behavior to the substance dependence criteria of the corresponding *DSM* edition of the time (Goodman, 2001; Sealy, 1995; Wines, 1997).

Neuroscience and biophysiological research are emerging fields of study seeking to validate the behavioral addiction construct. Gambling disorder was included in the *DSM-5* in the "substance-related and addictive disorders" section as the only nonsubstance disorder. The inclusion of this diagnosis reflects the "evidence that gambling behaviors activate reward systems similar to those activated by drugs of abuse and produce some behavioral symptoms that appear comparable to those produced by the substance use disorders" (APA, 2013, p. 481). Sexual addiction is among the many life preoccupations that theorists consider a behavioral, process or "natural" addiction (D. L. Hilton, 2013). D. L. Hilton (2013) draws on current understanding of pathological gambling and "food addiction" to support his hypothesis that a comparable mechanism underlies sexual addiction. Sexual behavior is seen as a powerful form of reward-based learning. He proposes that repeated viewing of sexual imagery alters neural receptivity and pathways that lead to observable behavioral change. Clinicians and researchers who endorse the SA framework are looking toward neuroscience to establish the etiology of SA with a particular focus on "pornography addiction." D. L. Hilton (2013) believes the contemporary understanding of neuroplasticity and the *DSM-5* inclusion of gambling disorder foretell the inclusion of SA as a biological and behavioral diagnosis. However, he concedes, "there is, of course, a lack of comparable functional and behavioral work in the study of human sexual addiction, as compared to gambling and food addictions" (p. 2). Reid, Carpenter, and Fong (2011) critique this biobehavioral foundation for SA. They state that there is no agreed-upon standard of what constitutes an addiction (which makes obtaining evidence of a sexual addiction challenging) and that assertions without similar studies within human sexual behavior are "speculative and unsupported" (p. 4). They add a cautionary note that the addiction model may limit our understanding by offering an overly simplistic view of the diverse issues encountered by this clinical population. There is little systematic research dealing directly with sex as an addiction and the epidemiology and treatment literature is "primarily anecdotal in nature" (Giugliano, 2009, p. 16).

Impulsive/Compulsive Sexual Behavior

ICSB is a "clinical syndrome characterized by the experience of sexual urges, sexually arousing fantasies, and sexual behaviors that are recurrent, intense, and a distressful interference in one's daily life" (Coleman, 2011, p. 376). People concerned about ICSB identify their behavior as excessive and struggle to stop. Coleman indicates that he prefers this term because of its descriptive nature and that it provides room to incorporate multiple pathological pathways and treatments. As the name suggests, sexual symptoms are seen as impulsive or compulsive, distinguished by the underlying motivations driving the behavior. Impulsive behaviors are intended to feel pleasurable, whereas compulsive behaviors intend to prevent or reduce subjective discomfort. These characteristics can also be seen in the sexual addiction model, but ICSB does not include the concepts of withdrawal or tolerance, which bedevil sexual addictions theorists (Giugliano, 2009).

ICSB distinguishes between two types: paraphilic and nonparaphilic. The primary difference is the former involves sexual behavior considered deviant and the latter involves normative behavior. Within each type are behavioral subtypes: paraphilic ICSB includes the paraphilias identified in the *DSM-5* and nonparaphilic ICSB subtypes. Coleman also proposes a sexual behavior continuum from healthy/problematic to impulsive/compulsive. A diagnosis of ICSB is made when sexual behaviors cross a threshold from problematic to impulsive/compulsive as determined by the provider. Because there is currently no clinically validated measure to diagnose ICSB, Coleman recommends using established psychiatric and medical diagnosis procedures and gathering a sexual history to determine the threshold for ICSB. Coleman acknowledges that the threshold between problematic sexual behavior and ICSB is subjective and that there is a potential risk of diagnosing both healthy and problematic sexual behaviors as pathologically disordered. He attributes insufficient clinician training as well as client and/or therapist disapproval of diverse sexual fantasies and sexual activities as significant factors in misattributing sexual behavior as ICSB (Coleman, 2011).

Hypersexual Disorder

HD is a sexual-desire disorder characterized by recurrent and intense sexual fantasies, urges, or sexual behaviors (Kafka, 2010). Motivations underlying hypersexuality are associated with relieving dysphoric emotions and experiencing multiple unsuccessful attempts to limit or control the amount of time spent engaging in sexual thoughts, urges, or behaviors. Kafka (2010) drafted the proposed disorder criteria for *DSM-5* with established medical and psychiatric terminology used in other sexual-disorder diagnoses. HD also includes the familiar psychiatric diagnostic threshold of time spent, response to dysphoric moods or stressful life events, unsuccessful efforts to control or reduce sexual symptoms, and engaging in sexual behaviors despite adverse consequences. As with sexual addiction and ICSB, HD delineates subtypes of sexual behavior such as masturbation, cybersex, or strip clubs.

Kafka (2010) suggests that there is sufficient data to consider HD a sexual disorder, one with both compulsive and impulsive features, or to classify it as a behavioral addiction. He advocates for clinical criteria that can incorporate dimensions across differing clinical samples and incorporating differ pathological pathways. Researcher and clinician Rory Reid has been instrumental in examining etiology, prevalence, and treatment of HD. He acknowledges the infancy of HD research and the need for more studies to clarify HD criteria. At this time, "little is known about the onset, clinical course, and trajectories of HD symptoms as they manifest in various populations and across gender" (Reid, 2013, p. 13). Moser (2013) cites Kafka's (Kafka & Hennan, 2000) research, suggesting that the treatment of co-occurring psychiatric disorders may often ameliorate the sexual symptoms and should be the preferred diagnostic frame used instead of "branding" clients with a disorder that can only be put in remission but not resolved.

Common Clinical Concerns With Existing Models

Before we can introduce our OCSB conceptual framework, we want first to clarify and discuss general topics and areas of clinical concern that are common within sexual dysregulation diagnoses.

Sexual Behavior Classification

Identifying clinical subtype classifications based on specific sexual behaviors or actions is a common feature among the proposed dysregulated sexual behavior diagnoses. Thus, observable sexual behaviors that share some common actions are either organized or diagnostically labeled based on their common features. The behavioral subtypes are all incorporated within a primary disorder of dysregulated sexual behavior. The categories do not identify distinct etiologies, but rather provide specificity for assessment and treatment. In our review of the literature, we found three general groupings for classifying sexual behavior problems. In one category, the specific sexual activity includes entertainment practices such as erotic literature, nongenital contact at strip clubs, and watching sexual videos. A second category centers on partnered sexual activities, including anonymous partners, multiple partners, pursuing sex partners, sex in bathhouses, or unconventional turn-ons. A third group focuses on sexual behavior symptoms that either violate (through dishonest or exploitive deception) or are nonconforming with traditional sexual monogamy (either honestly or deceptively) within marital or relationship agreements. Common behaviors within this category are love affairs, one-night stands, genital contact at strip clubs, paying for sex, as well as unacceptable masturbation practices within the couple's agreement.

Is the specific sexual activity or context a useful or clinically pertinent factor for diagnosis? No other clinical disorder includes typology based on specific behavioral symptoms. At this point, eating disorders do not require the clinician to identify behaviors beyond the restrictive or binge/purge behavior patterns. There are currently no subgroup clinical distinctions like group binge eating or solo binge eating (compulsive masturb-eating?), food-specific binge eating (e.g., desserts, snacks, or quinoa), or deviant eating patterns (e.g., only eating protein supplements, pathological use of the Paleo or Atkins diets). Pathological gambling does not currently include categories like online gambling, casino gambling, or compulsive lottery-ticket scratching. Furthermore, any categories that involve technology quickly become dated. Look at how phone sex has evolved in the past 10 years. Is sexual webcaming considered phone sex or online sex behavior? And, for diagnostic purposes, does it really matter? To be clear, we do agree with the value of assessing the sexual behavior details to develop the client's Unique Clinical Picture as well as to establish an effective treatment plan. However, delineating sexual behavior subcategories risks assuming a common etiology links these behaviors when they may be caused by unrelated phenomena (Cantor et al., 2013). Not to mention how the mere act of labeling specific sexual behaviors as diagnostic subcategories risks conflating unconventional or socially unacceptable sexual behaviors with pathology.

Nonconsensual Sex

Established SA therapist certification standards do not distinguish treatment approaches between consensual and nonconsensual sex. It is unclear under what circumstances CSAT may exceed their scope of practice in treating nonconsensual sexual behaviors. The professional literature is also unclear concerning when a therapist should refer a client to a nonconsensual sexual behavior specialist; also, the standards for treating nonconsensual sexual behavior within the current sexual dysregulation models remain underdeveloped.

In 1991, when developing his out of control behavior therapy specialization, Doug received referrals from San Diego psychotherapists who not did think their male clients with problematic consensual sexual behavior were a good fit for participating in therapy groups with sex offenders. Men concerned about their excessive masturbation or part-nered sexual behaviors were sitting in group therapy with men who were arrested for sex crimes, who had engaged in child molestation or nonconsensual public sexual exposure. When formulating his own treat-ment group, Doug considered the potential impact of mixing these pop-ulations within his future groups. Would men engaged in consensual sexual behavior benefit from a group that includes men who engaged in nonconsensual, illegal, or predatory sexual behavior? Or, are the treatment strategies for consensual and nonconsensual sexual behaviors different enough that a mixed group is not the best approach?

In 1993, Doug decided that his outpatient psychotherapy group and individual OCSB treatment program would only treat clients concerned about consensual sexual behavior. This meant men with a history of rape, sex with minors, exhibitionism, voyeurism, and frottage would be referred to nonconsensual specialists for further assessment and treatment. Of course, not all sexual behaviors fit easily into the consent/nonconsent binary. For example, Bill, a 42-year-old gay Californian, living with his husband of 5 years, wears wide-leg shorts without underwear to his gym. He is preoccupied with men glancing at his legs and being able to see his penis. When he returns home, he remembers their faces and masturbates to these visual images. He has never disclosed this behavior or that this is a peak erotic turn-on. Omar is a 37-year-old heterosexual man married for 12 years with two children. He has been taking women's underwear from dirty-clothes hampers in family and friends' homes since he was a teenager. During masturbation, he touches and smells the underwear and ejaculates on them and then puts them in the trash. During a recent social gathering, he was discovered taking underwear from a neighbor's bedroom hamper. Clients who report nonconsensual sexual behaviors require a clinical assessment to determine the most effective course of treatment. What is first disclosed should not be assumed to be the full breadth of the historical or current nonconsensual behavior. We address the role of consent/nonconsent in the OCSB protocol in Chapters 2 and 5 on sexual health principles and the screening procedure, respectively.

Paraphillic and Nonparaphillic Sexual Disorder

The mental health field has historically identified that non-normative sexual interests and behaviors are clinical disorders. Both deviancy and sexual dysregulation involve sexual behaviors and interests that are persistent, problematic, and frequently at odds with an individual's values, ethics, or desired self-image. *Paraphilia* is the current conventional medical term used to describe sexual behavior and arousal patterns that deviate from social norms (Bancroft, 2009). The Greek root of the prefix *para* means "besides," and, when added to the base word, indicates an abnormality. Together with *philia*, an ancient Greek word meaning "love" or "friendship," the term *paraphilia* can be understood as "outside of normal love" or "abnormal love." The history of the medical term *paraphilia* dates to the early 20th-century psychoanalysts and writers Wilhelm Stekel and his protégé, Benjamin Karpman (Money & Lamacz, 1989). The term was first introduced into the *DSM-III* in 1980 replacing the term *perversion*.

Paraphilia's definition was expanded at the end of the last century by sex researcher John Money (1999). He proposed a developmental process that rooted the origins of paraphillic sexual functioning within prepubertal antecedents. According to Money (1999), the forerunners of adolescent and adult paraphilias were to be found in threatened or actual childhood abandonment, separation, or loss in early life. These adverse childhood experiences influenced childhood sexual development by creating a need for a psychological splitting between relational attachments and sexual behavior or erotic imagery. Money (1999) explains paraphillia as an individual's triumph in salvaging his or her intense bodily sexual arousal, pleasure, and desire from the wreckage of derailed childhood developmental processes. He coined the term *lovemap* to describe the resulting personal schema of this compromised yet effective solution to keep both one's capacity to love and to experience sexual excitement.

The current *DSM-5* diagnostic criteria for paraphillic disorder emphasize Money's early distinction between a major pathological paraphilia (those listed in *DSM*) and a minor playful sexual variant. The *DSM-5* (APA, 2013) defines *paraphilia* as "any intense and persistent sexual interest other than sexual interest in genital stimulation or preparatory fondling with phenotypically normal, physically mature, consenting human partners" (p. 685). To receive a paraphilic disorder diagnosis, the paraphilia must cause distress or impairment to the individual or, if the paraphilia is personally satisfying, the specific sexual behavior does not entail personal harm or risk of harm to others. One can now have a paraphilia without meeting criteria for a clinical disorder.

The establishment of paraphilic disorder was not without controversy. Moser (2011) deconstructs the definition to illustrate how psychiatric diagnositic criteria do not reliably differentiate between paraphilic and normophilic conditions. For instance, is an intense and persistent sexual interest in surgically enhanced breasts or shaved hairless bodies considered "phenotypically normal"? Does a preference for being whipped rather than engaging in coitus constitute a paraphilia, whereas being whipped as fore-play to coitus is subsumed under normophilic criteria? He also observes the sexism evident in paraphilia evaluation when a woman wearing silk panties to feel sexy is privileged over the same behavior in a man. "It is possible that a scientific distinction between paraphilia and normophilia does not exist—only one based on shifting societal norms" (Moser, 2011, p. 484). Philosopher Robert Scott Stewart writes about the last century's focus on normative or perfectionistic sex as reciprocal, affectionate, and interpersonal and how these same values and normative standards remain the clinical thresholds for demarcating sexual perversions, paraphilias, and sexual disorders (Stewart, 2012). It is deeply problematic when failure to reach these socially constructed ideals is defined as a mental illness or sexual disorder.

Distinctions between paraphillic and nonparaphillic traits in dys-regulated sexual behavior vary depending on the model's current iter-ation. For example, the language of paraphilia is nonexistent in early sexual addiction writings. The framework describes three levels of devi-ancy described as culturally acceptable sexual behavior; nuisance sexual behavior; and dangerous, abusive, or life-threatening behavior. These categories are descriptive of progressive levels of risk, not progressive stages of addiction (Carnes, 1989). In this model of deviancy, what might be called paraphillic is instead organized around a person's escalating level of sexual risk-taking behavior. In this conceptualization, no distinc-tion is made between paraphillic and nonparaphillic behavior, rather the diversity of paraphillic behaviors is viewed through the lens of cul-tural acceptance/violation, legal consequences/risks, victimization, and degree of public dislike or outrage.

Separating paraphillic and nonparaphillic sexual behaviors has been discussed in the development of HD (Kafka, 2010; Reid & Kafka, 2014) and ICSB (Coleman, 2011). Although they conclude that the similarities between the paraphillic and nonparaphillic types of problematic sexual behavior far outweigh the differences, both Kafka and Coleman focus on the degree of deviance or unconventionality that are specific to paraphilia.

A Profession Divided

It is understandable why a consensus has yet to materialize regarding the etiological mechanisms or the establishment of a dysregulated sexual behavior disorder. The factors that contribute to sexual behavior problems are diverse and multivariate, and intertwined within a range of sociocul-tural influences and biopsychological factors. Over time, these models have gained prominence and undergone scrutiny in scientific and nonscientific venues, from peer-reviewed journals and conference presentations to blog posts and talk shows. SA is the prominent model in the consumer literature and a specific certification process has been developed around it. *Sexual addiction* is frequently the construct used when sexual behavior problems are discussed or criticized in the media, churches, courtrooms, hospitals, and therapy offices. Proponents of an SA, ICSB, and HD diagnosis critique the limitations, biases, or etiological mischaracterizations of the other models or opposing perspectives. Thought leaders presume the superiority of their conceptualization with a confidence unsupported by the accumulated scientific evidence and discussion between fellow practitioners devolves into rigid defensive postures at the expense of complex professional dialogue and critical thinking. As if it is not already difficult to discuss the wide array of client sexual problems among peers, discussions between colleagues devolve into rigid discourse in which professionals defend their positions at the expense of complex critical thinking. As practitioners in the field and consumers of the literature, we are discouraged by the tension that prohibits open dialogue about OCSB.

Charles Samenow, editor of the *Journal of Sexual Addiction and Compulsivity*, in an opening editorial for a volume that focused on HD, stated, "although there remains no unified model for what we and our clients call sex addiction, I think in reviewing the research presented in this journal one can only conclude that the similarities between the constructs and different research continues to outweigh the differences" (Samenow, 2013, p. 1). Samenow recommends that the "work must include developing grounded theories, research to illuminate the biological and neurochemical mechanisms associated with problematic sexual behaviors, and outcome research to find effective treatments (both pharmacological and psychosocial) to relieve the pain and suffering associated with this phenomenon" (p. 2). Samenow's introductory comments strike a professional collaboration tone. It is admirable to read his message in a journal dedicated to sexual addiction and compulsivity research in a special issue specifically examining HD research.

Most important, many of the current psychotherapists and researchers are united by their common interest in improving clients' lives. It is easy to get mired in debates about etiology, the latest fMRI research, or the perceived sex-negative cultural values in sexual dysregulation models. Frequently lost in the debate is the acknowledgment that, in the three decades since the term "sex addiction" was popularized, the benefits of the various treatment models coexist with their weaknesses. The main benefits include:

- A common language used to discuss the diverse range of behaviors under the umbrella of "sex addiction."

- Dysregulated sexual behavior shifted from a source of moral judgment and rejection associated with promiscuity to a medical problem allowing people access to treatment and empathy.
- The development of the HD diagnostic criteria (Kafka, 2010), which enabled the recent scientific inquiry for inclusion in the *DSM-5* (Reid et al., 2012).

Here are the main costs and limitations we have seen in practice or identified in the literature:

- Sexual addiction, ICSB, and HD risk reinforcing sociocultural disapproval of specific sexual behaviors (M. P. Levine & Troiden, 1988; Ley, 2012; Moser, 2013; Reay, Attwood, & Gooder, 2015b).
- Failure to behave within concepts of normative or conventional sex is defined as a sexual disorder (Stewart, 2012).
- SA carries the historical burden of labeling the adjustment symptoms of sexual identity development for gay and bisexual men as an addiction.
- Nonconsensual sexual patterns are inappropriately subsumed within SA, ICSB, and HD criteria.
- Sexual dysregulation appears in those reporting higher levels of sexual desire and it is unclear whether the additional features of proposed disease models add any explanatory power (Steele, Staley, Fong, & Prause, 2013; Winters et al., 2010).
- Data demonstrating that SA, ICSB, and HD are distinct mental disorders are lacking (S. Levine, 2010b; Moser, 2013; Reid, 2013).
- Prematurely framing a sexual problem as a clinical disorder pathologizes normative behavior, affects the individual's self-concept, and invites overly restrictive sexual interventions.
- Creating a disorder for sexual dysregulation or sexual excess risks mental health professionals inadvertently inducing symptoms related to that disorder (i.e., an iatrogenic illness; Bancroft & Vukadinovic, 2004; Giugliano, 2004).
- The popularization of the SA model has created a meme in the general public in which sexual behavioral problems are routinely evaluated through the lens of addiction despite the lack of scientific consensus.

We share S. Levine's (2010b) hope that the field may be ready to reexamine the concepts of sexual dysregulation disorders and no longer confuse the "utility in getting people into treatment with the validity of the idea that the men have a discrete disorder" (p. 274).

OUT OF CONTROL SEXUAL BEHAVIOR—A SEXUAL PROBLEM

S. Levine (2010a) organized sexual difficulties on a spectrum from worries to problems to disorders. Sexual worries are common, almost universal concerns people have about their sexuality that only reach an intensity level of distraction. Worries are the most frequently occurring sexual difficulty because they are "concerns that are inherent in the experience of being human" (S. Levine, 2010a, p. xi). Examples include: When will I have my first intercourse? Will my partner be less attracted to me if I am bald? Does my vagina smell funny? Is it normal to be less interested in sex now that I am breastfeeding? Sexual worries are unavoidable and evolve over the life span.

On the other end of the spectrum, sexual disorders are the most frequently studied and least prevalent of all sexual difficulties. These include the officially recognized medical and psychiatric diagnoses such as erectile dysfunction, vaginismus, or premature ejaculation. Despite their lower prevalence rate, sexual disorders are assumed to be more prevalent than health care professionals diagnose and have the greatest potential to disrupt one's life (S. Levine, 2010a). Sexual problems fall between common sexual worries and discrete sexual disorders. They are a source of suffering that afflicts groups of people, but attract little research due to the varied contributing factors and underlying causes inherent in sexual problems. Furthermore, "what is regarded as 'problematic' sexual functioning may be normative in a different cultural context" (K. Hall & Graham, 2013, p. 1). When evaluating the lens through which we label sexual behaviors as problematic, the role of sociocultural values is essential to consider. Western societies centered in Western Europe, Britain, Canada, and the United States have conducted most of the treatment research for sexual problems (K. Hall & Graham, 2013). Unfortunately, this means much of what is understood to be generalizable sexual problems may too often be a culturally defined problem. What is understood as normative in one culture can often be highly stigmatized in another. Social mores and stigma related to sexuality may skew statistical information gathering that informs sexual-disorder definitions (Giugliano, 2004). Sexual orientation, termination of pregnancy, differing levels of desire between couples, and notions of sexual pleasure in some contexts are sexual problems and symptoms of pathological disorders in others.

To understand the line between sexual problem and disorder, Bancroft and Vukadinovic (2004) pose a question that theorists and researchers have not answered: Is OCSB a problem on the extreme end of the "normal" range of sexual behavior or is it a distinct behavior that is "qualitatively different from the norm in ways that are problematic" (p. 225). We believe their recommendation remains an important contemporary position: It is premature and perhaps iatrogenic to establish a sexual dysregulation clinical disorder and instead we recommend using the phrase "out of control sexual behavior." Therefore, until such time that evidence supports the establishment of a sexual disorder, we view OCSB as a problem within the normal range of human sexual expression. We believe if disordered levels exist, they are extremely rare, comprising a much smaller segment of the men seeking treatment for OCSB.

We define OCSB as a sexual health problem in which an individual's consensual sexual urges, thoughts, or behaviors feel out of control. Some client symptoms may fit criteria of the previously discussed disorder proposals, but we are more interested in exploring the client's subjective experience. Men may report feeling out of control regularly or in different situations. Onset may be recent or decades in the past. We invite you to think of "out of control" as an expression of an individual's subjective experience. It is a personal description of the various sensations, thoughts, perceptions, and emotions contributing to their sexual behavior problems. Marty Klein (2012) makes a subtle, but significant distinction about this definition: *feeling* out of control is different than *being* out of control. It is unlikely that the client is pervasively without the ability to direct his sexual behavior. However, clients are communicating an affective experience that feels like they lack agency during certain sexual situations.

It is important to clarify our use of language. We define OCSB as a sexual health problem in which an individual's consensual sexual urges, thoughts, or behaviors feel out of control. Rather than repeating "out of control sexual urges, thoughts or behavior," we condense the string of words to OCSB or out of control sexual experiences. We are not excluding urges and thoughts when referring to OCSB. We also use the phrase "problematic sexual behavior" or "sexual behavior problems." Problematic sexual behaviors are behaviors that generate significant negative consequences, but the phrase is not meant to infer a felt sense of being unable to control sexual thoughts, urges, and behavior. In short, OCSB is likely problematic, but not all problematic sexual behaviors are considered OCSB. Problematic sexual behavior is usually discussed during the early stages of an assessment as we are clarifying the client's subjective experience.

Areas of Distinction

Several areas differentiate OCSB from the three primary models. HD, ICSB, and sexual addiction stem from a proposal that considers sexual dysregulation as a clinical disorder (e.g., psychosexual disorder or addictive disorder). HD and ICSB assume multivariate pathological pathways and SA assumes one etiological mechanism. With OCSB, we contextualize all sexual behavior within a general theory of human behavior. As with all behaviors, various factors influence a person's ability to satisfactorily assert control or feel satisfied in his choices and behaviors. Pathological pathways may contribute to OCSB as various clinical disorders have sexual consequences. We organize the various factors that contribute to a client's sense of feeling out of control, including established clinical disorders, personality traits, adverse experiences, and chemical dependency that has sexual symptoms. But, not all vulnerability factors are disordered pathways. As a result, we identify various vulnerability factors that contribute to OCSB. We consider the role of motivations that compete with sexual health and how these competing motivations create an internal struggle that affects self and attachment regulation and sexual/erotic-identity development. In our practice, we conduct a comprehensive assessment that leads to constructing each client's Unique Clinical Picture, which guides treatment planning and recommendations.

An empirically informed approach and clearly developed concept of sexual behavior problems are necessary to ensure quality treatment when faced with the sexual-disorder meme and sexuality misinformation, which overly influences the therapeutic interaction. Along with our OCSB definition and clinical model, we propose a sexual health assessment and treatment pathway to guide psychotherapy. One important disclaimer: Our OCSB conceptualization and protocol is currently limited to men. They are the primary demographic who present for sexual dysregulation in the United States and this model reflects our collective clinical experiences over the past 20 years. The OCSB conceptualization and protocol can inform a therapist's approach with women, but, as practitioners, we are currently not in a position to construct that bridge.

Consensual Sexual Behavior Problems

The OCSB Model makes a clinical distinction between nonconsensual sex and paraphilias. The OCSB protocol encourages clinicians to investigate possible sexual- and erotic-identity obstacles and propose "sexual and erotic conflicts" as one of three clinical areas for investigation and clinical response. We are interested in identifying the degree of "fixatedness" in a client's arousal pattern. OCSB treatment facilitates positive sexual- and erotic-identity development by integrating the man's arousal patterns into his self-concept. If a sexual or erotic conflict is present and involves a rigid arousal pattern, the goal of therapy is to expand a man's range of arousal and integrate his turn-on within his sexual or erotic identity.

This clinical emphasis on integration of erotic orientation within men's sexual lives is one of the reasons why clients with nonconsensual sexual urges, thoughts, or behaviors are excluded from OCSB treatment. This clinical distinction leads us to refer these individuals to nonconsensual specialists who are capable of assessing and treating men with nonconsensual sexual behavior and to provide the treatment interventions that differ from clinical work for men with consensual sexual behavior problems. In Chapter 5, we discuss how we assess and refer men who report nonconsensual sexual behavior.

Self-Discrepancy, Not Personal Distress

Client personal distress about sexual behavior is another clinical distinction within OCSB treatment. There is a clear segment of the population who report distress because of their sexual behavior. The reason you may be reading this book is that you have met with clients distressed about their sexual behavior. We began this chapter by introducing a range of clinical situations in which one or more people bring their distress to a professional. It is often a sudden client sexual crisis that precipitates a request for help. Each of the three proposal diagnoses, sexual addiction, ICSB, and HD, include aspects of personal distress either in its diagnostic criteria or clinical descriptions. Coleman (2011) indicates that people must reach a level of clinical distress to meet criteria for ICSB. Clinically significant distress or impairment in various areas of life is a criterion for HD (Kafka, 2010). The absence of distress does not preclude an HD diagnosis as long as personal impairment, occupational impairment, or social impairment is demonstrated. The role of distress in SA is more difficult to ascertain. Sexual addiction in its most basic definition focuses on a pattern of sexual behavior that causes problems in someone's life. The distress may be twofold, as an emotional consequence of the sexual behavior as well as the inability to reliably stop the pattern of behavior as a response to negative consequences (P. Hall, 2013).

The definition of OCSB intentionally excludes the mention of personal distress. We are interested in highlighting the concept of behavioral control and client motivation for change. We are less focused on a clinical threshold of distress to establish a psychiatric disorder in order for the client to access treatment. Client distress may be related to the external disapproval, disgust, or conflict about sexual behavior rather than the client's felt sense of his sexual control. Personal distress does not mean the same thing as a self-discrepancy about one's sexual urges, thoughts, or behavior. Clients may be distressed because their partner is upset about their masturbating with sexual imagery. Or, distress may arise out of unreasonable expectations or standards about sexual desires. These situations may cause a client distress, but may not motivate him toward sexual health. We focus on the individual's internal conflict and self-discrepancy when assessing sexual behavior problems and determining whether to recommend treatment. Because OCSB outpatient therapy focuses men toward changing their sexual health, we are more concerned about motivation for health behavior change than an arbitrary level of clinically significant distress.

No Sexual Behavior Categories

Finally, the OCSB Model and protocol eschews clinical sexual behavior subcategories. Instead, the OCSB protocol focuses on behaviors that violate sexual health principles (discussed in the following chapter). We believe categories based on specific sexual activity codify sociocultural sex negativity within the clinical models and privileges conventional sexual behavior as "healthy." By framing our OCSB protocol in a sexual health paradigm and grounding our conceptualization in a general theory of human (rather than a disease or disorder) behavior, we strived to create a less shame-based sexual behavior organization to help men change their self-discrepant sexual behavior.

REFERENCES

American Psychiatric Association. (1952). *Diagnostic and statistical manual of mental disorders*. Washington, DC: Author.

American Psychiatric Association. (1968). *Diagnostic and statistical manual of mental disorders* (2nd ed.). Washington, DC: Author.

American Psychiatric Association. (1980). *Diagnostic and statistical manual of mental disorders* (3rd ed.). Washington, DC: Author.

American Psychiatric Association. (1987). *Diagnostic and statistical manual of mental disorders* (3rd ed., rev.). Washington, DC: Author.

American Psychiatric Association. (2000). *Diagnostic and statistical manual of mental disorders* (4th ed., text rev.). Washington, DC: Author.

American Psychiatric Association. (2013). *Diagnostic and statistical manual of mental disorders* (5th ed.). Arlington, VA: American Psychiatric Publishing.

Bancroft, J. (2009). *Human sexuality and its problems* (3rd ed.). Edinburgh, UK: Elsevier Limited.

Bancroft, J., & Vukadinovic, Z. (2004). Sexual addiction, sexual compulsivity, sexual impulsivity, or what? Toward a theoretical model. *Journal of Sex Research, 41*, 225–234.

Barth, R. J., & Kinder, B. N. (1987). The mislabeling of sexual impulsivity. *Journal of Sex & Marital Therapy, 13*, 15–23.

Cantor, J. M., Klein, C., Lykins, A., Rullo, J. E., Thaler, L., & Walling, B. R. (2013). A treatment-oriented typology of self-identified hypersexuality referrals. *Archives of Sexual Behavior, 42*(5), 883–893.

Carnes, P. J. (1983). *The sexual addict.* Minneapolis, MN: CompCare Publishers.

Carnes, P. J. (1989). *Contrary to love.* Center City, MN: Hazelden Foundation.

Carnes, P. J. (1991). *Don't call it love.* New York, NY: Bantam.

Carnes, P. J. (1994). *Out of the shadows.* Minneapolis, MN: Hazelden Foundation.

Coleman, E. (1990). The obsessive–compulsive model for describing compulsive sexual behavior. *American Journal of Preventive Psychiatry & Neurology, 2*(3), 9–14.

Coleman, E. (2011). Impulsive/compulsive sexual behavior: Assessment and treatment. In J. E. Grant & M. N. Potenza (Eds.), *The Oxford handbook of impulse control disorders* (pp. 375–388). New York, NY: Oxford Press.

Coleman, E., Elders, J., Satcher, D., Shindel, A., Parish, S., Kenagy, G., Bayer, C. R., … Light, A. (2013). Summit on medical school education in sexual health: Report of an expert consultation. *Journal of Sexual Medicine, 10*, 924–938.

Edwards, W. M. (2011). *Life, liberty and the pursuit of sexual health.* Minneapolis, MN: Sexual Health Institute, LLC.

Edwards, W. M., Delmonico, D., & Griffin, E. (2011). *Cybersex unplugged: Finding sexual health in an electronic world.* CreateSpace Independent Publishing Platform.

Ford, M. P., & Hendrick, S. S. (2003) Therapists' sexual values for self and clients: Implications for practice and training. *Professional Psychology, Research and Practice, 34*(1), 80–87.

Giugliano, J. (2004). A sociohistorical perspective of sexual health: The clinician's role. *Sexual Addiction & Compulsivity, 11*, 43–55.

Giugliano, J. (2009). *Out of control sexual behavior—A qualitative investigation.* Saarbrücken, Germany: VDM Verlag.

Goldfried, M. R. (2013). What should we expect from psychotherapy. *Clinical Psychology Review, 33*, 862–869.

Goodman, A. (2001). What's in a name? Terminology for designating a syndrome of driven sexual behavior. *Sexual Addiction & Compulsivity, 8*, 191–213.

Hall, K., & Graham, C. (2013). Introduction. In K. Hall & C. Graham (Eds.), *The cultural context of sexual pleasure and problems: Psychotherapy with diverse clients* (pp. 1–20). New York, NY: Routledge.

Hall, P. (2013). *Understanding and treating sex addiction: A comprehensive guide for people who struggle with sex addiction and those who want to help them.* New York, NY: Routledge.

Harris, S. M., & Hays, K. W. (2008). Family therapist comfort and willingness to discuss client sexuality. *Journal of Marital and Family Therapy, 34*(2), 239–250.

Hertlein, K. M. (2004). *Internet infidelity: An examination of family therapist treatment decisions and gender biases.* Unpublished doctoral dissertation. Virginia Polytechnic Institute and State University, Blacksburg, Virginia.

Hilton, D. L. (2013). Pornography addiction: A supranormal stimulus considered in the context of neuroplasticity. *Socioaffective Neuroscience & Psychology, 3.* doi.org/10.3402/snp.v3i0.20767

Hilton, V. W. (1997). Sexuality in the therapeutic process. In L. Hedges, R. Hilton, W. V. Hilton, & B. Caudill (Eds.), *Therapists at risk: Perils of the intimacy of the therapeutic relationship* (pp. 181–220). Northvale, NJ: Jason Aronson.

Joannides, P. (2012). The challenging landscape of problematic sexual behaviors, including "sexual addiction" and "hypersexuality." In P. J. Kleinplatz (Ed.), *New directions in sex therapy: Innovations and alternatives* (pp. 69–83). New York, NY: Routledge.

Kafka, M. (2010). Hypersexual disorder: A proposed diagnosis for DSM-V. *Archives of Sexual Behavior, 39*(2), 377–400.

Kafka, M. P. (1997). Hypersexual desire in males: An operational definition and clinical implications for males with paraphilias and paraphilia-related disorders. *Archives of Sexual Behavior, 26*(5), 505–526.

Kafka, M. P., & Hennan, J. (2000). Psychostimulant augmentation during treatment with selective serotonin reuptake inhibitors in males with paraphilias and paraphilia-related disorders: A case series. *Journal of Clinical Psychiatry, 61*, 664–670.

Kaplan, M. S., & Krueger, R. B. (2010). Diagnosis, assessment, and treatment of hypersexuality. *Journal of Sex Research, 47*(2–3), 181–198.

Klein, M. (2012, July/August). You're addicted to what? Challenging the myth of sex addiction. *Humanist.* Retrieved from http://thehumanist.com/july-august-2012/youre-addicted-to-what/

Kleinplatz, P. J. (Ed.). (2012). *New directions in sex therapy: Innovations and alternatives.* New York, NY: Taylor & Francis.

Levine, M. P., & Troiden, R. R. (1988). The myth of sexual compulsivity. *Journal of Sex Research, 25*(3), 347–363.

Levine, S. (2010a). Preface to the first edition. In S. Levine, C. B. Risen, & S. E. Althof (Eds.), *Handbook of clinical sexuality for mental health professionals* (2nd ed., pp. xiii–xviii). New York, NY: Routledge.

Levine, S. (2010b). What is sexual addiction? *Journal of Sex & Marital Therapy, 36*(3), 261–275.

Ley, D. J. (2012). *The myth of sex addiction.* Lanham, MD: Rowman & Littlefield.

Magness, M. S. (2013). *Stop sex addiction: Real hope, true freedom for sex addicts and partners.* Las Vegas, NV: Central Recovery Press.

Maurice, W. L. (1999). *Sexual medicine in primary care.* London, UK: Mosby.

Miller, W. R., & Rollnick, S. (2013). *Motivational interviewing: Helping people change* (3rd ed.). New York, NY: Guilford Press.

Money, J. (1999). *Principles of developmental sexology.* New York, NY: Continuum.

Money, J., & Lamacz, M. (1989). *Vandalized lovemaps: Paraphilic outcome of seven cases in pediatric sexology.* Buffalo, NY: Prometheus Books.

Moser, C. (2011). Yet another paraphilia definitions fails. *Archives of Sexual Behavior, 40*, 483–485.

Moser, C. (2013). Hypersexual disorder: Searching for clarity. *Sexual Addiction & Compulsivity, 20*(1–2), 48–58.

Quadland, M. C. (1985). Compulsive sexual behavior: Definition of a problem and an approach to treatment. *Journal of Sex & Marital Therapy, 11*(2), 121–132.

Reay, B., Attwood, N., & Gooder, C. (2015a). Inventing sex: The short history of sex addiction. *Sexuality & Culture, 17*, 1–19.

Reay, B., Attwood, N., & Gooder, C. (2015b). *Sex addiction—A critical history.* Cambridge, UK: Polity Press.

Reid, R., Carpenter, B. N., Hook, J. N., Garos, S., Manning, J. C., Gilliland, R., Cooper, E. B., ... Fong, T. (2012). Report of findings in a DSM-5 field trial for hypersexual disorder. *Journal of Sexual Medicine, 9*, 2868–2877.

Reid, R. C. (2013). Personal perspectives on hypersexual disorder. *Sexual Addiction & Compulsivity, 20*(1–2), 4–18.

Reid, R. C., Carpenter, B. N., & Fong, T. W. (2011). Neuroscience research fails to support claims that excessive pornography consumption causes brain damage. *Surgical Neurological International, 2,* 64.

Reid, R. C., & Kafka, M. P. (2014). Controversies about hypersexual disorder and the DSM-5. *Current Sexual Health Reports, 6,* 259–264.

Rogers, C. (1980). *A way of being.* New York, NY: Houghton Mifflin.

Samenow, C. (2013). A word on this special edition … *Sexual Addiction & Compulsivity: The Journal of Treatment & Prevention, 20*(1–2), 1–3.

Schnarch, D. M. (1991). *Constructing the sexual crucible: An integration of sexual and marital therapy.* New York, NY: W. W. Norton.

Schneider, J. P., & Irons, R. R. (2001). Assessment and treatment of addictive sexual disorders: Relevance for chemical dependency relapse. *Substance Use & Misuse, 36*(13), 1795–1820.

Sealy, J. (1995). Pscyhopharmacological intervention in addictive sexual behavior. *Sexual Addiction & Compulsivity, 2*(4) 257–276.

Seem, S. R., & Johnson, E. (1998). Gender bias among counseling trainees: A study of case conceptualization. *Counselor Education and Supervision, 37,* 257–268.

Spenhoff, M., Kruger, T. H., Hartmann, U., & Kobs, J. (2013). Hypersexual behavior in an online sample of males: associations with personal distress and functional impairment. *Journal of Sexual Medicine, 10*(12), 2996–3005.

Steele, V. R., Staley, C., Fong, T., & Prause, N. (2013). Sexual desire, not hypersexuality, is related to neurophysiological responses elicited by sexual images. *Socioaffective Neuroscience & Psychology, 3,* 20770.

Stewart, R. S. (2012). Constructing perversions: The DSM and the classification of sexual paraphilias and disorders. *Electronic Journal of Human Sexuality, 15.* Retrieved from http://www.ejhs.org/volume15/DSM.html

Weiss, R. (2013). *Sex addiction 101: A basic guide to healing from sex, porn, and love addiction.* Dublin, OH: Telemachus Press.

Wines, D. (1997). Exploring the applicability of criteria for substance dependence to sexual addiction. *Sexual Addiction & Compulsivity, 4*(3), 195–220.

Winters, J., Christoff, K., & Gorzalka, B. B. (2010). Dysregulated sexuality and high sexual desire: Distinct constructs? *Archives of Sexual Behavior, 39*(5), 1029–1043.

CHAPTER TWO

ENVISION SEXUAL HEALTH

JAY

"I can't believe I am sitting here," I said to myself. My stomach felt sick. My back was tense. I looked across our therapist's waiting room at Veronique, my wife. I never thought she would find those porn files.

"David's here," Veronique said. I looked up and saw our therapist standing in the doorway. I concentrated on my wife's back as we headed into his office.

David closed the door and she started crying, telling him about finding my secret e-mail account, seeing all those pictures. Then, like a punch to the gut she said, "It makes me sick."

I looked at David and said what I had practiced all morning., "I got rid of it all, I don't want to do this anymore."

Then ... silence. I felt so alone. I just kept looking at David. I couldn't look at my wife. If I did, I would have fallen through the floor.

HECTOR

I thought I would stop going to adult bookstores to have sex with men after I got into rehab. Now, I'd just found out I had gonorrhea. I didn't want to lie anymore, so just as I had agreed in rehab, I told my partner about having a sexually transmitted infection (STI). He was furious ... disgusted. He didn't want to sleep in the same bed with me.

I went to my aftercare group and knew I had to tell them, too. I intentionally sat across from my favorite counselor, Susan, which meant I sat next to the latest student intern (I can never remember her name). I felt so relieved that I didn't use. After I told the group, I said, "I haven't used, but I am afraid of what to do next." I sat very still, staring at Susan for guidance.

FRANK

Two weeks ago, my boss called me into his office and showed me the IT (information technology) investigation about my online sex site history at work. He told me to stop or I would lose my job. So I figured I'd tell my psychiatrist about my porn problem and maybe an adjustment of my anxiety medications could help.

She asked, "How are you doing?"

"I'm doing OK. Except I have something to talk about." I sat silently for what seemed like an eternity. "I need to talk about what happened at work," I muttered. "My boss found out that I was downloading porn at my desk. I've been doing it for years. I can't believe I got caught. I'm so stupid! I can't lose my job."

I saw this look on her face, kind of still, calm, but not like she was disgusted or wanted to throw me out. So I just waited for her to talk.

PETER

I live in a pretty small town. My kids go to school down the street. My wife directs the church choir. I know a lot of people who talk. I parked a few blocks away and tried to walk in the door when the stoplight down the street was red so no one could see me walk in. I never dreamed I would go to see a therapist because I watch porn. Reverend John told me to go. What if she's a Christian? I've been masturbating since I can remember. I always knew it was wrong and not God's plan. I thought prayer and talking with the Reverend would be enough. I thought I would stop when I got married. I told this to the therapist, Lynn.

I told Lynn that masturbating is a betrayal of my marriage sacrament and that my wife said I had to stop or she would leave me. Cautiously, I asked, "Is that something you can help me with? To only have sex with my wife?"

WILL

What was I thinking? It's not like I don't know how people get infected with HIV. So I have no right to be upset. This was my fault. If you don't use condoms, you're probably going to get HIV. I was careless. Stupid. And now I'm finally what my mom always thought I would be: just another fag with HIV.

My counselor thinks I am a sex addict. A *sex addict* … what does that even mean? Am I addicted to sex like people are addicted to alcohol? I definitely overdo it occasionally. But, If I'm a sex addict, do I have to stop having sex? Is it like a disease? Great, now am I just another HIV-positive Black man who might also be a sex addict?

ANTHONY

I learned that I like being discovered jacking off when I was 12. That was when my babysitter walked in on me masturbating in my bedroom. When I saw her, she was startled and kept looking at me. I finally yelled, "Get out of my room," while hiding my dick so she couldn't see it. It was such a rush! Ever since, I like to jerk off in places a woman might see me. No one knows about this turn-on.

Today I was in the hospital recovering from a car accident and I pushed the limit a little too far. No one was around. No roommate and the nurse wasn't supposed to bring my meds for a while. I felt the urge and was really excited. So I started jacking off. Just then the nurse walked in the room and yelled, "Put that away!" I felt sick. She looked really mad. What was going to happen? This was what I fantasized, for someone to walk in on me?

A VISION FOR SEXUAL HEALTH

Begin with the end in mind.
—Stephen Covey

Men rarely ask a psychotherapist to help them improve their sexual health. They typically focus on changing the sexual patterns that lead to unwanted consequences. Either men want the consequences to stop or they want to stop the sexual behavior. But, we are interested in moving beyond just discontinuing unwanted sexual behavior. We are invested in helping men promote and maintain their sexual health. When men combine their motivation to change sexual problems with a vision for sexual health, they can imagine a meaningful life beyond the mere absence of their troubling sexual behaviors.

We frame out of control sexual behavior (OCSB) as an individual's struggle to live congruently within sexual health principles and the individual's sexual values. We set aside the contentious debate concerning sexual dysregulation diagnosis and, instead, direct the client to a different question: "What is your vision for sexual health?" Most clients respond quizzically or list the behavior patterns they want to stop. This response happens so frequently that the question has become less about gathering information and more about signaling the direction in which we want to point treatment. It is a question that invites clients to reflect on their destination and away from the amelioration of a sexual disorder. We view the request for OCSB treatment not only as an opportunity to help clients regain a sense of control, but also as an opportunity to facilitate a sexual health conversation that can ultimately shape their personal vision of sexual health. Because of the general lack of sexual health education in the behavioral health field, it is imperative that we review what we mean by sexual health.

The current working definition of sexual health that emerged from a 2002 World Health Organization (WHO) meeting is the working construct on which we based problematic and out of control sexual behavior assessment and treatment:

> A state of physical, emotional, mental and social well-being in relation to sexuality; it is not merely the absence of disease, dysfunction or infirmity. Sexual health requires a positive and respectful approach to sexuality and sexual relationships, as well as the possibility of having pleasurable and safe sexual experiences, free of coercion, discrimination and violence. For sexual health to be attained and maintained, the sexual rights of all persons must be respected, protected and fulfilled. (WHO, 2006, p. 5)

We begin our discussion about a sexual health approach with a brief history of the term *sexual health*.

Defining *Sexual Health*

Historically, religious institutions provided the first guidelines for human sexual behavior. Stayton (2007) conceptualized Judaic and Christian religious values systems into three types: act centered, relation centered, and a hybrid of the two. Act-centered theology judged "specific *acts* of sex as holding moral or immoral value" (p. 80). Act-centered approaches greatly influenced laws and social norms that were invested in reinforcing the procreative

•

value of sex. Relationship-centered values, on the other hand, "help individuals, families, and society to develop criteria for decision making regarding sexual matters, taking into account the motives and consequences of sexual acts" (Stayton, 2007, p. 82). The last values system, a combination of the first two, encouraged proclaiming the morality or immortality of specific acts, but relationship-centered values are seen as more relevant in one's private and personal decision making. This hybrid approach usually creates conflict because these two values systems are incompatible (Stayton, 2007).

By the mid-1970s, sexual health was primarily the domain of venereology and defined by the absence of STIs and unplanned pregnancy (especially while unmarried; Coleman, 2007). In 1975, the WHO stepped forward to expand the definition. At the time, it was a radical notion to conceptualize sexual health beyond treatment related to procreation or STIs (WHO, 1975). It is difficult to comprehend the importance of the historical shift from a focus on avoiding these two consequences to a robust definition that outlines fundamental human sexual rights (WHO, 1975).

In 1975, the WHO published *Education and Treatment of Human Sexuality: The Training of Health Professionals*. This document included the following definition of sexual health, which changed the direction of public policy strategies and health promotion for the latter part of the 20th century: "Sexual health is the integration of the somatic, emotional, intellectual and social aspects of sexual being, in ways that are positively enriching and that enhance personality, communication and love" (WHO, 1975, p. 6).

Freedom From/Freedom To

As the definition of sexual health expanded over the next 40 years, the field wrestled with the ethical dilemmas imbedded in the process of defining sexual health. The WHO convened a working group in 1987 to refine the concepts of sexual health by focusing on different groups of people from all life stages, considering sex, relationship status, sexual identity, and disabilities (WHO, 1987). This meeting articulated a specific danger in establishing a definition of sexual health. As a result, the definition of sexual health contains an ethical stance vital to OCSB treatment. It recognizes negative and positive sexual freedoms, acknowledging that people have the right to be *free from* undo constraints along with the *freedom to* act. The right to be *free from* undo constraints includes freedom from the restrictions of sociocultural discrimination and oppression, sexual violence, and the impairments caused by sexual disorders and diseases. The freedom to act in the context of sexual health means the *freedom to* enjoy and express one's sexuality within personal and social ethics (see Mace, Bannerman, & Burton, 1974).

Protecting client rights is a familiar ethical responsibility for mental health clinicians. Therapists are responsible for providing the most effective and least restrictive care. For example, therapists do not recommend inpatient hospitalization if outpatient treatment will sufficiently address a client's depression. When a depressed client would benefit from a higher level of care, but declines that recommendation, the client is free to remain depressed. It is our job to tolerate our countertransference in response to the client's choice and not overly assert our wants at the expense of client automony. Mental health professionals have acknowledged their responsibility to use their influence in a way that does not overly restrict client's freedom. However, as stated eloquently by John Locke (1690) in the *Second Treatise of Government*, "But though this be a state of liberty, yet it is not a state of licence [*sic*]" (Sect. 6). Client freedom is not a license for the client to do whatever he or she wants. If that depressed client is also imminently suicidal, clinicians are permitted to break client confidence to restrict the client's potentially suicidal behavior and ultimately suspend the client's autonomy through an involuntary commitment into an inpatient facility. Mental health providers balance the client's right to autonomy with the right to be free from restriction and, as a field, decided that restricting client liberty in acute cases of suicidality is necessary. We invite providers to apply a similar, albeit less extreme version of this ethical principle when treating sexual dysregulation: Honor client sexual autonomy and avoid overly restrictive interventions while providing the most effective treatment to promote client sexual health and well-being.

Sexual Rights

The Pan American Health Organization (PAHO), the World Association for Sexual Health (WAS), and a WHO Regional Office convened in Antigua, Guatemala, in 2000 to incorporate advances in sexual knowledge and changes in the sociopolitical environment to enhance the definition of sexual health (Coleman, 2007). Previous documents addressed cultural, religious, educational, and health care professional attitudes as obstacles to sexual health. The document *Promotion of Sexual Health: Recommendations for Action* emphasized the sexual science and research that emerged from the AIDS epidemic and discovery of pharmacological sexual-disorder treatments (PAHO/WHO/WAS, 2000; Zucker, 2002). Sexual health promotion as an interaction between the individual and specialized sexual health services emerged as a model for articulating individual and societal responsibility for maintaining sexual health. The proposal posited human sexuality as central to overall well-being and introduced sexual rights into the definition of sexual health. "The emphasis on sexual rights as an essential ingredient for the attainment of sexual health was stated clearly and emphatically" (Coleman, 2007, p. 9). Maintaining sexual health was inextricably linked with respect for basic and fundamental human rights. "The association of sexual health and sexual rights is part of a strategy for building an international consensus in favor of a new sexual morality based on the principle and ultimate objective of health" (Giami, 2002, p. 20). Emphasizing health as the moral rationale for changing sexual behavior replaced previously prominent sexual moral values founded within religion, psychiatry, and cultural tradition (Giami, 2002).

The WAS adopted a formal declaration of sexual rights in 1999 and recommends its recognition, promotion, respect, and defense throughout the world (Coleman, 2007). In 2000, the WHO supported the WAS Declaration of Sexual Rights and integrated these declarations within their own 2002 working definition of sexual health. The WAS declaration was updated in 2014 and included the following list of human rights pertaining to sexuality (WAS, 2014).

1. The right to equality and nondiscrimination
2. The right to life, liberty, and security of the persons
3. The right to autonomy and bodily integrity
4. The right to be free from torture and cruel, inhuman, or degrading treatment or punishment
5. The right to be free from all forms of violence and coercion
6. The right to privacy
7. The right to the highest attainable standard of health, including sexual health; with the possibility of pleasurable, satisfying, and safe sexual experiences
8. The right to enjoy the benefits of scientific progress and its application
9. The right to information
10. The right to education and the right to comprehensive sexuality education
11. The right to enter, form, and dissolve marriage and other similar types of relationships based on equality and full and free consent
12. The right to decide whether to have children, the number and spacing of children, and to have the information and means to do so
13. The right to the freedom of thought, opinion, and expression
14. The right to freedom of association and peaceful assembly
15. The right to participation in public and political life
16. The right of access to justice, remedies, and redress

Responsible Sexual Behavior

An important sexual health milestone occurred in the United States in 2001. The surgeon general of the United States, David Satcher, released a document that provides a framework for a national dialogue on sexual health: *The Surgeon General's Call to Action to Promote Sexual Health and Responsible Sexual Behavior* (U.S. Surgeon General, 2001). In the opening statement, Surgeon General Satcher proclaims sexuality as a fundamental part of human life and calls for a mature and thoughtful sexual health conversation. The report promotes a national conversation that includes the physical, mental, and spiritual aspects of sexuality. It also describes thoughtful sexual health conversation as a collaborative process that incorporates a wide range of experience, expertise, and perspectives and provides the best available science-based information to the American people. The report reflects previously identified sexual health definitions and adds a significant contribution to previous work. The surgeon general incorporates the importance of individual and community sexual responsibility. It is the U.S. federal government's position that each citizen has the responsibility to understand his or her sexuality, respect others' sexuality, and avoid harm to oneself or others. Respect included recognizing and tolerating sexual diversity and exercising reproduction responsibility (U.S. Surgeon General, 2001).

The surgeon general's report recommends three strategies to promote sexual health and responsible sexual behavior. First and foremost, the report recommends promoting sexual health awareness. We hope this book contributes to this strategy by proposing a new OCSB assessment and treatment protocol based on sexual health principles and a nonpathological conceptualization of sexual behavior problems. Second, the report encourages implementing and strengthening sexual health interventions. We believe this is a limitation in current sexual dysregulation models. With our sexual health emphasis, we hope to expand the conversation about understanding and treating symptoms of OCSB, much like the first WHO meeting in 1975, during which the conversation moved from the rudimentary focus on disease prevention to a wider understanding of health. Finally, the surgeon general emphasized the need for expanding research on a range of matters connected with sexual health. Our treatment protocol not only draws on sexual science, but is also shaped by the fields of health behavior change, neurobiology, self-regulation, attachment, mental illness, drug and alcohol addiction, public health, sexology, HIV prevention, and reproductive health, Because sexuality is interwoven within overall health and wellness, it is imperative to develop an OCSB construct and protocol that includes the research and insights from disparate but related fields.

OUT OF CONTROL SEXUAL BEHAVIOR AND SEXUAL HEALTH

The development of sexual dysregulation treatment models paralleled the 25-year international focus on sexual health. What has emerged during this time are models of dysregulated sexual behavior with disparate criteria and limited sexual health integration.

Despite the breadth of three decades of publications, recent sex addiction (SA) treatment manuals and client workbooks have not acknowledged or referenced the emerging definitions or scholarly publications regarding sexual health. Sexual addiction promotes "twelve dimensions of human sexuality" (Carnes, 2010, p. 315), healthy sex (Magness, 2011), a Health Sexuality Model (Earle & Earle, 1995), and "satisfying sexuality" (Hall, 2013, p. 156). Hypersexual behavior literature does not mention sexual health or the international development of sexual health. Kafka (2009) does discuss the values conflict imbedded in the medical distinction of "normal" and "pathological" sexual behavior when defining hypersexual behavior. Kaplan and Krueger (2010) review evidence-based articles concerning diagnosis, assessment, and treatment of hypersexual conditions and chose the term *hypersexual* because "it appears to be the most atheoretical and neutral term" (p. 181). Their comprehensive review does not mention the developing definitions of sexual health, nor does it mention sexual health as a specific focus within assessment or treatment.

In 2002, Beatrice "Bean" Robinson and colleagues at the University of Minnesota Program in Human Sexuality created and researched the Sexual Health Model in a long-term sexuality education intervention to prevent HIV infection (Robinson, Bockington, Rosser, Miner, & Coleman, 2002). They based the Sexual Health Model on the WHO *sexual health* definition to research health care outcomes when applied in a clinical setting. They hypothesize that a holistic view of sexual health would enhance sexual negotiation within the sexual relationships of people with long-term sexual HIV risk. The Sexual Health Model identifies 10 components that constitute crucial aspects of healthy human sexuality (Robinson et al., 2002). Elements of sexual health contained in the Sexual Health Model include knowledge, self-awareness, self-acceptance, internal congruence, intimacy, communication, sexual desire, sexual functioning, responsibility, respect for individual differences and a sex-positive approach to sexuality. Clinical application may have been too ambitious in practical application of all 10 of the elements of their model. The model was found to be unwieldy and abstract for generalizable utility within clinical or client education settings (Edwards & Coleman, 2004).

In a 5-year collaboration with Stepping Stone of San Diego, a residential and outpatient drug and alcohol treatment center, Doug Braun-Harvey developed a sexual health-based relapse-prevention intervention for clients with high levels of sex/drug-linked behavior. Braun-Harvey hypothesizes that "building sexual health skills within the recovery process will reduce the risk of relapse" (Braun-Harvey, 2009, p. 8). The Sexual Health in Recovery curriculum involves 12 different sexual health skills used for reducing relapse risk associated with sexuality and sexual behavior among men and women in recovery. Clinical application of all 12 sexual health skills in recovery has limitations, given the various levels of care available within drug and alcohol treatment. Sufficient time to complete all 12 skills is more feasible in long-term residential treatment programs than in intensive outpatient programs.

Robinson et al. (2002) and Braun-Harvey (2009) identify limitations for integrating comprehensive sexual health models into some clinical situations. In the zeal to base clinical applications on the complete *sexual health* definition and sexual rights, psychotherapy interventions risk becoming overly focused on an idealized understanding for sexual health and expected men and women to integrate every sexual health concept and principle. Robinson et al. concluded that it was impractical to include all 10 components of the Sexual Health Model within specific clinical population applications. For example, significant time and expense are needed to train staff not to confuse sexual health with client sexual activity approved of by the professional leading the training (Robinson et al., 2002). Since the publication of *Sexual Health in Drug and Alcohol Treatment* (2009), several clinical settings shortened the original 12-lesson curriculum to teach within a briefer outpatient treatment setting. Anecdotally, it seems that integrating sexual health into behavioral health care is more feasible when sexual health models provide a framework without the expectation of addressing every component of sexual health.

Professional discourse about problematic or out of control sexual behavior has evolved with limited sexual health integration. This omission seems particularly pertinent given a common critique of diagnosis-driven models for sexual dysregulation is their propensity to promulgate religious, cultural, or societal bias (Joannides, 2012). Without accepted sexual health principles from respected international and interdisciplinary health organizations, sexual behavior diagnoses unwittingly become the latest medical manifestation of an act-centered values system restricting the expression of socially disapproved sexual activity, attitudes, and desires. Early attempts to define sexual health were aware of the hazards of establishing overreaching concepts that restricted diversity of sexual expression (WHO, 1987). Despite this risk, the task of developing a useful sexual health construct through an open consensus led to a surprisingly wide acceptance with only small challenges (see Coleman, 2007). Unfortunately, the lack of a consensus for a working definition of sexual health within the narrower sphere of sexual dysregulation treatment leaves the clinical models vulnerable to sanctioning negative sociocultural sexual norms within their respective pathology thresholds.

SIX SEXUAL HEALTH PRINCIPLES

We propose a sexual health foundation to provide effective and ethical treatment for men with OCSB. We operationalized the public health consensus on sexual health into a framework to mitigate the influence of proscriptive, disapproving, or stigmatizing sociocultural sexual values within our model. We distilled the sexual health construct into six principles:

1. Consent
2. Nonexploitation
3. Protection from HIV/STIs and unintended pregnancy
4. Honesty
5. Shared values
6. Mutual pleasure

The construct of the sexual health principles was summarized beautifully in the 2000 proceedings of a regional consultation convened by PAHO and WHO in collaboration with the WAS:

> Responsible sexual behavior is expressed at individual, interpersonal and community levels. It is characterized by autonomy, *mutuality*, *honesty*, respectfulness, *consent*, *protection*, pursuit of *pleasure*, and wellness. The person exhibiting responsible sexual behavior does not intend to cause harm, and refrains from *exploitation*, harassment, manipulation and discrimination. (PAHO/WHO/WAS, 2000, p. 8)

We italicized the concepts to reveal what we harvested from this description of responsible sexual behavior. We have translated the language of responsible sexual behavior into a clinical formulation to guide and measure outcomes of OCSB treatment.

Our intention is to develop a useful application of the sexual health construct for a purpose similar to Stayton's (2007) definition of a relationship-centered sexual values system—"to help individuals, families, and society to develop criteria for decision making regarding sexual matters, taking into account motives and consequences of sexual acts" (p. 82). We refer to this approach as "principle centered" as opposed to Stayton's "relationship centered." By changing *relationship* to *principle*, we hope to avoid the possible misperception that we are privileging sex in romantic relationships.

Integrating sexual health principles into the OCSB protocol is our attempt to remedy the justified fears of sociocultural norms that stigmatize the frequency or content of sexual urges, thoughts, and behaviors from overly influencing clinical interventions. Simply put, integrating these principles into the psychotherapy treatment frame is how we "first, do no harm." The principles are intended as protection from interventions that overly rely on act-centered judgments while, at the same time, helping clients to make decisions that will benefit their health and well-being. The principles help navigate the "freedom from/freedom to" ethical tension by providing a framework to guide clinicians on when and why to assert influence.

The six sexual health principles provide the necessary conceptualization for addressing OCSB as a sexual problem because we do not rely on diagnostic criteria to guide treatment. When clients are introduced to the sexual health framework, they can choose to enter a process in which they are responsible for constructing and maintaining their sexual health through incremental alignment with these six principles. Clients are also able to access treatment without having to accept a clinical diagnosis; all they need is motivation to change.

If clients are motivated to change their out of control sexual experiences, then treatment begins by evaluating their current behavior with the sexual health principles. When client sexual behavior is within the sexual health framework, the specific sexual acts in which clients wish to engage are up to them. Like the global public health community's development of an inclusive *sexual health* definition, we believe sexual health principles provide a necessary construct to inform sexual health-based OCSB therapy. We briefly elucidate key aspects of each principle.

1. **Consent**: a "voluntary cooperation" and the permission to reach sexual satisfaction and intimacy with oneself and willing partners (Wertheimer, 2003, p. 124). Consent is a balance between one's

autonomy to give clear unambiguous consent for sex in combination with everyone's right to engage in sex with whomever he or she chooses (Wertheimer, 2003). "Safe, consensual sex is a human right" (Swartzendruber & Zenilman, 2010, p. 1006) and the essential sexual health principle that makes mutually positive sexual interactions possible.

2. **Nonexploitation**: Exploitation can be seen as leveraging one's power and control to receive sexual gratification from another person, which compromises that person's ability to consent. A person can increase the likelihood of nonexploitive sex when he or she remains highly motivated to ensure he or she is not taking unfair advantage to gain access to a sexual partner or sexual activity. Nonexploitative sex is likely when each person considers the risk of exploitation as it relates to the consent between partners, the potential for harm, and the mutual advantageousness for each person to enjoy the sexual situation (Wertheimer, 2003).

3. **Protected from STIs and unintended pregnancy**: This sexual health principle is evident when those involved in the sexual activity are capable of protecting themselves and their partners from an STI (including HIV) and unintended or unwanted pregnancy. This includes access to testing and medical care and to scientifically accurate information regarding disease transmission, reproductive health, and contraception resources.

4. **Honesty**: Sexual health involves direct and open communication with oneself and one's partners. Self-honesty involves being open to sexual pleasure, experiences, and sexual education. Honesty is a crucial building block for sexual relations with others and is necessary for effective communication to uphold all of the sexual health principles. Honesty in sexual relationships varies based on relational factors and contexts and is not to be confused with complete transparency and unlimited candidness.

5. **Shared values**: Sexual relations between partners involve clarifying underlying motives, sexual standards, and the meaning of specific sexual acts for each person. This principle promotes conversations between sex partners to clarify their consent for sexual relations, discuss their sexual values, and articulate motivations for having sex.

6. **Mutual pleasure**: The mutual-pleasure principle prioritizes the giving and receiving of pleasure. There are many ways for both giving and receiving sexual pleasure. Each moment of heightened pleasure can have many meanings that can change over time and with different partners. Valuing the pleasure of sex as a positive

and life-enhancing aspect of sex is vital for ensuring mutual pleasure. Mutually pleasurable sexual activity invites clients to consider their bodily, erotic, and emotional sensualities for themselves
and their partners.

SEXUAL HEALTH CONVERSATIONS

Learning the sexual health principles is central to the protocol, but insufficient for working with OCSB. Talking about the sexual health principles
as well as engaging in sexual health conversations with clients requires
a therapist to have a level of comfort and ability to integrate sexual
health concepts within the therapeutic process. A therapist's communication style that fosters honest and open discussions about potentially
uncomfortable aspects of sexuality provides clients with an opportunity
to develop their vision for sexual health. Just as we want to set up our
clients to successfully utilize therapy to achieve their sexual health goals,
we want to successfully prepare therapists to facilitate sexual health conversations. Before we get into the sexual content of the OCSB sessions, we
focus on psychotherapy process points for increasing clinician effectiveness in sexual health conversations.

To help illustrate our suggestions to successfully facilitate sexual
health conversations, we describe key dialogue moments with our case
example participants: David, Charmaine, Beth, Lynn, Danny, and Amy.
We left each situation at a choice point immediately after the client initiated a sexual health conversation. Each therapist was given little to no
notice that the discussion would swerve toward sexual problems, fears,
or heartbreak. When clients unexpectedly bring a sexual crisis to therapy,
therapists with basic sexual health conversation tools are better equipped
to encourage constructive and open sexual health conversations.

Suspending Judgment

Hector's drug and alcohol group therapy intern, Chamaine, felt an
immediate disgust after hearing him describe having sex with his partner without disclosing to him that he recently had condomless anal sex
with a stranger. Will's therapist, Danny, had a long-standing antipathy
for the entire conceptualization of sexual addiction. Now Danny is meeting with Will, who is explicitly asking him for help with a problem that
was described by another health care professionals as "sexual addiction."
Sexual health conversations benefit from practitioners suspending their

judgments—to temporarily set aside their personal judgments to protect the therapeutic relationship. We are not suggesting that professionals become free of all judgments. More realistically, therapists can develop the skill to acknowledge their judgments when they occur and set them aside. A therapist's ability to suspend personal judgments allows the provider to uphold the aspect of acceptance at the heart of person-centered psychotherapy. Sexual health-based psychotherapy is a forum in which all participants intentionally set aside their personal judgments to gain useful insight into the client's self-discrepancy about his sexual experiences. Therapist judgments will likely generate client defensiveness or shame and demotivate them for change. When professionals learn to suspend their judgments about their client's sexual lives, they improve their ability to empower clients to take responsibility for clarifying and maintaining their personal vision of sexual health.

Therapists need resources for supervision, training, and consultation to integrate sexual health conversation skills within their clinical practice. Suspending judgments is an important skill needed to address a negative judgment when it surfaces during a session. Suspending it, however, is only part of the therapists' task. The therapist also needs to evaluate that judgment after the session ends to prevent it from impacting future client rapport. Clinicians benefit from a safe, informed, and respectful place to resolve those negative judgments and the countertransference that arises when treating sexual problems.

Sexual Health Conversations: Focus on the Details

We left David in a painful couple therapy moment for Jay and Veronique. Jay's wife disclosed her feelings of disgust about Jay's sexual behavior. This brings new painful facts into the couple's therapy. In this moment, David was learning that the couple had failed to integrate fundamental components of sexual health within their marriage. The vignette ended with Veronique sobbing and Jay looking dazed. David was prepared to move the dialogue toward the details of Jay's sexual activity rather than let the specifics remain absent. Consider Veronique's pronouns and the absence of detail when she first disclosed her pain and disgust after learning about her husband's online sexual behavior.

"I found it all" she says, her voice louder and more angry. "He's been lying the whole time. I looked at his e-mail and found a secret account he has been hiding from me. Apparently, he goes online and looks at porn and talks to women. He has files of pictures. It makes me sick." Jay, sitting quietly, looks at me and says, "I got rid of it all, I don't want to do this anymore."

Several sexual activities were alluded to in vague language during this 15 seconds of dialogue. Vague language like "it," "porn," or "talks to women" could each be a focus for David to clarify. Specific details of sexual activity are typically not well described by psychotherapy clients. In a heightened emotional moment, limited skills for using specific sexual terms and descriptions increase the likelihood of opinions and judgments entering the conversation. Therapists have a choice to either let the vague language stand without clarification or slow the moment down and ask for clarification about the vague terms. Slowing down heated moments when sex is discussed in therapy allows the clarification of vague, judgmental language and provides an opportunity for clients to change their current avoidant approaches to talking about sex. Whenever clients change avoidant behaviors, they can experiment with experiencing and tolerating difficult emotions in the therapy session.

David could ask Veronique to clarify vague words or metaphorical language that obscures the meaning of what she wants to be understood. Clients commonly use phrases like, "slept together," "down there," or "hooked up" that fail to communicate what sexual activity or body part is a source of distress. When client and therapist agree to verbally describe actual sexual activities, they are collaborating to circumvent common interpersonal patterns about sex that too often obfuscate what is actually happened. Details of sex elicit both the general discomfort in talking about sex and the hurt feelings related to the current situation. The sexual health conversation skill is necessary for therapists to discern when to move toward the sexual details and invite the client to use terms that clarify important circumstances of the sexual situation. This clinical intervention also provides an opportunity for the client to practice tolerating the emotional activation that typically accompanies talk about the sexual details. Helping clients identify, label, and express descriptions of sexual activity and the emotions activated by this discussion is a curative element of psychotherapy.

David, like all therapists in his circumstance, had multiple options. To maintain sexual health conversation norms (a useful treatment frame), David could have asked Veronique what was the "it" that made her sick. Maintaining curiosity about specifics when the details are linked with the most intense emotion (e.g., revulsion), can be an important opportunity for Veronique's emotions to balance her intense judgments. We propose that the factual details about the online sexual imagery (i.e., what did she see that generated such feelings of disgust) will often move the clients to deeper and more complex feelings and thoughts beyond their initial reactive intensity.

Integrating the Sexual Health Principles Into Your Treatment Frame

The psychotherapy treatment frame is the mutually agreed upon set of boundaries and conditions for therapy that are clearly defined and maintained through treatment. "The treatment frame and treatment contract serve a variety of functions in the opening phase and throughout the course of treatment, and maintaining the treatment frame is an essential responsibility of both patient and therapist" (Caligor, Kernberg, & Clarkin, 2007, p. 99). Integrating the sexual health principles into the psychotherapy treatment frame is an effective technique used to monitor and prioritize client sexual behavior that circumvents or contravenes these principles. The sexual health principles can be viewed with similar importance of other treatment frame agreements for therapy. When clients cross the frame, examining the meaning of their behavior becomes a priority in the session (Caligor et al., 2007). Similar to how therapists are trained to maintain a framework for patient safety, vague or passive suicidal statements prompt a therapist's inquiry. Clients disclosing behavior that crosses or has the potential to cross the sexual health framework prompts a therapist's inquiry.

Anthony's scenario of masturbating in his hospital room illustrates the importance of the sexual health treatment frame. Absent in Anthony's story was the use of the word *consent*. Amy did not mention it when talking with him about his behavior. Anthony did not mention it when discussing what happened with his babysitter. Anthony said "discovered" to talk about his sexual behavior. Describing the situation does not clarify the degree of sexual consent in his actions. He also revealed a history of enjoying masturbating in public places. In the clinical sense, sexual exhibitionism involves exposing one's genitals to others without their consent. The sexual health treatment frame prepares therapists to listen for language and behavior that signals the possibility that a client is engaged in nonconsensual sex. Clarifying these possibilities becomes a priority in the session. Questions like, "When you said 'accidentally,' were you intending for someone to see you?" "How did you feel when you were seen masturbating?" "When was the last time you engaged in nonconsensual sex?" Using the term *nonconsent* explicitly communicates the aspect of the behavior that is the concern of treatment. Someone watching Anthony masturbate is not the issue; the issue is that Anthony did not receive permission from the other people to masturbate in front of them.

Process Client Initiation of Sexual Disclosure

Often what gets lost in the initial distress of disclosing a highly emotional sexual problem is reinforcing the client's decision to honestly and openly reveal it. For instance, Hector was honest with himself about his gonorrhea symptom and then was honest with the STI testing counselor about his current symptoms. He was motivated to stay sober and chose to be honest with his recovery community. It was very painful, but he was also honest with his partner.

Sexual health conversations in therapy remain rare. In the heat of the moment, client, therapist, or both may move away from the intimacy of the here-and-now contact when clients talk about sex. We often hear therapists talk about how they manage their own emotions with clients talking about sex by moving the conversation away from details and specifics. When clients succeed at describing those details and experiencing the accompanying emotions, the therapist has an opportunity to reinforce the client for engaging in the honest sexual health discussion. Therapists can slow the moment down and ask the client about his thoughts, feelings, and observations in response to talking about sex. Join the client by becoming interested in his experience both prior to the disclosure and while he was discussing the sexual problem. Attending to the process of the sexual health conversation deepens rapport and creates future opportunities for sexual health conversations in psychotherapy.

Susan or Charmaine could ask Hector to describe his thoughts and feelings about discussing his STI with the group and the fallout from being honest with his partner. "Hector, you just said a lot, and I want the group to return to the many thoughts and feelings they may be having right now. But I wonder if you could first let us in on what the last few minutes or hours have been like for you as you anticipated coming to group and telling us about your sexual health concern?" Hector is the only one in the room who has had preparation for this moment. He may bring clarity to the group about how he made sexual health decisions over the last few days. Starting with the most recent, when he chose to speak openly with the group. Inviting Hector to discuss his here/now process with the group is a potent reinforcement for Hector to feel rewarded for his effort as well as a model for future group members to consider when it is their time to have a sexual health conversation with the group.

Sexual Health Conversations Require Therapist Mindfulness

Beth needed to be present and aware the minute Frank turned his medication management meeting into a sexual behavior crisis. He was doing the best he could to manage his anxiety symptoms. Beth was approaching her treatment with Frank as a patient with an anxiety disorder, but now Frank disclosed online sexual behavior problems in the workplace. Beth knew how to focus on regulating her own affective state when Frank described the true extent of his sexual behavior. She first attended to her emotions before asking for more information about Frank's dilemma.

Even the most seasoned therapists experience negative judgmental thoughts and/or uncomfortable feelings in response to patient sexual disclosure. Professional sexual health skills involve a self-awareness and affect regulation tools that can be utilized when sexual content evokes an unexpected level of emotional activation. Pausing to sufficiently self-regulate your own affect before moving forward toward more clinical discussion is an important sexual health conversation skill. For Beth, her affect regulation tool was to focus on her breath. For other clinicians, the pause may contain a decision to suspend their judgmental thinking and to later discuss their reaction in more detail in a peer consultation or clinical supervision.

REFERENCES

Braun-Harvey, D. (2009). *Sexual health in drug and alcohol treatment: Group facilitator's manual*. New York, NY: Springer Publishing Company.

Caligor, E., Kernberg, O. F., & Clarkin, J. F. (2007). *Handbook of dynamic psychotherapy for higher level personality pathology*. Arlington, VA: American Psychiatric Press.

Carnes, P. (2010). *Facing the shadow: Starting sexual and relationship recovery* (2nd ed.). Carefree, AZ: Gentle Path Press.

Coleman, E. (2007). Sexual health: Definitions and construct development. In M. S. Tepper, & A. F. Ownes (Eds.), *Sexual health volume 1: Psychological foundations*. Westport, CT: Praeger.

Covey, S. R. (2004). *The 7 habits of highly effective people: Powerful lessons in personal change*. New York, NY: Simon and Schuster.

Earle, R., & Earle, M. (1995). *Sex addiction: Case studies and management*. New York, NY: Brunner/Mazel.

Edwards, W., & Coleman, E. (2004). Defining sexual health: A descriptive overview. *Archives of Sexual Behavior, 33*(3), 189–195.

Giami, A. (2002). Sexuality and public health: The emergence, development and diversity of the concept of sexual health. *Annual Review of Sex Research, 13*, 1–35.

Hall, P. (2013). *Understanding and treating sex addiction: A comprehensive guide for people who struggle with sex addiction and those who want to help them*. New York, NY: Routledge.

Joannides, P. (2012). The challenging landscape of problematic sexual behaviors. In P. J. Kleinplatz (Ed.), *New directions in sex therapy: Innovations and alternatives* (2nd ed.). New York, NY: Routledge.

Kafka, M. (2009). Hypersexual disorder: A proposed diagnosis for DSM-V. *Archives of Sexual Behavior, 39*, 377–400.

Kaplan, M., & Krueger, R. (2010). Diagnosis, assessment, and treatment of hypersexuality. *Journal of Sex Research, 47*(2–3), 181–198.

Locke, J. (1690). *Second treatise of government.* Retrieved from: http://www.gutenberg .org/files/7370/7370-h/7370-h.htm

Mace, D. R., Bannerman, R. H. O., & Burton, J. (1974). *The teaching of human sexuality in schools for health professionals (Public Health Paper No. 57).* Geneva, Switzerland: World Health Organization.

Magness, M. (2011). *Thirty days to hope and freedom from sexual addiction.* Carefree, AZ: Gentle Path Press.

Pan American Health Organization, World Health Organization & World Association of Sexology. (2000). *Promotion of sexual health: Recommendations for action.* Washington, DC: Pan American Health Organization. Retrieved from: http://www2.paho.org/hq/dmdocuments/2008/PromotionSexualHealth.pdf

Robinson, B., Bockington, W., Rosser, S., Miner, M., & Coleman, E. (2002). The sexual health model: Application of a sexological approach to HIV prevention. *Health Education Research: Theory and Practice, 17*(1), 43–57.

Schmidt, G. (1987). *Sexual health within a societal context. Concepts of sexual health: Report of a working group.* Copenhagen, Denmark: World Health Organization, Regional Office for Europe.

Stayton, W. R. (2007). Sexual values systems and sexual health. In M. S. Tepper & A. F. Owen (Eds.), *Sexual health volume 3: Moral and cultural foundations.* Westport, CT: Praeger.

Swartzendruber, A., & Zenilman, J. (2010). A national strategy to improve sexual health. *Journal of the American Medical Association, 304*(9), 1005–1006.

U.S. Surgeon General. (2001). *The Surgeon General's call to action to promote sexual health and responsible sexual behavior.* Rockville, MD: The Office of the Surgeon General. Retrieved from: http://www.ncbi.nlm.nih.gov/books/NBK44216/

Wertheimer, A. (2003). *Consent to sexual relations.* New York, NY: Cambridge University Press.

World Association for Sexual Health. (2014). *Declaration of sexual rights.* Retrieved from: http://www.worldsexology.org/resources/declaration-of-sexual-rights/

World Health Organization. (1975). *Education and treatment in human sexuality: The training of health professionals.* Report of a WHO Meeting (Technical Report Series No. 572). Retrieved from: http://whqlibdoc.who.int/trs/WHO_TRS_572.pdf

World Health Organization. (1987). *Concepts of sexual health: Report of a working group.* Copenhagen, Denmark: WHO Regional Office for Europe.

World Health Organization. (2006). *Defining sexual health: Report of a technical consultation on sexual health 28–31 January 2002* (pp. 1–35). Geneva, Switzerland: Author.

Zucker, K. (2002). From the editor's desk: Receiving the torch in the era of sexology renaissance. *Archives of Sexual Behavior, 31*, 1–6.

CHAPTER THREE

WHAT IS OUT OF CONTROL SEXUAL BEHAVIOR?

I can resist anything except temptation.
—Oscar Wilde

PREMATURE LABELS

As we mentioned in Chapter 1, Bancroft and Vukadinovic (2004) published a small study on self-identified "sex addicts" that included a critical review of sexual addiction, compulsivity, and impulsivity. It was an article that heavily influenced the design of the out of control sexual behavior (OCSB) protocol. They conclude:

> While acknowledging the importance to both the individual and society of patterns of sexual behavior that are out of control and have problematic consequences, we think it likely that such patterns are varied in both their etiological determinants and how they are best treated. For that reason, we consider it to be premature to attempt some overriding definition relevant to clinical management until we have a better understanding of the various patterns and their likely determinants. (p. 233)

Our early protocol development was inspired by several of Bancroft and Vukadinovic's (2004) conclusions. Phrases like "sexual addiction" and "compulsive sexual behavior" describe the sexual behavior problem using diagnostic labels that fuse a disease model with a description of a human behavior problem. Bancroft and Vukadinovic's (2004) recommendations remain an important contemporary position. Because various factors separately and collectively contribute to problematic and out of control sexual behavioral patterns, it is premature to promote a clinical disorder, especially when a disease model does not add an explanatory value in most cases.

People are motivated to change when the benefits of change outweigh the benefits of the status quo (or the costs of the status quo outweigh the costs of change; Miller & Rollnick, 2002). When treating OCSB, clinicians can learn to tolerate a diagnostic gray zone and focus on what is motivating the client to change his sexual behavior. This treatment direction is set by one of the first questions we ask during a consultation appointment: "What is your vision of sexual health?" It is a simple yet frequently absent question in sexual dysregulation therapy. Too often, the bigger picture of sexual health is lost in the storm of painful consequences and a focus on diagnosing a clinical disorder.

The Problem With Labels

Bancroft and Vukadinovic (2004) ask a question that is still unanswered: Is OCSB a problem on the extreme end of the "normal" range of sexual behavior or is it a distinct behavior that is "qualitatively different from the norm in ways that are problematic" (p. 225). Until this distinction is clarified, they recommend the term "out of control sexual behavior." We adopted this phrase and define it as a sexual health problem in which an individual's consensual sexual urges, thoughts, or behaviors feel out of control. Labels are not without their problems and OCSB is no exception. The phrase *out of control* implies that clients have no power to direct or manage their behaviors, which has been criticized as a justification for remaining unaccountable for the consequences of their actions. This critique is linked with the assumption that being an addict or "out of control" means the person has no agency. Under this assumption, labeling sexual behavior as out of control risks reinforcing a disempowered, victim-like position in which a person is overtaken by an external or internal force greater than himself. Don't get us wrong, sex can be magical ... metaphorically. But, one's drive to have sex is not literally stronger than one's ability to choose or direct behavior, and we have yet to treat a client whose sexual experiences were pervasively out of control. We invite you to think of "out of control" as a reflection of an individual's internal sense of agency that does not introduce a reason why the individual feels that way.

Reveal or Conceal?

There is a long history of diagnostic labels and specific treatment paradigms for sexual dysregulation disorders (see Bancroft, Graham, Janssen, & Sanders, 2009; Cantor et al., 2013; Joannides, 2012). Unfortunately, current sexual dysregulation labels imply scientific certainty where none exists, and a client will frequently initiate therapy after coming to the conclusion that he is a "sex addict." After 30 years of consumer-based literature, media sensationalism, and the sociocultural forces evident since the 1980s (Reay, Attwood, & Gooder, 2013), sex addiction is the dominate lens through which sexual behavior problems are evaluated and the cultural meme that is present in the therapeutic relationship. Unfortunately, when clients self-identify as "sex addicts" or "hypersexuals," they have not revealed much about their experiences. Without further inquiry into the meaning of the client's language, therapists risk prematurely organizing their clinical interventions around a yet-to-be-established clinical disorder and may overlook a host of potential contributing factors. In our professional trainings, we often illustrate this dilemma with a medical parallel. A patient walks into his doctor's office and says, "Doc, I have cancer." And, the doctor says, "Well, at least we don't have to run all those tests. Let's start treatment."

When a client's chief complaint is sex addiction (SA), impulsive–compulsive sexual behavior (ICSB), or hypersexuality, this label may inaccurately describe the core issues causing his problems, because client perception rarely evolves independently from cultural or environmental influences (religiosity, social media, family values, etc.; Reid, 2013). From the start of psychotherapy, it is crucial to understand the client's meaning and utility of his sexuality language and maintain a persistent curiosity about his subjective "out of control" experiences. In developing our OCSB protocol, we intended to create a process that encouraged a conversation about the client's internal world. Providers protect the therapeutic space for client curiosity and honest self-reflection when they avoid prematurely endorsing the client's (or the spouse's) diagnostic conclusions. Maintaining this nonjudgmental stance can be difficult for therapists because of the aforementioned sociocultural forces influencing the conversation or when they are faced with clients in distress because of their sexual behaviors. Clients often contact mental health professionals while in the midst of the storm of a sexual consequence and press for an immediate resolution. Their solutions? "I don't have time for any tests—treat my 'sex addiction'!" The OCSB process challenges the therapist to establish a therapeutic alliance while tempering the client's wish to excise his disordered agency.

Sexual Urges, Thoughts, and Behaviors

Our OCSB definition includes the phrase "sexual urges, thoughts, or behaviors." They are the components of sexuality that are continually assessed and monitored to understand the intrapersonal and interpersonal sexual experiences of each client. But, what are sexual thoughts, urges, and behaviors? How are they related and distinct from each other?

- *Sexual urges* are the embodied sensations and activation that motivate sexual action. Nancy Raymond, coauthor of the *Sexual Symptom Assessment Scale*, describes urges as "having both a visceral and affective component" (N. Raymond, March 19, 2014, personal communication). An urge may be generated before or after a thought or behavior, but is not dependent on either (N. Raymond, March 19, 2014, personal communication). A sexual urge can feel like a force pushing the self from within or like a force pulling the self from without.
- *Sexual thoughts* are the ideas, mental pictures, and fantasies that contain sexual themes. Sexual scenes run through people's minds in response to a limitless supply of external and internal stimulation. Sexual thoughts are can also be the stimulus that evokes sexual urges and behaviors.
- *Sexual behaviors* are outward sexual expressions and are not limited to the actions that surround sexual intercourse. Any sexual expression involving one or more people is subsumed under sexual behavior (e.g., masturbation, sensual touch, vaginal and anal intercourse, oral sex, online sexual chatting, etc.). Sexual behaviors are also not dependent on sexual thoughts or urges. They can precede and follow or influence and be influenced by urges and thoughts.

Sexual urges and thoughts are products of a person's mind and are understood as subjective internal experiences. Sexual behavior is the observable action with oneself or others.

Dual-Process Model of Human Behavior

From Plato's Chariot Allegory to neuroscientific research, philosophers and scientists have attempted to explain the complexities and contradictions of human behavior. The mechanisms that produce human behaviors are often described as a combination of rational, goal-directed processes interacting with a reflexive process compelled by emotions, drives, and motivational states. The rational components influence behavior through restricting or directing the unpredictable, erratic, and complex affective system. To operationalize this interaction, dual-process models have been developed in the fields of psychology (Chaiken & Trope, 1999; Evers, Hopps,

Gross, Fischer, Manstead, & Mauss, 2014; Hoffmann, 2014; Kahneman & Frederick, 2002; Metcalfe & Mischel, 1999; Sherman, Gawronski, & Trope, 2014), economics (Andersen, Harrison, Lau, & Rutström, 2014; Benhabib & Bisin, 2005; Brocas & Carrillo, 2014; Fudenberg & Levine, 2006), and sexology (Bancroft et al., 2005, 2009; Janssen & Bancroft, 2007; Janssen, Vorst, Finn, & Bancroft, 2002). These differing dual-process models share the notion of two distinct systems of the mind that motivate human behavior and decision making. Each dual-process model describes an interaction between a programmed, unconscious, quick, evolutionarily older system balanced with a rule-based, conscious, and slower system (Evans & Frankish, 2009). Neuroscience suggests that numerous specialized systems interact within the multifaceted brain to generate human behavior. In his book *Incognito*, Eagleman (2011) observes the neurological oversimplification of condensing brain functioning into two systems. He likens the brain to a team of rivals made up of an entire parliament of pieces and parts and subsystems: "We are collections of overlapping, ceaselessly reinvented mechanisms, a group of competing factions" (p. 148). Consequently, a dual-process model seems reductionist. The most natural neurophysiological division within the brain, however, is the evolutionarily older brain structures and the prefrontal cortex (Loewenstein & O'Donoghue, 2007). We adopted Loewenstein and O'Donoghue's (2007) dual-process model of human behavior to conceptualize how sexual experiences feel out of control and answer our question, "Why are people repeatedly sexual in ways that are problematic?"

In the dual-process model of human behavior (see Figure 3.1), human behavior is seen as "the joint product of a *deliberative system* that assesses options in a consequentialist fashion and an *affective system* that encompass emotions such as anger and fear and motivational states such as hunger, sex, and pain" (Loewenstein & O'Donoghue, 2007, p. 3). The *affective system* houses our potential for action in any given situation.

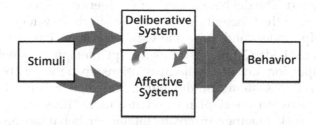

Figure 3.1 *Dual-process model of human behavior.*
Source: Loewenstein and O'Donoghue (2007).

The potential for action is generated by changes in physiological activation that include:

- *emotions*, such as standard emotions (e.g., mad, glad, sad, etc.) and emotions that are immediate, experienced "in the heat of the moment"
- *drives* (e.g., survival, hunger, thirst, sex, romantic love)
- *motivational states* (e.g., physical pain, discomfort, drug craving, attachment)

The affective system contains the automatic processes that run without conscious control and includes our sense of wanting, our desire to acquire something or to engage in an action.

The deliberative system houses the executive functions. It has the capacity to assess the consequences of behavior and influences behavior by asserting energy (i.e., willpower) over the affective system. "Executive functions are hypothesized to consist of a constellation of mental processes associated with adaptive behavior that function to assist an individual to interact with his or her environment in an efficient and acceptable way" (Reid, Karim, McCrory, & Carpenter, 2010, p. 120). The deliberative system contains processes that provide conscious control as well as remembering how much someone actually enjoys or finds pleasure in a particular action. This system critically considers various choices with a particular focus on the emotional consequences of an action. These consequences include predicted or expected emotions used to determine the best course of behavior.

The affective system, with its sensitivity to immediate situations, is constantly running and is primed to assert dominance over the deliberative system to protect the whole person (e.g., fight, flight, freeze response). The deliberative system, on the other hand, transcends the immediate situation from as little as the next few minutes to days or even years afterward. The deliberative system influences responses to stimuli without altering the inherent primacy of the affective system.

To help understand how these two systems interact to generate behavior, Haidt (2006) describes an apt metaphor to help visualize the proportionality of this joint relationship between the affective and deliberative systems of the mind: the dual process is like the interaction between an elephant and its rider. "Reason and emotion must both work together to create intelligent behavior, but emotion (a major part of the elephant) does most of the work. When the neocortex came along, it made the rider possible, but it made the elephant much smarter, too" (Haidt, 2006, p. 13). Although these interconnected subsystems were evolutionarily designed to promote our survival, reproduction, and wellness, they influence behavior through unseen internal conflicts between competing elements of the self. In other words, the motivations of the affective and deliberative systems are usually compatible. Other times, their motivations compete.

Competing Motivations

Here is an example of competing motivations: You are staring at a dark-chocolate cake in the bakery window. It looks soft and sweet, covered with your favorite icing. A familiar feeling rises from your stomach and your mouth starts to water. You can taste the cake without having put the first moist piece in your mouth. "But wait!" a thought pierces your consciousness. "You promised! No more sweets until you lose 20 pounds." Your doctor's voice rings in your head, "You need to lose weight. You have a family history of diabetes and your blood pressure is creeping up." So, there you are in the bakery lost in thought, pulled in two directions. Satisfy the urge or forgo temptation?

Decisions big and small can be an outgrowth of competing motivations. Each day is filled with mundane rituals like getting out of bed, commuting to work, and selecting foods to eat. Within our daily routines, there are infinite moments of choice. Somehow, in each of these moments, we consciously and unconsciously make decisions. Opportunities to choose elicit forces in our bodies that motivate us toward action or inaction. Choosing is a complicated mixture of priorities that frequently split the mind into short-term versus long-term interests. Much of the time, our immediate priorities and future concerns are consistent. Other times, short- and long-term goals are contradictory or, more specifically, our immediate desires run counter to our long-term interests. Because the affective and deliberative systems respond differently to environmental stimuli, disparate motivations are incited (Loewenstein & O'Donoghue, 2007). Thankfully, people have the capacity to see the long-term consequences of their decisions. Individuals know the outcomes of persistent smoking on health or tardiness on job evaluations. However, awareness of consequences does not stop actions that contradict long-term interests. Predicting long-term consequences does not always lead to avoiding them. And yet, people are often surprised or disappointed when they act inconsistently.

A dual-process model of human behavior is a useful model for understanding the complexities and contradictions in sexual behavior.

It accounts for the central tension in OCSB: *being of two minds*—wanting to do one thing while doing another. Peter was motivated to have sexual fantasies only about his wife but continued to masturbate watching online videos of other people having sex. Hector wanted to stay married but he continued to meet men at sex shops for anonymous sex, which violated his relationship agreements. Will was not interested in contracting HIV but continued having condomless anal sex with men. Envision these situations as internal conflicts that occur within the dual-process construct. Peter, Hector, and Will's deliberative system attempted to steer their behavior, evidenced by their conscious boundary settings and stated intentions. There were emotional consequences that they did not like and made efforts to avoid. However, other motivations were present and steered their behaviors in another direction. This internal tension over their sexual behavior is the out of control feeling frequently disclosed by our clients in OCSB treatment.

We encourage therapists to place sexual urges and thoughts within the broader construct of the physiological and psychological systems that comprise the embodied mind. In his book, *Mindsight*, Daniel Siegel (2011) defines health as the integration or linkage of differentiated parts; a systemic wholeness that honors both the difference between distinct parts and their connectedness. Conversely, nonhealth can be seen as a lack of integration within or between systems. An integrated wholeness is a concept applied in other areas of sexual health and wellness. For incidence, think of the systems involved in achieving a full and satisfying erection. Physiological systems like the nervous, vascular, and endocrine systems work in concert to activate male sexual response. When interconnected and functioning properly, erectile response will likely be excellent but when these systems are disconnected or impaired, they will likely produce a weak erection. A similar dynamic interplay of internal and external systems also influence one's sexual urges, thoughts, and behavior.

Jim, a heterosexual man, was married for 6 years. In group therapy, he described how 3 days earlier he had paid for sex on his way home from work. When a group member asked him to elaborate on what he recalled about driving home, he sheepishly replied, "I don't really know. I was driving home and, all of a sudden, I found myself driving down 10th Avenue looking to hook up. I left work and it was like my addict brain took over." Jim's felt sense of being "out of control" was described with metaphors like "addict brain," or reports of lost time like "all of a sudden." These phrases allude to a force that he perceives has hijacked his behavior in such a way that he no longer believes or remembers having any significant volition. Using the dual process to frame Jim's experience, either his affective system was overactive or his deliberative system was under-responding to a stimulus that resulted in sexual behaviors he later regretted. Jim's difficulty remembering what happened prior to driving down 10th Avenue is common among men in treatment for OCSB. When executive functions are disengaged, recalling what motivated the behavior becomes challenging. For Jim, 10th Avenue was a familiar location and he relied on habit to steer his actions. Unfortunately, with a disengaged rider, Jim was unprepared to assert the energy needed to steer the elephant toward his long-term goals when he became sexually activated.

Conceptualizing Jim's experience as an interaction between his affective and deliberative systems allows the therapist and group members to explore the client's internal experience without perpetuating the client's belief that he was not in control of his sexual behavior. The day Jim drove down 10th Avenue, his boss told him that management would not replace several coworkers who had recently quit. He immediately realized that this decision meant that his strenuous workload was not going to change. Jim recounted more details about the time from walking to his car after work and eventually propositioning a sex worker. Memories that initially he implied were absent with the words "all of a sudden" revealed a series of motivations that influenced his behavior. He remembered how angry he felt after the conversation with his boss. He was particularly hurt by management's decision and the casual manner with which his boss told him that his workload would remain high. Jim thought his boss ignored his rationale for replacing the vacated positions and remembered feeling stressed and resentful when he reached his car.

Jim's motivation to change his affective discomfort (e.g., anger, resentment, and disappointment) was competing with his deliberative goals of honoring his marital commitments. With the help of the group, Jim identified these competing motivations and recalled the rationalizing thoughts that represented a disengaged deliberative system. "My wife will not find out." "Paying for sex is a victimless crime." "I'm just going to see if anyone is out there." Jim's thoughts diverted his focus from future consequences and away from exerting willpower to balance his highly activated state. This ceded control to his affective system. When faced with a moment in which his long-term goal of remaining married by restricting his sexual behavior competed with his desire to feel something other than his heated resentment, he chose the short-term goal of regulating his uncomfortable activation. This "heat of the moment" decision did not mean Jim was disinterested in being married or no longer believed in honoring his marital commitments. The competing motivations coexisted and shifted Jim's priority in response to his workplace distress and environmental cues.

Clients often judge themselves as being weak, perverse, or disordered for knowingly and repeatedly engaging in sexual behaviors that risk negative consequences. They often develop erroneous conclusions based on their contradictory behaviors. "I must want to lose my job if I repeatedly violate the Internet policy about watching porn." "I must not love my husband if I keep watching sexual videos despite being asked to stop." They assume the contradictory behavior is indicative of their most authentic desires. Observable behavior is often thought to be the best resource to discern intent underlying contradictory behaviors. As if behavior is the real story. Do actions speak louder than words? Possibly. But, louder does not mean accurate. Alternatively, framing OCSB within the dual-process model conceptualizes contradictory behavior as quintessentially human, seen in the same imperfect and dynamic process that describes human behavior and its problems.

A BROAD PICTURE OF SELF-REGULATION

Self-regulation research suggests "most of the social and personal problems that afflict people in modern western [sic] society have some element of self-regulatory failure at their root" (Baumeister, Schmeichel, & Vohs, 2007, p. 2). Sexual behavior problems are no different. How does a client behave when his sexual excitation, desire, and lust are pushing him toward actions with significant negative consequences? How does a client proceed in situations in which the temptation is not chocolate cake but condomless sex or an extrarelational affair? Sexual health is inextricably linked to one's capacity to regulate feelings and direct behavior when internal motivations compete. In this section, we apply self-regulation theory and research to our OCSB conceptualization.

Self-regulation (also called *self-control*) is a capacity that has evolved to help humans to survive and thrive. Dunbar and Schultz (2007) review evolutionary trends of primate brains and suggest that the survival and reproductive benefits of primate social lives and pair bonding drove the evolution of the human brain. They conclude that the chances to survive predation and the ability to reproduce improved when living in groups. As a result, the ability to manage group cohesion and the demands of complex social networks was an important dynamic for people to manage.

Self-control is required to remain attuned, to work together within groups to achieve broader goals, and to manage one's behavior to avoid being removed from the group. (As any group therapist can attest, maintaining group cohesion with a member who is rambunctious, interruptive, impulsive, reactive, or combative is challenging work.) To survive and reproduce meant that the individual must forgo immediate gratification for the long-term benefit of group cohesion, especially when social network goals conflicted with an individual's immediate needs and desires. Fortunately, just as the affective system is constantly evaluating for environmental threats, the deliberative system is constantly monitoring our thoughts, emotions, and sensations to warn us of an impending regrettable behavior (McGonigal, 2012).

Our self-regulation capacity, developed to manage membership to our small social groups, is now adapting to the demands of larger, complex societies. Advances in agriculture, science, and medicine reduced threats to health and wellness. Individual time spent on satisfying basic needs for food, clothing, and shelter has decreased. People in modern Western societies find themselves with more time on their hands than our ancestors ever imagined. These successes of collective living have created social conditions that test self-control like no other time in human history.

Two large investigations of a broad range of human behavior compared people with "good" versus "poor" self-control (Tangney, Baumeister, & Boone, 2004). A variety of positive individual and interpersonal outcomes correlated with high rates of self-control (Tangney et al., 2004). Benefits included stronger academic performance, fewer impulse control behaviors like binge eating or drinking, and positive psychological adjustment in self-report psychopathology measures. Interpersonal benefits included better family cohesion, less conflict, better perspective taking (i.e., empathy capacity), being less apt to wallow in distress, and a greater likelihood of secure attachment styles. Tangney et al. (2004) also found that people with higher rates of self-control reported less anger and were more effective at managing the anger they did feel. Studies suggest people with high self-control experience the beneficial aspects of guilt and the less destructive consequences of shame. "Thus, self-control is associated with emotional patterns that seem beneficial both to the individual and to other people associated with the individual" (p. 42).

Living in the Age of Sexual Temptation

The diversity and accessibility of sexual opportunities for people living in the 21st century is unprecedented. Economies that provide millions of people with smartphones, tablets, and laptops carry with them extraordinary access to sexual activities and partners. Employees with smartphones can watch sexually explicit, high-definition video in their workplaces. People sex chat on electronic tablets with their partners sleeping beside them. The unconventional sexual interests that were previously difficult to find can now be privately explored without interacting with anyone. People carry pornography production studios in their pockets, ready to record any sex act with their mobile devices. Subsequently, these images or videos can be viewed privately, with another person, or quickly uploaded for anyone on the planet (with Internet access) to see. Mobile applications take advantage of GPS (global positioning system) technology to link people in close proximity for instant sexual hook-ups. A society that brought the convenience of fast-food drive-up windows has delivered a menu of people for sexual consumption.

Does society expect everyone to adapt and succeed with the saturation of sexual technology without harm to self or others? Twenty-four-hour/ 7-days-per-week sexual access stretches people's self-control capacities. From individuals in the first social networks huddled around fires with stirred loins to cruising digital social networks for naked pictures, some people have not faired well in balancing sexual pleasure seeking with communal norms, personal values, or relationship commitments. LaTour and Henthorne (2003), who study the use of sexuality in advertising, remind us that "for many decades, psychophysiological reactions to environmental stimuli have been looked to as a logical nexus for understanding the complexities of the mind–body interface" (p. 94). We frame sexual behavior regulation in the construct of the dual-process model to understand the interaction among stimuli, the embodied mind, and behavior. The influence of environmental stimuli on the mind is central to sexual behavior and decision making. Desirable behavioral outcomes involve the direct effects of environmental stimuli on the deliberative and affective systems and the reciprocal influences of each system on the other. In this section, we explore four distinct stimuli characteristics that influence deliberative–affective interaction and how they relate to regulating sexual urges, thoughts, and desires: *proximity, novelty, habituation*, and *vividness*.

Proximity

Emotional reactions are felt through physiological changes in heart rate, blood pressure, hormone secretions, muscle tension, and other bodily events. These sensations are labeled as emotions, drives, or motivational states. The intensity of these affective responses is significantly influenced by the juxtaposition between the environmental stimulus and the behavioral outcome. For example, it is early morning, you are hungry and are driving by your favorite bakery. The growing urge to eat your favorite scone is linked to the specific stimulus of the bakery. The environmental factor that intensified the emotional activation was proximity—you are a mere 100 feet from the bakery display case. Both the nearness and the visual immediacy of stimuli influence the strength of the emotional reactions to stimuli (Loewenstein & O'Donoghue, 2007).

Temporal proximity
Although certainly not the only factor, Loewenstein and O'Donoghue (2007) propose that the most important stimulus factor affecting behavior is the juxtaposition between the timing of the reward and the cost. The proximity in time between an event and a proceeding action is called *temporal proximity*. "Affective motivations are intense when rewards and punishments are immediate but much less intense when they are temporally remote. Deliberation is, in contrast, much less sensitive to immediacy" (p. 11). The rewards of sex are usually more temporally proximate than the costs, although both can be experienced during and after sexual experiences. Rewards range from the anticipatory excitement of sexual pursuit, the boost to one's self-confidence when sexual attention is reciprocated, or the pleasure of touch and orgasm from solo or partnered sex. In contrast, some more proximal costs are the emotional consequences of an unreciprocated sexual advance, dull sex, or the inability to maintain a firm erection for intercourse. The delayed, and thus less proximal, postcoitus costs may be the symptoms of a sexually transmitted infection (STI) that emerge days or weeks later. The full blowback of an affair may occur only if the secretive relationship is discovered. The financial consequences of paid sex may only surface when paying bills at the end of the month.

Visual proximity
Visual proximity is another factor that affects the activation. "Stronger responses to visual sexual stimuli in men have been reported frequently, and the assumed reasons are numerous, including biological as well as sociocultural factors" (Wehrum et al., 2013, p. 1338). A man's early response to visual sexual stimuli is driven, in part, by his initial affective reaction. A positive affective reaction directs men to focus toward the sexual content. A negative affective reaction directs visual attention away from sexual content (Samson & Janssen, 2014). Studies that demonstrate this visual link between sexual attraction and arousal suggests visual sexual stimulation notably evokes a man's physical sensations and feelings. In addition to sight, think about the difference between watching a person strip off his or her clothes alone or surrounded by other people. The proximity of seeing someone enjoy the same sexual activation is a form

of visual proximity that is more likely to evoke sexual feelings. People respond with increased sexual activation from stimuli that is physically close, in sight, or being consumed by someone near (Loewenstein & O'Donoghue, 2007).

The "marshmallow test" is a famous demonstration of the association between physical proximity and self-control (Mischel & Underwood, 1974). A quick Internet search of "marshmallow test" brings up videos of young children attempting to restrain themselves from eating a marshmallow that is in front of them because they were promised a second marshmallow if they waited 2 minutes. Now change the scenario. Switch toddlers to adults and marshmallows to smartphone sexual imagery or cruising for a sex partner. The smartphone scenario combines temporal and physical proximity. One's mobile device possesses temporal and visual proximity of an "always open" retail outlet for sexual expression.

Numerous studies have compared the life-course implications for men and women with differing early self-regulatory abilities (see Mischel et al., 2010). Milkman, Rogers, and Brazerman (2008) synthesized studies that looked at adult responses to analogous marshmallow test situations by examining the two sides that compete for supremacy in any given moment. Will adults behave responsibly or indulge impulsively? In these studies, they describe the adult internal conflicts as a tension between "a *want* self [affective system] fighting for whatever will bring more short term pleasure, and a *should* self [deliberative system] representing an individual's long-term interests" [brackets added] (p. 324). When the stimulus is visibly present, the affective system may activate and override the deliberative system. "People are considerably more likely to favor *should* [deliberative] options over *want* [affective] options when making choices that will take effect in the future than they are when making decisions that will take effect immediately" (Milkman et al., 2008, p. 326). This dilemma is often observed in the contradiction between what a client says during group and what happens afterward. A group therapy client who has no immediate sexual opportunity is more likely to confidently state his intention for maintaining his boundaries based on his deliberative process ("I am not going to have extramarital sex."). But later, when faced with the immediate opportunity for extramarital sex away from his therapist and the group, he makes a different choice ("I want to have sex now.").

Novelty

The affective system is highly responsive to novel and unfamiliar stimuli. Without newness, our bodily sensations and emotions acclimate to constant stimuli (whether rewarding or punishing) by deintensifying responsiveness. Growing accustomed to an unchanging stimuli over time alters the affective system, which starts to operate in response to the cue as if "nothing can be done about the situation, and that it is not worth devoting further attention or motivation to it" (Loewenstein & O'Donoghue, 2007, p. 12). The action tendencies of our affective system are principally focused on changes in circumstances and much less responsive to routine, mundane, or what was once novel and is now expected. It would be too difficult to remain sensitive to new and immediate changes in circumstances without the ability of our affective system to acclimate to continuous and predictable stimuli. However, there is the possibility of a thinking error within this adaptive response to novelty. If a novel stimulus leads to a positive response, people assume this desirable outcome will be sustainable and lasting. The desirability of the response to the novel stimuli can turn into a wish for longevity.

Morin (1995) studied peak erotic turn-ons to understand men and women's erotic preferences and desires. His work in eroticism supports these cross-disciplinary studies of novelty as powerful stimuli for our affective system responses. Morin's (1995) investigation of human eroticism identified categories of reliable and memorable sources for arousal and excitation. According to Morin (1995), sexual firsts, sexual surprises, and spontaneity contributed to peak erotic experiences. In his research, nearly a third of the participant's peak erotic stories contained a sexual first or intensely pleasurable surprise. His research suggests that novelty amplifies sexual and erotic pleasures in both partnered and solo sex. A novel stimulus may be memorable as a peak erotic turn-on, but it rarely prevents the inevitable habituation of the erotic system. Even the most spontaneous and hot encounter, if repeated enough times, loses its luster. Sexual response and erotic expression, even when intensely pleasurable, are not immune to habituation.

Habituation

Repeated exposure to life events or circumstances, whether pleasurable or painful, reduces psychological or behavioral responses. "Negative affective states alert us that something is wrong and motivate us to change. Positive affective states provide immediate reward when we rectify whatever is wrong" (Loewenstein & O'Donoghue, 2007, p. 12). Over time, we acclimate to the change in affective states—the body no longer alerts us and returns to our previously established homeostasis. This return to the set point (i.e., baseline response) is frequently labeled as *hedonic adaptation* or *habituation*. Happiness research that studied people after winning the lottery and getting married or losing a job or getting into a car accident looked at the tendency of people to return to their happiness set point after these life-changing events (Easterlin, 2003; Lucas, 2007). Easterlin (2003) acknowledges that a full return to baseline may not occur after extreme negative events such as getting divorced or becoming disabled. However, as Lucas (2007) concludes, adaptation occurs, but it is not inevitable and the intensity or quality of the life event does matter.

Habitation and sexual imagery

What happens when people habituate to the sexual media in their possession? Acquiring new sexual media used to take more effort and energy. Prior to the Internet, men interested in viewing a sexual video had to find the time to travel to the nearest sex shop and muster up the courage to enter (hoping no one would seeing them). Once inside, they would grab a VHS (video home system) tape with an appealing cover photo (no free previews!) and exchange awkward pleasantries with the cashier. If sexual imagery was unwelcomed at home, then they had the added pressure of sneaking it home and hiding it until it was discarded. In the Internet age, people still habituate to sexual imagery. But, they only have to wait as long as their Internet speed requires to download a new image. Cooper (1998) coined the term *Triple A Engine*—affordability, accessibility, and anonymity—to capture the appeal of online sexual images. Young, Griffin-Shelley, Cooper, O'Mara, and Buchanan (2000) describe a similar conceptualization using the *ACE model*: anonymity, convenience, and escape. Both view the Internet as the principal change that has occurred in proximity and access to sexual imagery. Inconvenience and emotional and financial costs were significant external barriers to sexual media in the pre-Internet period.

There is limited research on sexual response habituation (Dawson, 2012). Recent studies find similar patterns in male and female participants' habituation to sexual stimuli. Habituation was measured by participant distraction by nonsexual stimulus elements and less attention and absorption in the sexual aspects of an image. Becoming distracted by nonsexual visual elements was measurable by a decrease in genital response of successively smaller magnitudes (Dawson, Suschinsky, & Lalumière, 2013). When subjects who had exhibited sexual habituation were given a novel stimulus their sexual response returned. Of more interest to Dawson and her colleagues was the response that occurred when the previously habituated image was reintroduced after viewing the arousing novel image: the previously habituated image returned to providing sexual excitement (Dawson et al., 2013). Without awareness of their habituation, men who mindlessly pursue online sexually explicit materials may label habituation as a symptom of an addictive process or an Internet porn addiction. They may describe pursuing the images that are more "extreme" or "intense," moving into areas of sexual expression that they judge negatively and fear is evidence of a sexual addiction. These labels, however, reveal two different things. First, they indicate that the clients may harbor negative judgments regarding images that they found erotic. Second, the clients are also describing the process they underwent to feel sexual pleasure after they had habituated to the images they were previously viewing. They may be unaware that their behavior was an attempt to prolong the experience of sexual pleasure in spite of their adaptive tendencies and evaluate their behavior using the cultural lens of addiction. But their internal conflict about what aroused them is not a symptom of a disorder, but rather suggests a values conflict about their erotic attractions.

Vividness

The final stimulus quality is *vividness* or the ability to conjure the experience of the stimuli in one's mind. Mental imagery, which may include the sense memory or emotions connected to past experiences, influences affect intensity. It is the individual's ability to summon lucid, luminous, here/now imagery (the stimulus) from previously erotically charged memories that activate the sexual sensation system. The more memorable the factors associated with a peak erotic pleasure, the more likely the individual will feel the sensations associated with engaging in the imagined behavior. This mental vividness, conjured from life experience and harvested in sexual situations, intensifies affect. We frequently see vividness activation when clients deconstruct their thoughts and levels of excitement prior to engaging in a sexual behavior that they want to change. Men report a cognitive focus on the pleasure they anticipate feeling when they engage in the sexual boundary-crossing behavior. They remember the times when it felt exciting and fun. They often edit the negative events associated with the behavior and focus their thoughts on the positive, pleasure-intensifying moments that eventually tip the scale toward action. They replay scenes from partnered sex or sexual videos that are reliable turn-ons that lead to an orgasm. Their affective intensity (e.g., horniness or anticipatory excitement) fixes their sexual motivation for action and diminishes the balancing influence of their deliberative system.

How to Apply the Dual-Process Model to Sexual Health Treatment

OCSB outpatient psychotherapy helps men change and maintain sexual health by recalibrating their deliberative and affective interactions. It does not involve a new theoretical orientation or novel form of psychotherapy.

In the next few chapters, we walk through our assessment and treatment protocol for sexual behavior problems and OCSB. If you have been conducting therapy for a while, we suspect you will find the sexual health interventions similar to your own work. The OCSB Model incorporates a range of diverse factors that contribute to sexual behavior problems, providing therapists an opportunity to integrate a holistic health approach and their well-developed clinical expertise.

The OCSB treatment protocol provides therapists with a process to facilitate gradual improvement in men's balance between their affective and deliberative systems. Improved balance between these two systems does not mean equal influence between the two systems. It is unlikely that psychotherapy will affect the evolutionary development of affective primacy. Our older brain system continues relatively unchanged in obtaining nutrition, maintaining body temperature, and reproducing under favorable conditions. Instead, OCSB treatment evaluates client stimulus and explores how an individual's affective and deliberative sexual behavior system responds. Over time, clients either increase or decrease deliberative involvement or intensify or deintensify affective involvement; in a sense, it retrains the elephant and better uses the rider. One primary objective is to facilitate a change process that motivates clients to change their behavior to fit within the sexual health principles. This requires a process that evaluates and addresses the factors that influence the affective–deliberative system interaction. Figure 3.2 illustrates this goal.

At the heart of the OCSB Model is the concept of competing motivations. Miller and Rollnick (2013) describe four variations of internal conflicts that contribute to our conceptualization for understanding OCSB. First, the *approach–approach conflict* occurs when a person is faced with a choice between two attractive options. What we may jokingly refer to as a good problem to have. Second, an *avoidance–avoidance conflict* involves choices in which all options have negative consequences, the proverbial, either-option-sucks moment. Or, as we often say to our clients, "Which

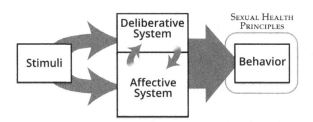

Figure 3.2 *Dual-process model of human behavior with sexual health principles.*

disappointment do you want to choose?" Third is the *approach–avoidance conflict*. In this scenario, one is "both attracted to and repelled by the same object" (Miller & Rollnick, 2013, p. 14). "I want to buy that new sex toy, but where would I put it so the kids won't find it?" The *double approach–avoidance conflict* is really tormenting and may have much in common with OCSB. Both options have significant positive and negative attributes. When leaning toward one, the negative aspects are more salient while enhancing the longing for the other.

We find that defenses among our clients are similar to Miller and Rollnick's description of "the discomfort of conscious ambivalence" (p. 157). Clients do not want to think about their moments of acute ambivalence ("I forgot to tell you that I crossed a boundary last week, just slipped my mind"). Others begin the slow deliberative justification that maybe things are just fine the way they are ("What's really so bad about masturbating to sexual videos anyway?"). We particularly draw attention to men who manage ambivalence by defensively fleeing to hopeless or helpless. ("It's no use, nothing works. I tried everything.")

Figure 3.3 illustrates the role of competing motivations on the affective–deliberative interaction. The up and down arrows represent the affective–deliberative interaction that is set in motion when one is exposed to a stimulus. We are careful to avoid simplifying competing motivations as merely a conflict between the pleasure and rational centers or a repackaged conflict between the id and ego. The *competing motivations* that are specific to OCSB encircle both affective and deliberative systems. Each system may contain congruent or conflicting motives. The *wants* of the affective system may be contradictory. Or, the deliberative system can be locked in a contemplative pro/con loop. In the OCSB Model, feeling out of control describes the difficulties resolving these competing motivations in a manner that produces satisfactory sexual behavior.

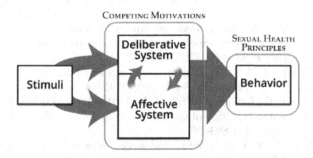

Figure 3.3 *Dual-process model of human behavior with sexual health principles and competing motivations.*

Hence, *competing motivations* encircle the entire system of the mind to represent the proposed origins of this conflict and depict an imbalanced affect affective–deliberative interaction.

With the dual process as an organizing concept for OCSB, therapists can listen with an organized map as clients describe their internal conflicts and competing motivations about their sexual lives. Out of control sexual experiences may represent the honorable attempts by clients to solve the complex imbalance between their affective and deliberative systems of the mind. They may result from how some men regulate the pervasive struggle between instant sexual gratification and long-term sexual rewards, between the sexual "wanting" of their affective systems and the "disliking" of their deliberative system. The dual-process model and the sexual health framework offer a compassionate alternative for clients to examine their sexual problems and promote their sexual health.

REFERENCES

Andersen, S., Harrison, G. W., Lau, M. I., & Rutström, E. E. (2014). Dual criteria decisions. *Journal of Economic Psychology, 41*, 101–113.

Bancroft, J., Graham, C. A., Janssen, E., & Sanders, S. A. (2009). The dual control model: Current status and future directions. *Journal of Sex Research, 46*, 121–142.

Bancroft, J., Herbenick, D., Barnes, T., Hallam-Jones, R., Wylie, K., Janssen, E., & Members of BASRT*. (2005). The relevance of the dual control model to male sexual dysfunction: The Kinsey Institute/BASRT Collaborative Project. *Sexual and Relationship Therapy, 20*(1), 13–30.

Bancroft, J., & Vukadinovic, Z. (2004). Sexual addiction, sexual compulsivity, sexual impulsivity, or what? Toward a theoretical model. *Journal of Sex Research, 41*, 225–234.

Baumeister, R., Schmeichel, B., & Vohs, K. (2007). Self-regulation and the executive function: The self as controlling agent. In A. W. Kruglanski & E. T. Higgins (Eds.), *Social psychology: Handbook of basic principles* (pp. 516–539). New York, NY: Guilford Press.

Benhabib, J., & Bisin, A. (2005). Modeling internal commitment mechanisms and self-control: A neuroeconomics approach to consumption–saving decisions. *Games and Economic Behavior, 52*(2), 460–492.

Brocas, I., & Carrillo, J. D. (2014). Dual-process theories of decision-making: A selective survey. *Journal of Economic Psychology, 41*, 45–54.

Cantor, J. M., Klein, C., Lykins, A., Rullo, J. E., Thaler, L., & Walling, B. R. (2013). A treatment-oriented typology of self-identified hypersexuality referrals. *Archives of Sexual Behavior, 42*(5), 883–893.

Chaiken, S., & Trope, Y. (Eds.). (1999). *Dual-process theories in social psychology.* New York, NY: Guilford Press.

Cooper, A. (1998). Sexuality and the Internet: Surfing into the new millennium. *CyberPsychology & Behavior, 1*(2), 187–193.

Dawson, S. J. (2012). *The habituation of sexual responses in men and women* (Unpublished doctoral dissertation). University of Lethbridge, Lethbridge, Alberta, Canada.

Dawson, S. J., Suschinsky, K. D., & Lalumière, M. L. (2013). Habituation of sexual responses in men and women: A test of the preparation hypothesis of women's genital responses. *Journal of Sexual Medicine, 10*(4), 990–1000.

Dunbar, R. I., & Shultz, S. (2007). Evolution in the social brain. *Science, 317*(5843), 1344–1347.

Eagleman, D. (2011). *Incognito: The secret lives of the brain.* New York, NY: Pantheon Books.

Easterlin, R. A. (2003). Explaining happiness. *Proceedings of the National Academy of Sciences, 100*(19), 11176–11183.

Evans, J. S. B., & Frankish, K. E. (2009). *In two minds: Dual processes and beyond.* New York, NY: Oxford University Press.

Evers, C., Hopp, H., Gross, J. J., Fischer, A. H., Manstead, A. S., & Mauss, I. B. (2014). Emotion response coherence: A dual-process perspective. *Biological Psychology, 98*, 43–49.

Fudenberg, D., & Levine, D. K. (2006). A dual-self model of impulse control. *American Economic Review, 96*(5), 1449–1476.

Haidt, J. (2006). *The happiness hypothesis: Finding modern truth in ancient wisdom.* New York, NY: Basic Books.

Hoffmann, J. P. (2014). Religiousness, social networks, moral schemas, and marijuana use: A dynamic dual-process model of culture and behavior. *Social Forces, 93*(1), 181–208.

Janssen, E., & Bancroft, J. (2007). The dual-control model: The role of sexual inhibition and excitation in sexual arousal and behavior. *Psychophysiology of Sex, 15*, 197–222.

Janssen, E., Vorst, H., Finn, P., & Bancroft, J. (2002). The sexual inhibition (SIS) and sexual excitation (SES) scales: I. Measuring sexual inhibition and excitation proneness in men. *Journal of Sex Research, 39*(2), 114–126.

Joannides, P. (2012). The challenging landscape of problematic sexual behaviors, including "sexual addiction" and "hypersexuality." In P. J. Kleinplatz (Ed.), *New directions in sex therapy: Innovations and alternatives* (pp. 69–83). New York, NY: Routledge.

Kahneman, D., & Frederick, S. (2002). Representativeness revisited: Attribute substitution in intuitive judgment, In T. Gilovich, D. Griffin, & D. Kahneman (Eds.), *Heuristics and biases: The psychology of intuitive judgment* (pp. 49–81). Cambridge, UK: Cambridge University Press.

Klein, M. (2012, July/August). You're addicted to what? Challenging the myth of sex addiction. *Humanist.* Retrieved from www.thehumanist.com

LaTour, M., & Henthorne, T. (2003). Nudity and sexual appeals: Understanding the arousal process and advertising response. In T. Reichert & J. Lambaise (Eds.), *Sex in advertising: Perspectives on the erotic appeal* (pp. 91–106). New York, NY: Routledge.

Loewenstein, G., & O'Donoghue, T. (2007). The heat of the moment: Modeling interactions between affect and deliberation. *Unpublished manuscript.* Retrieved from: https://odonoghue.economics.cornell.edu/heat.pdf

Lucas, R. E. (2007). Adaptation and the set-point model of subjective well-being: Does happiness change after major life events? *Current Directions in Psychological Science, 16*(2), 75–79.

McGonigal, K. (2012). *The willpower instinct: How self-control works, why it matters, and what you can do to get more of it.* New York, NY: Penguin.

Metcalfe, J., & Mischel, W. (1999). A hot/cool-system analysis of delay of gratification: Dynamics of willpower. *Psychological Review, 106*(1), 3.

Milkman, K. L., Rogers, T., & Bazerman, M. H. (2008). Harnessing our inner angels and demons: What we have learned about want/should conflicts and how that knowledge can help us reduce short-sighted decision making. *Perspectives on Psychological Science, 3*(4), 324–338.

Miller, W., & Rollnick, S. (2002). *Motivational interviewing: Preparing people for change.* New York, NY: Guilford Press.

Miller, W. R., & Rollnick, S. (2013). *Motivational interviewing: Helping people change* (3rd ed.). New York, NY: Guilford Press.

Mischel, W., Ayduk, O., Berman, M. G., Casey, B. J., Gotlib, I. H., Jonides, J., ... & Shoda, Y. (2010). "Willpower" over the life span: Decomposing self-regulation. *Social Cognitive and Affective Neuroscience, 6*(2), 252–256.

Mischel, W., & Underwood, B. (1974). Instrumental ideation in delay of gratification. *Child Development, 45*(4), 1083–1088.

Morin, J. (1995). *The erotic mind: Unlocking the inner sources of sexual passion and fulfillment.* New York, NY: HarperCollins.

Reay, B., Attwood, N., & Gooder, C. (2013). Inventing sex: The short history of sex addiction. *Sexuality & Culture, 17*(1), 1–19.

Reid, R. (2013). Personal perspectives on hypersexual disorder. *Sexual Addiction & Compulsivity: The Journal of Treatment & Prevention, 20*(1–2), 4–18.

Reid, R. C., Karim, R., McCrory, E., & Carpenter, B. N. (2010). Self-reported differences on measures of executive function and hypersexual behavior in a patient and community sample of men. *International Journal of Neuroscience, 120*(2), 120–127.

Samson, L., & Janssen, E. (2014). Sexual and affective responses to same- and opposite-sex stimuli in heterosexual and homosexual men: Assessment and manipulation of visual attention. *Archives of Sexual Behavior, 43*, 917–930.

Sherman, J. W., Gawronski, B., & Trope, Y. (Eds.). (2014). *Dual-process theories of the social mind.* New York, NY: Guilford Press.

Siegel, D. J. (2011). *Mindsight: The new science of personal transformation.* New York, NY: Bantam Books.

Siegel, D. J. (2012). *Pocket guide to interpersonal neurobiology: An integrative handbook of the mind (Norton Series on Interpersonal Neurobiology).* New York, NY: W. W. Norton.

Slovic, P., Finucane, M. L., Peters, E., & MacGregor, D. G. (2007). The affect heuristic. *European Journal of Operational Research, 177*(3), 1333–1352.

Tangney, J. P., Baumeister, R. F., & Boone, A. L. (2004). High self-control predicts good adjustment, less pathology, better grades, and interpersonal success. *Journal of Personality, 72*(2), 271–324.

Wehrum, S., Klucken, T., Kagerer, S., Walter, B., Hermann, A., Vaitl, D., & Stark, R. (2013). Gender commonalities and differences in the neural processing of visual sexual stimuli. *Journal of Sexual Medicine, 10*(5), 1328–1342.

Young, K. S., Griffin-Shelley, E., Cooper, A., O'Mara, J., & Buchanan, J. (2000). Online infidelity: A new dimension in couple relationships with implications for evaluation and treatment. *Sexual Addiction & Compulsivity: The Journal of Treatment and Prevention, 7*(1–2), 59–74.

CHAPTER FOUR

THE OCSB CLINICAL AREAS

A man can do what he wants, but not want what he wants.
—Arthur Schopenhauer

COMPETING MOTIVATIONS IN THREE CLINICAL AREAS

We view out of control sexual behavior (OCSB) as a sexual health problem related to how people resolve their competing motivations. We divide the assessment of their unresolved competing motivations into three clinical areas.

    I. Self-regulation
   II. Attachment regulation
  III. Sexual and erotic conflicts

These distinct and interrelated clinical areas comprise the primary focus of OCSB assessment and treatment. We move from individual coping strategies to relational strategies and then into the final area, which involves both. The self-regulation clinical area explores how self-control capacities may affect out of control experiences. The area of attachment regulation explores how sexual behaviors may reflect the emotional needs or attachment patterns in romantic relationships. Finally, we explore the impact of sexual and erotic conflicts on out of control sexual experiences.

I. SELF-REGULATION

Self-regulation refers to one's capacity to alter behavior or activation in response to particular stimuli (Baumeister, Schmeichel, & Vohs, 2007;

Baumeister & Vohs, 2007). As described in Chapter 3, activation is an umbrella term that describes the internal response to stimuli that is commonly labeled as emotions, motivational states, or drives. An individual's capacity to take action and change how he or she feels, to self-regulate, is an integral component of navigating the world and is seen during the first weeks of life (Greenspan & Greenspan, 1985). In the classic book, *First Feelings: Milestones in the Emotional Development of Your Baby and Child*, Stanley Greenspan and Nancy Greenspan describe how infants respond to the new stimulation outside of the womb. Newborns regulate their activation through a choreography of reaching out to novel sensations and retreating from overstimulation, only to reengage and retreat again in an ongoing dance toward and away from a stimulus (e.g., mother's face). The ability to alternate movement toward and away from a novel situation (even when highly pleasurable) is correlated with the ability to create a state of relaxation. The infant's early-life activation regulation may support the development of a self-concept and lays the groundwork for sexual regulation.

Optimal Activation

One of our implied goals for OCSB treatment is helping clients develop flexible and adaptive behaviors to effectively manage their lives. In general, people are less flexible and adaptive when their affective responses are disproportional or unrelated to the current situation. For instance, in a life-threatening circumstance, survival may depend on the affective system's fast processing, which elicits a hyperactivated (i.e., excessive or above normal incitement) or hypoactivated (i.e., excessively or slightly below normal incitement) response. In the absence of that threat, however, high- and low-activation levels are unnecessary and may lead to undesirable or ineffective behaviors because the deliberative system is less engaged and is not guiding behavior significantly. Maintaining an optimum level of activation between hypo- and hyperactivation, in which both the affective and deliberative systems are collaborating toward a common goal, is more likely to produce flexible, adaptive, and effective behavior. Siegel (2011) refers to the optimum level of activation as the window of affect tolerance—the space in which a balanced affective–deliberation interaction is maintained. Depending on the individual, the window is a narrow or wide band of arousal within which an individual can function well. "If an experience pushes us outside our window of tolerance, we may fall into rigidity and depression on the one hand or into chaos on the other. A narrow window of tolerance can constrict our lives" (p. 137).

OCSB treatment is designed to provide a process to experience, investigate, and expand a client's window of affect tolerance. There are two learning objectives when working with the window of affect tolerance. One objective is to increase the client's ability to maintain states of optimum activation. The second is to expand the range of affect that is tolerable. These two objectives help clients reduce chaotic reactivity or unwanted consequences attributed to an overly rigid, narrow window of affect tolerance. Combined individual and group OCSB therapy, in part, is intended for clients to practice maintaining optimum levels of activation and provide a laboratory to expand their range of tolerable affect.

Four Ingredients of Self-Regulation

"Perhaps the most widely agreed-on function of self-regulation is to bring thoughts and behavior in line with goals and intentions" (Wagner, Heatherton, & Todd, 2015, p. 805). However, self-regulation is a skill that can break down in numerous ways. It is a complex and multifaceted process, which makes it impossible to identify one cause or causal sequence to explain all instances of self-regulation failure. A combination of four ingredients is likely needed to effectively align thoughts and behaviors with goals and intentions: *standards*, *monitoring*, *willpower*, and *motivation*. These components suggest possible pathways for underregulation or misregulation as well as a formula for effective self-regulation (for a review, see Baumeister & Heatherton,1996; Baumeister, Heatherton, & Tice, 1994; Baumeister & Vohs, 2007; Carver & Scheier, 1981).

Self-regulation *standards* are the meaning and importance people place on their behavior. "Effective self-regulation requires a clear and well-defined standard. Ambiguous, uncertain, inconsistent, or conflicting standards make self-regulation difficult" (Baumeister & Vohs, 2007, p. 117). The second self-regulation ingredient is *monitoring*. Monitoring is the capacity to compare the behavior or state of the self against one's standards and expectations. When the action falls short, a motivational process is initiated to better align the self with one's standards (see feedback loop theory; Carver & Scheier, 1981). People also transcend the immediate moment to predict how they might feel after taking an action. In a sense, they are monitoring how they think they will feel in the future. It is a monitoring feature that helps people to maximize positive outcomes and minimize negative outcomes based on how they felt in a similar situation or how they expect to feel given what is known. To generate or replicate desirable behavior, people must have the capacity to learn from their choices and behavior, which entails an internal process of applying that information to choices in the moment.

The next self-regulation ingredient is the strength to restrict or direct behavior away from one's immediate wants, frequently labeled as *willpower*. The energy expended to change the self to align with standards is limited and requires replenishment after expenditure. Willpower is not considered a trait, but rather a potential based on available energy in the moment of self-restraint that becomes temporarily depleted afterward (aka ego depletion; Muraven & Baumeister, 2000; Vohs & Heatherton, 2000). If the self does not have the normal energy resources, it is suggested that the self is rendered less able and willing to function optimally (Baumeister & Vohs, 2007).

The last ingredient is *motivation*. "Even if the standards are clear, monitoring is fully effective, and the person's resources are abundant, he or she may still fail to self-regulate due to not caring about reaching the goal" (Baumeister & Vohs, 2007, p. 117). People are not going to change their behavior if they are unmotivated or not ready to do so. However, if one is motivated, that motivation may offset impaired capacity to self-monitor and compensate during states of ego depletion (Baumeister & Vohs, 2007).

Self-Regulation Clinical Questions

Jim, whom we met in Chapter 3, was initially unable to describe how he ended up paying for sex. In therapy, he identified the motivations that influenced his self-regulation. He was motivated to change his anger and resentment toward his job. His primary strategy was paying for sex, but that behavior clashed with his motivation to avoid arrest or lose his marriage. Jim's decisions and actions, like those of all OCSB clients, can be explored through the lens of self-regulation and the motivations that influence behavior. To organize the assessment, we examine four clinical questions about client self-regulation patterns related to sexual self-control:

1. How are OCSB symptoms related to self-regulation ingredients?
2. How are sexual urges, thoughts, or behaviors solutions to regulating uncomfortable activation?
3. Are the OCSB symptoms an outcome of a hyperactivated or hypoactivated state?
4. How does the client regulate sexual activation?

1. How are OCSB symptoms related to self-regulation ingredients?

Standards

Regulating behavior may be difficult and lead to feeling out of control when sexual standards are vague and underdeveloped or overly precise and rigid. Frank's underdeveloped standards were apparent in his casual attitude about accessing online sexual videos on his workplace computer. His standards about using his employer's equipment for sexual pursuits were too vague to elicit a motivation to regulate his behavior. His unclear standards left his affective system operating without much deliberative involvement. Like so many people without clear standards, Frank found himself in sexual situations overly directed by his pleasure-seeking systems and forces of habit. He was unable to think clearly about his internal values against which he could evaluate his actions and thus build motivation to change his behavior.

On the other end of the spectrum, "highly restrictive sexual attitudes can result in inability to conform, starting off a cycle of guilt, mental pain, and the urge to act out" (Bancroft, 2013, p. 859). Failing to meet idealistic expectations can lead to a variety of emotional and relational consequences (Coleman, 1986). Peter's case is an example of inconsistent ability to conform to restrictive and idealistic standards. His cultural and religious beliefs shaped his rigid and narrow sexual standards into a fidelity expectation that prohibited solo sex and sexual fantasies involving women who were not his wife. As a result, Peter expected that all of his sexual energies would be directed into his marriage and that he would never masturbate. After repeated episodes of dishonoring his standard, he hoped OCSB therapy could resolve his masturbation dilemma by increasing his strength to avoid solo sex and fantasizing about other women. He was motivated to restrict any sexual urge, thought, or behavior that violated his religious beliefs and marital commitments but was ultimately frustrated when his sexual drive was not contained within his high expectations. He judged his inability to follow his sexual standards as a symptom of an addictive disorder and moral failing and less motivated to evaluate the effect of restrictive sexual standards on his difficulties following them.

Self-monitoring

Self-regulation benefits from an ability to look inward and identify internal affective states. Without self-monitoring, the feedback loop is interrupted and people are less able to direct their behavior toward more desirable outcomes. This capacity varies among people and can be compromised in a variety of ways. We organize factors that undermine self-awareness into a list of screening criteria that are reviewed during the first client appointment (see Chapter 5). Factors that may impair self-monitoring include untreated mental health disorders, active drug and alcohol abuse, and unresolved medical problems. Psychological undercurrents related to personality traits or disorders, adjustment to adverse life experiences, and posttraumatic stress affect self-monitoring abilities. Clients should be screened for factors that impair self-monitoring before drawing conclusions about their ability.

For some clients, a limited ability to transcend a sexually activating moment often results in failing to maintain relationship agreements or their own sexual self-standards. In general, resisting the pull of instant gratification is more challenging when in the mists of a sexual urge. Heightened sexual excitement lessens the inhibiting influence of distal consequences. For instance, Will's sexual behavior problems were linked with self-monitoring failures. Outside of a sexual situation, he expressed a strong desire to maintain a negative HIV status and was well-informed of the risks of condomless anal sex. When Will was in the "heat of a moment," he was less motivated by his long-term goal of avoiding HIV infection. His attention was focused on his immediate gratification and he minimized whatever might inhibit his proximate sexual pleasure. He would often fail to transcend the moment and thus lose sight of his health goal.

The role of habit in OCSB is also useful to identify and explore. In general, habits free the deliberative system during routine and familiar behaviors. When behaviors are on "autopilot," mental energy is available for novel and less familiar situations that benefit more from self-awareness and conscious intention (Wood & Neal, 2007). However, what happens when sexual behaviors are habits? Clients commonly report limited self-monitoring regarding masturbation to sexual imagery. They routinely masturbate before falling asleep or when waking up in the morning. With time and repetition, client's sexual behaviors become less intentional and more habitual without realizing the progression. Regulating sexual routines requires the reintroduction of conscious monitoring and, ultimately, forming new sexual health habits. By definition, new behaviors are not habits and take conscious effort to change and sustain. With time and repetition, new sexual health habits develop and the effort to maintain these sexual boundaries decreases, indicating that the affective–deliberative interaction has been recalibrated to maintain the new sexual behaviors.

Willpower
Baumeister and Vohs (2007) suggest that willpower is like a muscle; it relies on a finite source of energy that is exhausted after use and needs to be ecologically managed. Exhausting willpower energy resources creates

a state of "ego depletion" that results in someone being temporarily less willing and able to function optimally (Baumeister & Vohs, 2007). The more clients assert willpower, the less ego strength is available for balancing the affective system. Ego depletion leaves some men vulnerable to feeling sexually out of control. For instance, clients who are struggling to regulate masturbation to sexually explicit media frequently contend with the loss of willpower. Because sexual videos are easily accessible from multiple technology platforms, they persistently confront the opportunity and the urge to cross their boundaries. If they have not established environmental controls, then they are likely relying on their internal capacity to restrict their urges to watch a sexual video. Over time, clients deplete their energy resources and are less able or willing to maintain their boundaries in the next opportunity. By reducing the amount of temptation in their environment (e.g., establishing Internet filters or technology-free zones in the home), they can reduce the amount of energy needed to restrict their impulses.

The good news for men with OCSB is that willpower can be strengthened. Research suggests that people can improve their willpower by committing to small and consistent acts of self-control (Baumeister, Gailliot, DeWall, & Oaten, 2006; Muraven, 2010; Muraven, Baumeister, & Tice, 1999). McGonigal (2011) points out that the "muscle" being trained was not getting better at restricting a problematic behavior. It was improving the capacity to observe when an old behavior pattern was returning and then choosing a new behavior instead. Over time, the practice of pausing before acting became easier.

Motivation
Motivation is the initiation and maintenance of goal-directed behavior; it causes people to act and behave in a manner they believe is congruent with their goals. Motivation is also an outcome of an interaction between people, thus adding interpersonal processes as an essential aspect of motivation (Miller & Rollnick, 2002). The first of the six screening criteria for assessment of OCSB examines the client's motivation and stage of readiness for change. Our assessment process, in part, is a lengthy interpersonal exchange over weeks, sometimes months, during which the client and therapist slowly identify the discrepancy between the client's current sexual behavior and his emerging vision for sexual health. OCSB assessment invites the client to clarify his motivation for sexual health and welcomes his readiness to change throughout each stage of treatment. We devote more attention to this self-regulation ingredient in Chapter 5.

2. How are sexual urges, thoughts, or behaviors solutions to regulating uncomfortable activation?

Everyone experiences feelings that are uncomfortable, but labeling it as uncomfortable does not indicate what the emotion is or why it is uncomfortable. At most, it indicates that an emotion, urge, or drive is unwanted or disliked. Reasons for not liking a specific activation are varied and idiosyncratic. The emotion can be painful, distracting, or just incongruent with how one wants to feel. The individual may want to upregulate his or her activation because he or she does not want to feel so low. Or, the individual wants to downregulate the intensity of his or her affect because he or she feels too agitated. Whatever the specific quality that makes an activated state uncomfortable, it prompts the drive to change the feeling. To override the emotion or alter the level of activation is the most common type of emotional self-regulation (Baumeister & Vohs, 2007).

Uncomfortable activation presents each client with a choice. Does he continue feeling the uncomfortable emotion, the low mood, or whatever feeling he would rather not have or does he change it? If it is the latter choice, sexual expression or fantasy is an easy and effective strategy to use to change internal activation or to modulate affect intensity either up or down. Miller and Rollnick remind us, "human beings seem to have a built-in desire to set things right" (2002, p. 20). When people's activation moves outside of their tolerance window, they usually respond to bring themselves back into optimum activation. If they are feeling something they would rather not feel, they usually act to change it. Their intention to self-regulate is honorable, but the sexual solution (e.g., hours spent masturbating or sex that risks HIV/unintended pregnancy) may have negative consequences.

3. Are the OCSB symptoms an outcome of a hyperactivated or hypoactivated state?

Self-regulation ingredients, such as monitoring, willpower, and motivation, are mechanisms for maintaining optimal activation. Once outside the window of optimal activation, self-regulation is more difficult because *self-monitoring* is impaired, more *willpower* is needed to counterbalance hyper- or hypoactivated states, and *motivation* to behave within one's *standards* is lower. Rather than using a strategy to restore optimum activation, out of control sexual experiences may be the result of limited agency during hyper- or hypoactivated states.

Hector expected his pattern of sex at adult bookstores to stop when he was sober from alcohol. However, when he was not drinking and continued his old patterns, he was confused. One area of inquiry we recommend assessing is the possible link between Hector's hyper- or hypoactivation and out of control sexual experiences. Was anonymous sex a regulation strategy to self-soothe uncomfortable activation? Or, was his anonymous sex a symptom of a hyperactive state stemming from an untreated mood disorder that was camouflaged by his drug and alcohol use? Unfortunately, client and clinician can be distracted by sexual symptoms and fail to spot a wider range of factors that influence affect intensity. In Chapter 5, we outline screening criteria for conditions that may elicit hyper- or hypoactivation states with sexual symptoms.

4. How does the client regulate sexual activation?

The two previous sections reviewed how men might use sex to regulate uncomfortable activation and how impaired agency during high and low activation might result in sexual behavior problems. In this section, we discuss how clients regulate activation that is sexual. The sexual motivational system is typically activated when a person notices a stimulus (e.g., another person) and subjectively appraises attractiveness and sexual interest (Fisher, 2004). This engagement of attraction and sex generates arousal and excitement. Bancroft (2013) describes the subsequent sexual arousal as a complex state, involving automatic and conscious processes, incentive motivations and general arousal, and genital response. This complexity is conceptualized within the dual control model of sexual response: "The occurrence of genital response and, with it, the characteristic sequence of general arousal, incentive motivation, and relevant information processing, which combine to produce the experience of sexual arousal, are determined by the interaction between excitatory and inhibitory mechanisms" (Bancroft, 2013, p. 856).

We previously noted the widespread application of dual-process models in contemporary psychology (Loewenstein & O'Donoghue, 2007). The dual control model of sexual response and the dual-process model of human behavior share several traits. The dual control model describes response as a weighted relationship between sexual excitation and inhibition (Janssen & Bancroft, 2007). Both the dual-process model and dual control model are interactional models focusing on the relative influence of these two systems on each other. Just as behavior is a joint product of the interaction between the affective and deliberative systems of the embodied mind, sexual response is an outcome of the interaction between embodied excitatory and inhibitory mechanisms. In other words, sexual response is also the result of internal opposing forces. And, just like the affective and deliberative systems of the mind, the excitatory and inhibitory mechanisms in sexual response have physiological and psychological ramifications.

When Janssen and Bancroft (2007) set out to study their dual-control hypothesis, they expected to find one overriding distinct sexual inhibitor. Instead, they found two inhibiting factors within their study population. The first factor was threat of sexual-functioning failures during a sexual situation or encounter. Colloquially referred to as "performance anxiety," a man's worry, anxiety, or fear about his sexual function inhibits his level of sexual excitation. The second distinct inhibiting factor they found was the threat from a perceived or actual consequence of the sexual activity (e.g., contracting an STD or getting arrested). A man's worry, anxiety, or fear about a potential negative consequence during or preceding a sexual encounter also inhibits his level of sexual excitation. They label the first inhibitor a sexual-performance threat and the second a sexual-consequence threat. Each inhibitor counterbalances the man's excitation level within a given sexual situation. Both inhibition factors are shaped by the sociocultural context in which men live and vary significantly among men.

Therapists can apply the dual control model to frame cases involving male sexual disorders and sexual behavior problems. For example, when thinking about a client's sexual dysfunction, his propensity for high sexual inhibition and/or low sexual excitation may lead to difficulties achieving or sustaining an erection. High sexual excitation and/or low inhibition may lead to rapid ejaculation. The likely profile for out of control sexual behavior is a propensity for high levels of sexual excitation and/or insufficient sexual inhibition (Bancroft & Vukadinovic, 2004). There are two OCSB profiles within their dual control model that exemplify men whose inhibition mechanism does not balance their sexual excitation propensity. One profile is men whose sexual inhibition level is lower than their excitation level. The second are men with high levels of inhibition who disinhibit in problematic ways in order to be sexual (e.g., using drugs or alcohol to regulate negative emotional consequences that make sex less enjoyable). The other version involves someone with moderate or average levels of sexual excitation, but who has a low sexual inhibition propensity. In both profiles, the OCSB psychotherapy objective is to adjust men's sexual inhibition mechanism to more effectively balance their sexual excitation patterns. Psychotherapy is unlikely to affect a client's capacity for sexual excitation, but it can modulate the client's sexual inhibition levels through reappraisal of sexual-performance threats or consequences.

We hypothesize that sexual health can be improved by enhancing client self-regulation ingredients to rebalance the sexual excitation and inhibition interaction. Men with self-regulation deficits and higher than average sexual excitation levels are more likely to make an in-the-moment decision that contradicts their sexual and relationship agreements. For instance, people with low traits for self-control also report having low dispositional sexual restraint (Gailliot et al., 2007). Motivations for STD (sexually transmitted disease) protection and upholding fidelity agreements may significantly decrease when participants are sexually motivated by partner attractiveness (Ariely & Loewenstein, 2006). Some OCSB symptoms are explained by sexually excited men with underdeveloped inhibiting capacities.

II. ATTACHMENT REGULATION

The second OCSB clinical area concerns the association between out of control sexual behavior experiences and attachment patterns. We explore how men's sexual symptoms may reflect their regulation of emotional proximity and the various ways men resolve their competing motivations within their romantic relationships. As in self-regulation, men's competing motivations associated with attachment arise from internal drives and expectations. However, when men are attempting to change or alter how they feel in their sexual or romantic relationships, they must also give attention to the drives and expectations of their partners. Both the client and partners engage in a dance of emotional proximity as a method to alter their personal feelings. As men regulate their feelings by creating emotional distance or closeness, they encounter intimate partners who engage in similar relationship strategies and who are attempting to satisfy their own sexual and intimacy needs. If that is not complicated enough, these relationship dynamics occur within sociocultural contexts that shape people's expectations about sexual and romantic relationships.

To make sense of this complexity, we first focus on the internal drives. Fisher (2004) discusses three different, but entwined, internal drives that propel people toward connection and sexual relationships. According to Fisher, romantic love, lust, and attachment share a common evolutionary purpose for mating, but travel different neurological pathways. Fisher describes how each component of this trio instructs different aspects of reproduction and carries additional purposes beyond ensuring procreation that are equally as important. At times, romantic love, lust, and attachment drives interact in ways that stimulate or enhance each other. Other times, love, lust, and attachment act to dampen or diminish each other (Fisher, 2004). It is another example of how the goals of the rider and elephant may compliment or compete with each other as well as within each other.

External forces, such as the socioculture norms that shape relationship expectations and values, complicate the interplay of the three relationship drives. Perel (2006) explores how these drives are affected by overburdened intimacy standards on contemporary pair-bonded relationships. She describes the consequences for long-term couples in which one potentially lifelong partner is expected to satisfy drives of romantic love, attachment, and lust. Current Western cultural values idealize relationships that combine these drives into long-term attachments between two people. These ideals are not only a relatively recent marital expectation, they have infiltrated most aspects of how partners (and clinicians) interpret and respond to relationships that struggle to uphold this standard. For instance, partners, family, and clinicians often privilege love and attachment drives over the lust drive and, as a result, negatively judge those who are motivated to satisfy their lust drive as an equal or perhaps more valued need.

Perel (2006) also highlights a common thinking error found in many couples seeking therapy (as well as in the therapists from whom they seek guidance). Both members of the couple (as well as many couples' therapists) may assume that lust will follow as long as the couple secures their emotional attachment. The assumption that emotional security is linked with lustful sexual attraction may derive from the onset of the relationship, when romantic love and lust drives effortlessly overlap. The intertwined drives of this relationship stage, commonly referred to as limerence, gradually disentangles as the couple moves into the next stage of their relationship. As limerence fades, it allows other needs from each partner to surface. Sometimes limerence is replaced by the serenity of a loving attachment. Other times, the relationship ends. Fisher and Perel assert that these current sociocultural expectations of romantic love, lust, and attachment did not evolve among humans to maintain contemporary Western ideals of long-term, pair-bonded, monogamous attachments. Some long-term couples may feel frustrated and disappointed that their relationships do not live up to this ideal couple after limerence has faded. When the cross-purposes of lust, love, and attachment emerge within the couple, many seek help to manage their internal tensions and process the unmet ideals of their long-term relationship.

How can therapists integrate the knowledge about the internal and external dynamics that influence behaviors without sending the impression that they are endorsing sociocultural norms about ideal relationship expectations and configurations? Sex outside of a committed romantic relationship is one of the most common forms of sexual behavior men report when seeking OCSB treatment. But the problem is not that they were having sex outside of a committed relationship. The issue is their pattern of not honoring the sexual agreements of their relationship.

Imbedded in their treatment request is an unknown combination of competing motivations between the internal forces of love, lust, and attachment and the external forces of the partner's needs and sociocultural expectations. Without judging relationship agreements or structures as good or bad, healthy or unhealthy, we encourage therapists to instead investigate the behavioral discrepancy that exists between establishing those agreements and not honoring them. At one time these men were motivated to enter into their current relationship agreements and, evidenced by their request for OCSB treatment, experienced a competing motivation that threatens or leads to dishonoring their agreements. By grounding the clinical inquiry within the clients' contradictions, therapists have an opportunity to explore the details of the out of control sexual experiences without promoting the current sociocultural ideal of romantic relationships.

Understanding the complex forces involved in contradictory relationship patterns is a challenging task. To organize the investigation, we briefly review attachment theory and then discuss these three OCSB assessment and treatment attachment-related questions.

1. How do OCSB symptoms reflect attachment styles?
2. How does the client maintain his sexual relationship agreements?
3. Does the client display traits of sexual narcissism?

Attachment Theory Review

Attachment refers to the emotional bond between people. John Bowlby and Mary Ainsworth originated attachment theory to explain how parental relationships influenced child development (Ainsworth, Blehar, Waters, & Wall, 1978; Bowlby, 1969, 1973, 1980). Attachment, like other motivational systems such as pain avoidance or drug-craving mechanisms, compels mainly subconscious, goal-directed actions to seek a protective attachment figure when threatened (Mikulincer & Shaver, 2007). "Bowlby viewed the healthy functioning of this behavioral system as crucial for emotional stability, mental health, and satisfying, close relationships" (p. 28). The quality of interactions with a previous and current attachment figure differentially activates the attachment system in the current relationship and is reflected in relationship behaviors that regulate primary proximity-seeking behaviors. When the primary proximity-seeking behavior does not bring about the desired feeling of security, secondary activation responses of the attachment system either intensify proximity-seeking strategies or cause one to disengage from the relationship (see Mikulincer and Shaver [2010] for a detailed review of attachment theory).

Caregiver emotional and physical availability influences how a child learns to depend on relationships to reduce anxiety, feel more secure, and seek soothing. Childhood attachment patterns that develop from the caregiver relationship are called *attachment styles*, which develop from the interplay of the child's neurobiology and caregiver behavior (Shore, 2003).

Both self-regulation and attachment theories contain a feedback-loop system. Self-regulation and the attachment system are goal-directed behaviors that monitor progress and disengage from unproductive behaviors. Mikulincer and Shaver (2007) suggest that attachment security allows people to maintain a calm, coherent, and confident state of mind when handling challenges and investing their cognitive resources toward important tasks. In contrast, they contend that attachment insecurities:

> motivate defensive distortions of perception, helpless or unrealistically confident stances toward problem solving, and feelings of being threatened or endangered that interfere with realistic planning and effective action. Over time, these insecurities impair self-regulation and interfere with close relationships, important life projects, and personal growth. (p. 222)

Attachment research progressed over time to include the influence of the attachment mechanism on adult pair bonding (Hazan & Shaver, 1987). *Adult attachments styles* are the patterns of relational expectations, needs, emotions, and behaviors that develop in response to a person's attachment history (Mikulincer & Shaver, 2007). Although attachment theory stems from parent–child relationships, adult romantic relationships differ in significant ways. For instance, adults in romantic relationships switch roles between the dependent position of needing security and comfort and the caregiver position of providing the security and comfort. Both romantic partners share in exchanging sexual roles. Despite the differences between child–parent attachment patterns and adults, core principles of attachment can be applied and inform how we understand adult relationship behavior (see Mikulincer and Shaver [2007] for a review for adult attachment theory).

Adult attachment styles comprise two dimensions: attachment-related avoidance and attachment-related anxiety. *Avoidance* is an attachment dimension that focuses on discomfort with closeness and dependency, whereas the *anxiety* component focuses on fears of abandonment (Brennan, Clark, & Shaver, 1998). People who prefer to rely less often on others and choose independent coping strategies will likely score higher on measures that evaluate attachment-related avoidance. Those who feel more comfortable with intimacy and search out others when in need of solace or emotional support will likely score lower on measures for attachment-related avoidance. People who worry about their part-ner's attention, availability, and responsiveness typically score higher on levels of attachment-related anxiety. An adult's attachment style is determined by combining one's individual predilection for relationship avoidance with one's predisposition for relationship anxiety. Securely attached adults are characterized by a combination of low scores in both attachment-related anxiety and avoidant coping strategies. The pre-occupied attachment style combines high scores in relationship anxiety and low frequency of relationship avoidance patterns. Dismissive attach-ment styles are reflected in a low score of attachment-related anxiety and high scores on avoidance and fearfulness; the fourth attachment style is composed of high scores on both dimensions (Fraley, Heffernan, Vicary, & Brumbaugh, 2011). Attachment style scores can be visually depicted using the anxious and avoidant dimensions as vertical and horizontal axes, respectively, and then plotting a person's scores on a four-quadrant graph (see Figure 4.1). Fraley developed a multiple relationship con-text measure that evaluates attachment propensities in relationships

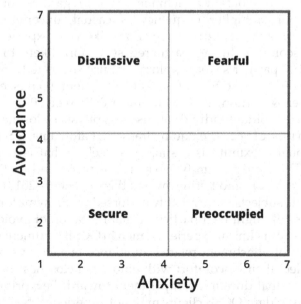

Figure 4.1 *Attachment style graph.*

with romantic partners, as well as relationships with mother, father, and friends. Assessing attachment dimensions in multiple contexts using relationship-specific measures more accurately predicted intrapersonal and interpersonal relational outcomes than broader attachment measures (Fraley et al., 2011).

1. How do OCSB symptoms reflect attachment styles?

Attachment research suggests that sexuality is interrelated with attachment mechanisms and is an important dimension in understanding sexual health problems. "Attachment styles may reflect an important source of differences in the way people generate, experience, and express their sexual emotions" (Dewitte, 2012, p. 118). People with different attachment styles regulate their sexual urges, thoughts, and behaviors differently, mainly because they hold different meanings and goals for sexual encounters. Conversely, attachment mechanisms may amplify or inhibit sexual feelings, which can influence sexual regulation (Dewitte, 2012). Furthermore, research suggests that insecure attachment styles contribute to sexual problems in predictable and distinct ways (Mikulincer & Shaver, 2007). Sexual patterns of OCSB treatment-seeking clients may reflect their discomfort with emotional closeness in their romantic relationship or their propensity to sexually soothe relationship anxieties.

People with avoidant attachment styles, regardless of sexual orientation, report a higher frequency of casual, uncommitted sexual partners. Avoidant individuals are more likely to experience various forms of discomfort during partnered sex, more likely to be dismissive of mutual partner sexual exploration, use sex to reduce stress, and experience sex as a source of self-enhancement (Davis et al., 2006; Davis, Shaver, & Vernon, 2004; Mikulincer & Shaver, 2007; Schachner & Shaver, 2004). Avoidant individuals use less physical closeness to soothe partners in a time of need (Péloquin, Brassard, Lafontaine, & Shaver, 2013).

Emotional proximity is a subjective feeling that is unique to the individual. The same proximity can be felt as warm and soothing by one person and cold or smothering by another. Crocker (2013) found that avoidant male subjects more reliably endorsed OCSB symptoms and suggests that OCSB might be a particular manifestation of avoidant attachment styles. In our clinical experience, men in OCSB treatment who exhibit high degrees of attachment-related avoidance engage in sexual behaviors that reflect their discomfort with emotional closeness or experience a sexual drive that does not compel them toward their primary romantic partner. Avoidant OCSB clients may not experience the same motivation to connect with their primary partner when they feel distressed or sexually excited as do securely attached men. They tend to create emotional distance to regulate the discomfort with the emotional closeness of their primary romantic partner. Emotional distance achieved through sexual behavior may be evident in using solo sex practices or extrarelational, non-romantic partnered sex. We observed that when anxiously attached men's motivational systems were activated during stressful periods, they often attempted to create emotional closeness through sexual encounters. If their primary partners were not available because the partners were not interested in sex or the clients were single, they tended to seek soothing through sexual expression via online sexual encounters or casual/anonymous sex with others.

As a reminder it is important to find the individual experience that lies within the attachment-style generalizations. Securely attached individuals are not necessarily free from sexual problems and insecurely attached individuals do not always experience sexual problems. Dewitte (2012) raises the main point we want to highlight in the relationship between attachment and sexuality: "Attachment relationships may provide a context for regulating sexual emotions and sexual interactions may be involved in regulating attachment emotions" (p. 118). When clients present with OCSB, it provides an opportunity to become curious about how their sexual problems are related to their attachment patterns and the attachment function of their sexual experiences. Out of control sexual experiences may stem from struggling to rectify competing love, lust, and attachment drives. Some men pay for sex, seek out casual or anonymous partners, masturbate or engage in online erotic sex chat as their conscious or unconscious remedy for regulating emotional proximity or relationship anxiety.

2. How does the client maintain his sexual relationship agreements?

Motivations for dishonoring sexual relationship agreements are numerous and elude a singular generalization. Broken sexual agreements within committed romantic relationships are nearly universal among the nonsingle OCSB treatment-seeking men. Too often clinicians insufficiently explore the client's commitment process and focus attention on the specific and often stigmatized sexual behaviors that violate the agreement. We suggest that clinicians assist clients to verbalize and clarify their motivation for agreeing to their current relationship boundaries before exclusively focusing on the commitments they crossed. We often find that behind all the emotional turmoil surrounding a sexual agreement violation lies a man's unsuccessful strategy to resolve his conflicted motivations between his intimate relationship expectations and his sexual interests.

Couples of every configuration (i.e., monogamous, nonmonogamous, polyamorous, etc.) implicitly and explicitly agree to a range of sexual boundaries and expectations. These spoken and unspoken agreements form the couple's rubric for sexual fidelity, loyalty, commitment, honesty, and responsibility. Sexual behavior that is congruent with the couple's sexual agreements is the demonstration of how each member of the couple expresses and perceives partner loyalty and devotion. Sexual agreements can establish a sense of trust and security designed to protect the intimate core of romantic relationships. The specifics of these agreements depend on the individual and collective values and sense of emotional security of the intimate partners within monogamous, nonmonogamous, and polyamorous relationships. The assessment is a space for clients to get curious about the contradiction between making and dishonoring their agreements without privileging one sexual agreement over another.

Because OCSB treatment-seeking clients regularly present with extra-relational sexual behavior, it is important for therapists to evaluate their assumptions about this behavior. The most common sexual agreements among the men in our OCSB practice is the agreement to have a monogamous sexual relationship. At some point in the relationship, an expectation of monogamy was implicitly or explicitly established and this agreement was to be honored from that moment onward. Monogamy, however, is only one sexual agreement among many possible commitments and it is important to avoid equating monogamy with fidelity, or more specifically, nonmonogamy with infidelity. Therapists cannot assume that clients are dishonoring their relationship agreements simply because they are sexually nonmonogamous. Nor should therapists view nonmonogamy as a symptom of an unhealthy romantic relationship. The WHO (2006) working definition of *sexual health* and our sexual health principles do not proffer monogamy as a component of sexual health. Instead, we recommend assessing OCSB from the perspective of honoring commitments, which commonly cross the sexual health principle of honesty. All romantic relationships, including nonmonogamous and polyamorous couples, have sexual agreements. Just knowing whether a client is in a monogamous, nonmonogamous, or polyamorous relationship does not provide enough details about the client's propensity to honor those agreements and the motivations for dishonoring them. We recommend that clinicians clarify the sexual agreements into which clients have entered, their motivations for agreeing to those commitments, and their history of maintaining those commitments.

How the couples understand the agreement complicates the inquiry of the client's pattern of (dis)honoring the commitment. Agreements may be established with limited discussion and lack clear definitions of the sexual acts that are excluded. Or, couples may have a clear prohibition against extrarelational sexual intercourse, but the precipitating crisis involved online flirtations with anonymous people: The client followed the agreement, but violated the spirit of his commitment. Maintaining an inquisitive, nonjudgmental space is further complicated by the relationship dynamics that occur after infidelity. Commonly, the injured partner hopes that the OCSB assessment will prove culpability, sanction responsibility, and assign blame, establishing the partner as the moral voice of the couple. The partner's goals and influence may compete with the clinical goal of a nonjudgmental inquiry into the patterns of dishonoring relationship agreements. Although the OCSB assessment is a self-reflective process designed to help clients take responsibility for their behaviors, the end result is not meant to entrench the unequal power dynamics that occur immediately after an agreement violation (Moller & Vossier, 2015). The OCSB assessment objectives are to uncover and address the factors that contributed to violating his sexual relationship commitments, which, one hopes, will help the couple heal and develop a more explicit, clear, and egalitarian relationship.

Focusing on how clients honor sexual agreements has other treatment functions. It raises client self-awareness about the internal discrepancy, an important process for enhancing motivation for health behavior change (Prochaska & DiClemente, 2005). Explicit sexual agreements within a couple increase the likelihood of men seeking help when they are unable to stop behaviors that violate these agreements. Combining situational clarity with feelings associated with failing to keep his commitment provides an opportunity for the clinician and client to better understand the internal conflicts and unseen or unspoken function of his sexual behavior. Linking men's emotions with their contradictory sexual behavior provides an opportunity for the client to reevaluate his motivation to maintain his current relationship commitments. Are they still relevant for the client? Are they too rigid? Is this rigid standard contributing to attachment disruptions in a similar manner in which overly restrictive standards impair self-regulation? In these moments of introspection, clients have an opportunity to find alternative, sexual health-informed solutions to their attachment binds. With implicit sexual agreements, clinicians have an opportunity to explore how clients entered into unspoken arrangements and how implicit agreements function for the client.

This line of inquiry sets up post assessment interventions. After identifying the client's relationship patterns, therapists have the opportunity to identify how the client recreates these patterns in the therapeutic relationship. Does he not honor the therapeutic relationship agreements? Is there a pattern of relating in group therapy similar to the attachment style used in his romantic relationship? Therapists can apply the attachment information to here-and-now interventions that can raise the client's awareness about his relationship patterns and subsequently stretch into new ways of coregulating emotions.

Hector's case had an attachment-regulation component. He and his partner, Phil, had implicitly agreed to only have sex with each other. Nonetheless, Hector was certain that the unspoken expectation was that penetrative sexual intercourse outside the relationship must include condoms. Phil had a lower sex drive and when Hector initiated sex, Phil frequently declined. Hector often felt a mixture of resentment and rejection. His attachment scores indicated a propensity for high attachment-related anxiety and avoidance in his romantic relationship and he often pursued nonrelational, anonymous sex with other men. In treatment, Hector reported "feeling trapped" in his resentments toward Phil and Hector had a distressing inability to talk with Phil about how he felt. These thoughts and feelings were closely followed by sexual urges and thoughts to masturbate at an adult bookstore. His intentions were usually to masturbate alone, but if a man found him desirable, he did not decline, which, in the "heat of the moment," often led to disregarding his sexual health boundary regarding using condoms. Hector chose to relieve his resentment through sex rather than upholding his sexual agreement.

3. Does the client display traits of sexual narcissism?

Widman and McNulty (2010) examined whether cognitive components of narcissistic personality can be measurably more activated in sexual situations. They developed a domain-specific sexual narcissism measure to ascertain associations between sexual situation-specific behaviors and measurable activation of narcissism. Their study results mirrored our clinical experiences and led us to include the influence of sexual narcissism within the clinical picture of OCSB. Before discussing sexual narcissism, we review personality theory, how it fits within our OCSB construct, and how we clinically approach personality disorder (PD) diagnoses.

"*Personality* refers to the pattern of thoughts, feelings and behavior that makes each of us the individuals that we are. This is flexible and our behavior differs according to the social situations in which we find ourselves" (Gask, Evans, & Kessler, 2013, p. 1). Personality is a construct that relates to how people cope with their everyday stresses. As with any human quality, however, there is variability in an individual's capability to repeatedly generate desirable behavior over time or in diverse settings. Most people have personalities that allow them to be effective enough in their lives. People are less adaptive and suffer emotional, interpersonal, and mental health problems when their personalities are inflexible or underdeveloped.

According to the American Psychiatric Association's *Diagnostic and Statistical Manual of Mental Disorders,* Fifth Edition (*DSM 5*; American Psychiatric Association, 2013), a *personality disorder* [PD] is an inner experience and behavior that deviates from the norms and expectations of the person's culture. It is pervasive and inflexible, is stable over time, begins in adolescence or early adulthood, and leads to distress or impairment. PD within the *DSM-5* is a persistence of traits set apart from mental illness. The APA considers mental illness a morbid process, which, in theory, has a recognizable onset and ending (American Psychiatric Association, 2013; Gask et al., 2013). A meaningful or clear distinction between personality and mental disorders is not without criticism (see Krueger, 2005; Widiger, Simonsen, Krueger, Livesley, & Verheul, 2005).

PD is not a construct or a term that is generalizable as a correlate for OCSB treatment-seeking men. In one study, participants in treatment for hypersexual disorder displayed modestly higher risks for comorbid PD along with rates of PD greater than that found in the general population but lower than what is typically found in people who seek psychiatric treatment (Carpenter, Reid, Garos, & Najavits, 2013). Narcissistic PD was the most common personality diagnosis found within this study and the only diagnosed PD to meaningfully exceed the general population prevalence rate with an occurrence typically found among outpatient mental health treatment populations. This study found prevalence rates of PD within hypersexual treatment-seeking populations similar to some studies (Lloyd, Raymond, Miner, & Coleman, 2007; Reid & Carpenter, 2009) and less than the rates seen in other studies (Black, Kehrberg, Flumerfelt, & Schlosser, 1997; Raymond, Coleman, & Miner, 2003).

Narcissism is a multifaceted personality style characterized by a tendency to exploit others, a general lack of empathy, and a pervasive confidence in one's abilities (Campbell, Foster, & Finkel, 2002). People with high narcissistic traits tend to be oriented toward sexual relationships that may lead them to pursue sex with people other than their primary partner (Hurlbert, Apt, Gasar, Wilson, & Murphy, 1994; McNulty & Widman, 2014; Wryobeck & Wiederman,1999). A possible explanation for why narcissistic individuals tend to be less committed to their romantic partners and exhibit a higher likelihood to engage in infidelity is characterized by their tendency toward a certain individuality that places a greater value on agentic rewards (e.g., physical pleasure) while tending to devalue shared intimacy (DeWall et al., 2011; Drigotas, Safstrom, & Gentilia, 1999; Foster, Shrira, & Campbell, 2006). Finally, research suggests that people who display limited empathetic ability often perceive their romantic relationships as dissatisfactory, leading to marital difficulties and increased risk for infidelity (Bravo & White Lumpkin, 2010; McNulty & Widman, 2014). Studies find men and women with avoidant styles, which narcissistic individuals tend to have at elevated levels, demonstrate less empathic concern (Feeney & Collins, 2001; Joireman, Needham, & Cummings, 2002; Mikulincer & Shaver, 2007). People with avoidant attachment styles are also less inclined to take the perspective of a distressed person (Corcoran & Mallinckrodt, 2000; Mikulincer & Shaver, 2007) and those with high-avoidant styles have reported less ability to share other's feelings (Trusty, Ng, & Watts, 2005).

Similar inconsistences found within narcissistic PD and hypersexual behavior comorbidity are reported in studies looking at narcissism and infidelity (see Jones & Weiser, 2014). These inconsistencies led Widman and McNulty (2010) to research the predictability of infidelity only in situations (e.g., when sexually activated) in which the narcissistic personality system is activated (McNulty & Widman, 2014). They created the Sexual Narcissism Scale (SNS) to measure four specific sexual domains of narcissism to operationalize men's narcissistic motivations in sexual situations: (a) sexual exploitation, (b) sexual entitlement, (c) lack of sexual empathy, and (d) grandiose sense of sexual skill. Their outcomes suggest that sexual exploitation, sexual entitlement, and lack of sexual empathy are negatively associated with sexual satisfaction and sustained marital satisfaction (McNulty & Widman, 2013) and positively correlated with infidelity (McNulty & Widman, 2014). "Taken together with the facts that it was sexual, but not global narcissism that was associated with infidelity, these findings highlight the importance of sexual motivations, rather than more general interpersonal motivations, to infidelity" (McNulty & Widman, 2014, p. 8).

Although McNulty and Widman were not specifically studying correlations between sexual narcissism and sexual behavior control, we find their sexual narcissism construct helpful in understanding the complexities with men who consistently dishonor their sexual agreements or violate sexual health principles. Over the years of conducting individual and group therapy, we have observed a subset of OCSB clients who display narcissistic traits in their interpersonal relationships and have observed sexual narcissism more frequently than narcissistic PD. In particular, we observed a sense of entitlement to sexual expression and gratification that guided sexual decisions. They displayed a tendency to exploit their romantic partner's trust and assumptions of fidelity or exploited their sexual partners in paid sex encounters.

And, their empathy capacity was too underdeveloped during sexual activation to provide a countervailing force against dishonoring their relationship sexual agreements or sexually exploiting another person. By focusing on situation-specific personality traits within OCSB treatment, therapists can explore the common internal dynamics that contribute to the client's sexual behavior patterns.

III. SEXUAL AND EROTIC CONFLICTS

The interaction between what compels people to take action and the forces that restrict action is central to our OCSB conceptualization. In the first clinical area, we discuss the effects of competing forces on self-regulation and expand the scope to the dynamics between intimate partners. In this last clinical area, we discuss a sexological subject that involves both intra- and interpersonal competing motivations. In the area of *sexual and erotic conflicts*, we examine the obstacles to sexual and erotic self-acceptance and satisfaction. Out of control sexual experiences are often connected to a client's unresolved conflicts with the clients' sexual and erotic selves; what is sexually and erotically compelling competes with what the client thinks he should want or contradicts who he wants to be. These conflicts between the real and ideal selves create shame, fear, and disgust and may carry the threat of interpersonal judgment and rejection. People often defend against these negative emotional and relational consequences with coping strategies that split the unwanted aspects of their sexuality from their self-concept and shield them from their loved ones. However, no matter how much effort is expended to ignore components of their sexual and erotic template, sexuality persists and may be experienced as out of control. In this section, we review the basic concepts of sexual and erotic orientation and identity development to understand the connections with OCSB. We explore these connections during the assessment with the following clinical questions:

1. Are the OCSB symptoms related to sexual or erotic conflicts that clients have with themselves?
2. Are the OCSB symptoms related to sexual or erotic conflicts that clients have with others?
3. Does the client exhibit fixed or unconventional arousal patterns?

1. Are the OCSB symptoms related to sexual or erotic conflicts that clients have with themselves?

Sexual Orientation

Sexual orientation is the term that loosely describes a person's emotional and sexual attraction to members of the same or other sex. For basic understanding of sexual orientation, we recommend organizing one's capacity for same-sex and other-sex sexual attraction as a two-dimensional precept that defines sexual orientation. Storms (1980) was the pioneer sex researcher who proposed that same-sex and other-sex attractions were separate dimensions rather than poles on a binary dimension, as described in the Kinsey scale (Kinsey, Pomeroy, & Martin, 1948). Storms's model can be depicted by a graph with two intersecting axes where the horizontal axis represents the degree of other-sex attraction (low to high) and the vertical axis represents same-sex attraction (low to high). The intersecting axes create four quadrants that represent how a person may describe his or her general sexual orientation at any given time: homosexual, heterosexual, bisexual, and asexual.

The degree of flexibility in a person's sexual responsiveness is also important to consider. Diamond (2014) proposes that women have a greater tendency for changes in same-sex attractions than men, are less exclusive to one gender in their attractions over the life span, have less specific and consistently definable genital responses, and experience more nuance in the interpersonal and situational factors associated with their sexual desires. She calls this combination of "situation-dependent flexibility in sexual responsiveness" a woman's capacity for sexual fluidity (p. 641). Sexual-fluidity research suggests that men experience less change in their attractions and identity over the life span; however, some studies show that teen and young adult and lesbian, gay, and bisexual youth may have more fluidity than other men (Katz-Wise & Hyde, 2014). Savin-Williams and Ream (2007) found significant migration within sexual attraction, sexual behavior, and sexual identity among the adolescents and young male participants who identified themselves as other-than-exclusively heterosexual.

Sexual-Identity Conflict

Because most people are raised under the assumption of heterosexuality, individuals may adopt a sexual identity before they fully realize the direction of their sexual attractions. For those whose sexual attractions are heterosexually orientated, developing an affirming and integrated sexual identity in which sexual attractions, behavior, and identity are congruent, may not be an issue. Internal conflicts occur, however, when sexual attraction or sexual behavior are incongruent with an individual's self-concept. Most cultures privilege heterosexuality and the fear, shame, and anxiety among individuals who discover their sexual orientation is not exclusively heterosexual may delay or avoid integrating that awareness into their sexual identity. The terms *gay, lesbian, bisexual,* and *straight* are the terms generally used to describe one's sexuality, but the limitations of language can constrict or confuse identity development. Sexual identity is also informed by one's romantic attractions, but the terms do not communicate the nuances in flexibility, intensity, or diversity of these attractions. Furthermore, diversity in gender orientation challenges the fundamental concepts of same and other sex that serve as a reference point in the definition of sexual orientation. Determining same or other sex may be unclear if the individual or the person to whom that individual is attracted does not fit neatly into the gender binary of same or other sex.

In our clinical experience, OCSB treatment-seeking clients occasionally mistake sexual-identity crises as a sexual dysregulation disorder. These clients have realized their sexual and romantic attractions are incongruent with their sexual identity, which is usually exclusively heterosexual. The conflict may be related to an attraction they have denied their entire lives or they have not integrated the changes in their sexual and romantic capacities that have occurred over time into their self-concept. A reevaluation of the sexual identity typically carries implications that the client does not want, such as loss of significant relationships, rejection from important religious or social groups, or the mourning of the heterosexual life he thought he would lead. Although the attractions may feel out of control because the client, for whatever reason, does not want to consider himself other than exclusively heterosexual, the solution is not to change his attraction. A client may be motivated to label this sexual-identity crisis a sexual addiction or compulsion as a solution to change his orientation, but the treatment recommendation for these cases is to help the client integrate his sexual and romantic attractions into his self-concept.

Erotic Orientation

We dedicate sections in Chapters 1 and 2 to prepare clinicians to facilitate sexual health conversations about OCSB because diagnostic ambiguity and negative sociocultural sexual values complicate the therapeutic alliance and treatment planning. In this section, we add another complication—the complexities, unpredictability, and paradoxical nature of eroticism (Morin, 1995). This an area where anything that inhibits arousal (e.g., anxiety, guilt, or fear) can amplify it in another circumstance; where intensely arousing and gratifying human sexual actions can also frighten, shame, or cause harm (Money, 1999). This is an area in which the developmental struggles in life and love also shape the richness of erotic passion (Morin, 1995).

The term *erotic orientation* is less familiar than *sexual orientation* and first appeared in the sexological literature in the middle of the last century (Kinsey et al., 1948; Money, 1988; Storms, 1979, 1981). Whereas sexual orientation refers to one's capacities to be attracted to a particular gender profile, we view erotic orientation as an individual's pattern of sexually arousing content. The template includes the content of the individual's fantasy and the external stimuli that is sexually arousing (Storms, 1981). Research suggests that sexual orientation develops through processes separate from an individual's erotic orientation. It is likely, for instance, that the gender of the desired partner (sexual definition) formed during critical periods in sexual differentiation and gender-role development, and is then reinforced through social and emotional attraction and the genital arousal connected to the gender of the individual who evoked it (Pfaus et al., 2012). On the other hand, the content of sexual desires (erotic orientation) may be shaped and focused through a learning process in which early formative experiences with sexual arousal are ascribed sexual meaning. Researchers and theorists suggest that erotic development is a learning process between an individual's sensual and sexual systems and the contexts in which the individual feels the reward of sexual pleasure and excitement (Bader, 2002; Bancroft, 2009; Morin, 1995; Pfaus et al., 2012). "Reward gives us the power to know what we like, and directs our attentional mechanisms to focus on cues that predict the reward" (Pfaus et al., 2012, p. 55). The dynamic interaction between the individual's feeling of sexual reward and his or her continually changing developmental contexts focus and alter the content of an individual's erotic desires. This learning process is significantly influential in the developmental trajectory of sexual desires and the diverse erotic worlds of humans.

Larger than a collection of sexual thoughts and physical sensations, the gestalt of eroticism portrays a process in which sex becomes meaningful (Morin, 1995). The transformation of stimulus to arousal involves an intermediary step of the mind (Bader, 2002). The meaning of the event endows the sensation or situation with sexual excitement (Bader, 2002). It captures why one person is turned-on by gentleness and another is not. Or, why medical examination of one's genitals does not generate the same excitement as the genital touch of a romantic partner. "When it comes to sexual arousal, psychology makes use of biology, not the other way around" (p. 6).

Although an individual's sexual desire can be activated by all kinds of stimuli and situations, the most passionate responses launch from the interaction of two competing forces (Morin, 1995). The first is the attraction that compels a person toward the erotic object and the second is an obstacle to overcome. Morin (1995) summarized this dynamic in his erotic equation: attraction + obstacles = sexual excitement. By its nature, he posits, "the erotic experience is shaped by the push–pull of opposing forces and is therefore engergetic, interactive, and potentially dangerous" (p. 51). The irony therefore is that the negative consequences of an individual's actions might have also been the ingredient that enhanced sexual excitement, which motivates future sexual choices. Because eroticism resides in the friction created by restriction and impulse, sexual excitement requires a degree of operational tension that is not too restrictive (which would shut down passion) in order to generate heat (Morin, 1995).

Negative consequences from sexual behavior are a common oppositional force. The erotic equation is vital in helping OCSB treatment-seeking clients frame the inherent contradictions of their erotic excitement without judging this paradox as pathological. We propose the nature of feeling sexually out of control describes the dilemma of competing motivations—wanting to do one thing while doing the other. This oppositional process also describes the generation of erotic pleasure and may be the experience clients identify as feeling out of control. In other words, what they are describing as pathological is the genesis of erotic pleasure.

Erotic-Identity Conflict

Developing an affirming sexual identity is a psychological process in which an individual strives to align his or her sexual self-concept with his or her sexual attractions and behavior. Erotic identity is a similar psychological process in which individuals strive to align their erotic self-concept with the content of their desires, fantasies, and sexual activities. Erotic-identity conflicts occur when individuals judge their sexual desires as deficient, immoral, or disgusting or they may fear rejection from significant attachments. When left unresolved, managing these negative emotions competes with integrating the erotic orientation into one's self-concept. While obstructed in a manner similar to sexual-identity development, erotic-identity development has different sociocultural taboos and contexts that discourage expressing erotic interests, especially those that are unconventional. Variability in erotic orientations is less visible and valued than sexual orientation and advances in lesbian and gay civil rights and social acceptance have not translated into a celebration of erotic diversity. In their seminal book, *The Ethical Slut*, Easton and Liszt (1997) warn of the harmful consequences wrought by sexual deprivation used to cope with the internal and external sex-negativism directed toward erotic diversity. "We see ourselves surrounded by the 'walking wounded'—by people who have been deeply, if not irrevocably, injured by fear, shame and hatred of their own sexual selves" (p. 19).

Men with erotic conflicts quietly feel shame at the thought of revealing their most precious and vital source of sexual and erotic pleasure. In *Coming Out of Shame*, Kaufman and Raphael (1996) vividly describe the experience of shame:

> To experience shame is to feel *seen* in a painfully diminished sense. Our eyes turn inward in the moment of shame, and suddenly we've become impaled under the magnifying gaze of our own eyes. Even when other people are present and watching, we are watching ourselves; but we actually mistake the watching eyes as belonging only to others. Exposure is what we feel in the instant shame strikes: our face burns hot, we blush, we lower our head or eyes, yearn to disappear, to escape all those watching eyes, to find cover. But we can never hide from ourselves, from those watching eyes *inside*, not entirely. (p. 17)

When shame is connected to one's sexuality, it creates a troubling bind. Either pursue what feels sexually and erotically fulfilling or avoid the painful feeling of shame. To avoid feeling shame, individuals hide from exposure and expend tremendous energy to prevent shameful characteristics from being seen by others and, ultimately from themselves. Shame defenses may effectively obstruct an affirming erotic identity, but they do not extinguish sexual or erotic desire. The erotic desires remain intact, but the shamed individual must contend with motivations to avoid experiencing shame that is coupled with those desires. Frequently, these conflicts feel out of control and solutions lead to difficulties with regulating sexual behavior and avoidant attachment strategies. These defenses allow individuals to remain conflicted about their erotic nature and they suffer negative health consequences from hiding the source of their deepest sexual pleasure (Williamson, 2000).

In OCSB assessment and treatment, sexual and erotic orientation maladjustment is a common profile for OCSB treatment-seeking men. Clients who express feeling sexually out of control may be describing distress about the content of their sexual fantasies and urges, or perhaps disappointment and fatigue for failing to change what arouses them. These clients have developed an adversarial relationship with their sexual and erotic orientations, which has created disharmony in their affective and deliberative system interaction. Frequently, the internal distress regarding persistent sexual and erotic thoughts that impinge on attachment and love is erroneously applied to criteria of a sexual addiction or compulsion. By treating this conflict as a disorder, the client and therapist unwittingly collude to maintain this psychological split rather than work toward a more reasonable process of change. Splitting is a shame defense in which sexual and erotic desire is psychologically separated from one's self-concept. In circumstances involving intense self-contempt, the coping strategies used to maintain a split are frequently destructive and can lead to a fracture of the self. This severing defense is more than denial; it is an action to permanently disconnect a shameful characteristic from the self (Kaufman & Raphael, 1996). In some circumstances, the client's investment in maintaining the split is extreme. Clients may want to extinguish their urges to pursue their sexual or erotic desires or stop feeling the pleasure of their unwanted turn-on or even disallow their erotic fantasies to be enlivened their sexual thoughts. These clients tend to be greatly disappointed when we explicitly communicate that erotic-ectomies are not performed in our psychotherapy offices (nor do we believe it is possible). As reparative therapies that attempt to change same-sex attractions are ineffective, unethical, and harmful, so are erotic orientation conversion therapies. Therefore, the goal is never to change to whom a client is attracted, what arouses the client, or to excise what he knows already turns him on. The goal is to facilitate positive identity development by fully integrating sexuality into one's self-concept.

2. Are the OCSB symptoms related to sexual or erotic conflicts that clients have with others?

Developing self-acceptance and maintaining romantic relationships may be complicated by the nature of one's erotic orientation. Imagine, during the course of a man's life, he discovers a secret pleasure for having his most intense, enjoyable, and reliable orgasms. An orgasm that electrifies his body leaves him exhausted and fulfilled at the same time. He learns that the sexual stimulus that led to his intense orgasm was something that other people find disgusting, revolting, or sinful. He fears that a current or future sexual partner will reject, dismiss, or abandon him if he reveals the secret to his highly pleasurable orgasms. He might project onto others his own judgments as a pervert, sinner, or unfit partner. What is a solution to this bind? Should he take the risk and disclose the details of his erotic orientation? Or, is it better to withhold this private pleasure while attempting to extinguish it from his nature? The answers to this conflict are not obvious, especially because some of his fears of rejection are rational. Many people seeking OCSB treatment are in the midst of such conflicts.

A common resolution to shame about erotic turn-ons within OCSB clients is to hide highly pleasurable erotic desires. The consequence for the secrecy is similar to an avoidant attachment style that prevents intimacy and perpetuates a distant attachment. OCSB clients often report a history of sly or indirect methods for gauging their partner's attitude or potential reaction to one of their peak erotic interests. They may accidently leave an image on the computer that shows a specific sex act or a highly arousing body part. The client waits for his partner to discover the image and, once discovered, the partner's immediate reaction becomes the data men use to evaluate their partner's short- and long-term attitude and openness to his erotic interest. Partners often have no idea they are the subject of this erotic compatibility research. The partner's facial expression, look of disgust, surprise, or admonition is generalized as an overarching repudiation of the client's entire erotic orientation. Clients often extrapolate from this one-time occurrence (which may have happened very early in the relationship) any future attempts to introduce this erotic turn-on. They avoid shame, rejection, and disgust by hibernating further in their hidden erotic den. Revulsion or fear about revealing erotic turn-ons to long-established or new sexual partners, no matter how common or unconventional, may indicate the existence of an unresolved erotic conflict. These clients may also have to manage the consequences of a double disclosure—crossing their sexual agreements along with revealing their hidden erotic interests. The shock of the discovery combined with the partner's judgmental reaction to the specific erotic interest may activate a flood of distressing emotions and thoughts.

The client, in a rush to save his relationship and fix his erotic conflict, may erroneously label these erotic interests a sexual compulsion or addiction. Clients who are in a rush to save their relationship may erroneously label these erotic interests a sexual compulsion or addiction for a few reasons. In our cultural landscape, the immediate narrative of "I have a sex addiction" offers a comforting medical road map with clearly defined treatment tasks. Second, the clinical focus on healing the interpersonal betrayal staves off the difficult work of erotic-identity development and conflict resolution. Partners, in turn, may feel comforted, vindicated, or absolved of their contribution to the cocreated relational dynamics that avoided erotic integration. The flight to "sex recovery" often masks the reality of a sexual turn-on that disinterests or disgusts either or both members of the couple. The partner may demand treatment specifically for sexual addiction as a condition for the couple to even consider remaining together with the assumption that the person will abstain from the erotic interest.

Not all OCSB treatment-seeking clients avoid the erotic conflict. Some men just have a specific or very narrow range for erotic arousal. They may feel shame or embarrassment about their limited range of sexual pleasure and avoid partnered sex by immersing themselves in solo sex, where they can easily find their erotic interests without the interpersonal negotiation or judgments. We find that the narrower a man's range of arousal, the lower the probability of finding a partner with a reciprocal turn-on. These individuals may also be highly likely to avoid partner disclosure and lack experience exploring the particular sexual pleasures of partnered sex. Reciprocal matches for any particular fixed or unconventional erotic template are not plentiful (Money, 1999).

Perel (2006) explores the consequences that exist within couples overburdened by unrealistic contemporary intimacy standards for long-term relationships. One standard she explores is the expectation that each member of the couple will be a lifelong source of emotional security and a source of sustained sexual passion. This 21st-century marital expectation to find security and passion with the same partner for a lifelong relationship is challenging for most couples. They frequently struggle with the tensions between the need for dependency and autonomy or security and freedom as well as familiarity and novelty (Perel, 2006). As couples move toward emotional security, they often collapse the space between the individual and the other, the very space in which eroticism thrives. Erotic desire requires recognizing the partner as an *other*, someone who is outside of oneself (Morin, 1995). "The breakdown of desire appears to be an unintentional consequence of the creation of intimacy" (Perel, 2006, p. 24).

In the theories of sexual and erotic development, Money (1999) and Morin (1995) propose that people find ways to preserve and express their erotic selves. If clients and their partners have not protected their sense of separateness in the relationship, their erotic expression may represent a reemergent self, but not in the manner one or both members of the couple expected or wanted. Sexual behaviors that violate relationship agreements or direct sexual energy away from a primary partner is a common hidden and unilateral solution to keeping the erotic self alive. This erotic solution successfully preserved their erotic selves but had the terrible relationship consequences that tend to prompt a referral to OCSB treatment.

3. Does the client exhibit fixed or unconventional arousal patterns?

Fixed Arousal

Forming a positive erotic identity may also involve coming to terms with a fixed arousal pattern. We think of a fixed arousal pattern as a sexual stimulus that is reliably arousing and necessary for achieving a satisfying or deeply pleasurable orgasm. We agree with Money's (1999) assessment that the degree of "fixedness" in a client's arousal pattern is relevant, but we do not use the term *paraphilia*. In our attempts to use sexual health terms that limit a moral judgment or tone, we discuss fixed turn-ons from the perspective of normalizing the diversity of sexual turn-ons and arousal patterns. The OCSB assessment process assists men in becoming sexually educated about fixated sexual turn-ons and then developing a realistic and sexologically informed sexual health plan for integrating these turn-ons into their overall sexual lives. (This is a primary reason OCSB treatment is only for men concerned about consensual urges, thoughts, and behaviors. The goal for men with fixated nonconsensual sexual arousal is not to integrate their turn-ons into their sexual lives because it violates the sexual rights of others.) To determine fixatedness, OCSB assessment explores how predictable, persistent, and reliable the stimulus is in generating sexual arousal, as well as the range of sexual stimuli that elicit satisfactory levels of sexual excitement. The more fixed and narrow a man's arousal pattern, the more complications he will likely experience forming a positive self-concept and reciprocal sexual or romantic relationship.

The prevailing assumption is that there is a critical period in young men's lives in which some connection is established between a stimulus and sexual response (Bancroft, 2009). Pfaus et al. (2012) corroborate this assumption in their social constructionist theory of sexual development: "at certain critical ages and during certain critical events … the sensory, cognitive, affective, and motoric aspects of sexuality become fundamentally integrated, organized by direct experiences of reward and pleasure" (p. 52). These critical events are milestones in sexual development ranging from first stirring of desire, first solo-sex experimentation and orgasm, first shared orgasm with another person (consensual or nonconsensual), first consensual partnered sexual relationship, and so on (Tolman & Diamond, 2014).

For some men, the sexual stimulus is so specific, preferred, and persistent they become more preoccupied with the presence of the sexual signal and less focused on the loved one with whom they are having sex (Bancroft, 2009). These fixed arousal patterns become troubling when they "weaken rather than strengthen the sexual bond with the sexual partner and, in its most extreme form, makes the sexual partner, as a person, virtually redundant in sexual terms" (Bancroft, 2009, p. 283). Brancroft (2009) describes three principal categories of sexual signals that can organize the range of fixed turn-ons: a specific body part; an object that is an extension of a body (clothing, etc.); or a specific texture, material, or other source of tactile stimulation.

Morin (1995) discusses erotic conflicts from a different perspective. When the balance between love and lust in partnered relationships is fused or in opposition, erotic conflicts emerge from the "twin beliefs that love is good and lust is bad" (Morin, 1995, p. 193). Morin identifies two common strategies of the erotic mind to deal with love–lust conflicts. One approach, termed love–lust fusion, seeks to purify or control lust by fusing it with love. Sensations that would be considered lustful are interpreted as loving or affectionate, infusing even casual sex with emotions and significant meaning. According to Morin, merging love with lust impairs sexual judgment and can contribute to loneliness when a sex partner does not share their affection. In the second strategy to manage love–lust conflicts, Morin describes a strategy used to protect "the purity of love by creating an invisible barrier between it and lust so that a person becomes unable to feel both at the same time or with the same person" (p. 193). This aptly named love–lust split detaches tenderness and affection from one's erotic attention and contributes to difficulties in maintaining long-term romantic and sexual relationships. This division between romantic affection and sexual arousal leads to hotter sexual excitement, but to the exclusion of the attachment and intimacy components of sexual relationships. Over time, the affection and love felt toward a partner eventually intrudes, reducing or ending the erotic charge with the partner. The unfortunate outcome of both of these love–lust split scenarios is that lust or erotic energy becomes a source of disgust that is incompatible with love (Morin, 1995). Commonly, the disgust or deep disappointment surrounding a love–lust conflict is mislabeled as an erectile dysfunction, ejaculatory control problem, low sexual desire, or a sexual addiction. The person feels out of control because he cannot force himself to lust after the loved one in the same way as experienced earlier in the relationship or that is idealized in society.

Unconventional Arousal

Not only do people struggle to integrate fixed erotic orientations into their erotic identities, they also experience difficulty integrating unconventional erotic pleasures into their dating, love, or partnered relationships.

We use the term "unconventional" to refer to an urge, thought, or behavior that does not conform to the trends characteristic of the vast majority of people (O'Sullivan & Thompson, 2014). Just as nonexclusively heterosexual men comprise a subgroup of sexual orientation minorities, men with unconventional erotic turn-ons, whether adventurously pleasurable or rigidly specific, are a subgroup whose erotic orientation may differ from sociocultural expectations. Unlike sexual minorities, there are few resources for men to collectively integrate unconventional erotic turn-ons. The Internet has expanded sexual options yet has not coalesced to create a social or cultural process for men to use to emerge from their hidden erotic conflicts. The full range of possible erotic interests is likely available on the web, which has allowed even the most unconventionally erotic interest to find an expression. It has also added yet another sexual activity that is promoted as Internet sex addiction (Perelman, 2014).

We include unconventional arousal along with fixed arousal because atypical, socially judged, and less common sexual interests are an additional source of vulnerability that contributes to sexual problems. Fixed arousal patterns are an internal process that generates difficulties because a specific sexual stimulus must be present in some manner to feel sexual arousal or achieve sexual pleasure. Consequently, partners may perceive the individual as emotionally distant when he shifts focus to an erotic object to reach orgasm. The concept of unconventionality is a broad range of sexual arousal patterns that conflict with sociocultural norms and personal sexual values. Clients who internalize sociocultural norms and are highly motivated to conform with socially approved sexual urges, thoughts, and behaviors may restrict their unconventional erotic turn-ons as a defense against shame or rejection. Here, as well as with the fixed turn-on, OCSB clients may historically avoid asking for what they want. They diverted themselves toward sexual activity that is free of partner rejection and attempted to preserve their erotic selves through watching specific online sexual imagery, hookups, or paid sex.

REFERENCES

Ainsworth, M. D. S., Blehar, M. C., Waters, E., & Wall, S. (1978). *Patterns of attachment: A psychological study of the stranger situation*. Hillsdale, NJ: Lawrence Erlbaum.

American Psychiatric Association. (2013). *Diagnostic and statistical manual of mental disorders* (5th ed.). Arlington, VA: American Psychiatric Publishing.

Ariely, D., & Loewenstein, G. (2006). The heat of the moment: The effect of sexual arousal on sexual decision making. *Journal of Behavioral Decision Making, 19*(2), 87–98.

Bader, M. J. (2002). *Arousal: The secret logic of sexual fantasies*. New York, NY: St. Martin's Press.

Bancroft, J. (2009). *Human sexuality and its problems* (3rd ed.). Edinburgh, UK: Churchill, Livingstone & Elsivier.

Bancroft, J. (2013). Sexual addiction. In P. M. Miller (Ed.), *Principles of addiction* (pp. 855–862). San Diego, CA: Academic Press.

Bancroft, J., & Vukadinovic, Z. (2004). Sexual addiction, sexual compulsivity, sexual impulsivity, or what? Toward a theoretical model. *Journal of Sex Research, 41*(3), 225–234.

Baumeister, R. F., Gailliot, M., DeWall, C N., & Oaten, M. (2006). Self-regulation and personality: How interventions increase regulatory success, and how depletion moderates the effects of traits on behavior. *Journal of Personality, 74,* 1773–1801.

Baumeister, R. F., & Heatherton, T. F. (1996). Self-regulation failure: An overview. *Psychological Inquiry, 7*(1), 1–15.

Baumeister, R. F., Heatherton, T. F., & Tice, D. M. (1994). *Losing control: How and why people fail at self-regulation.* New York, NY: Academic Press.

Baumeister, R., Schmeichel, B., & Vohs, K. (2007). Self-regulation and the executive function: The self as controlling agent. In A. W. Kruglanski & E. T. Higgins (Eds.), *Social psychology: Handbook of basic principles* (pp. 516–539). New York, NY: Guilford Press.

Baumeister, R. F., & Vohs, K. D. (2007). Self-regulation, ego depletion, and motivation. *Social and Personality Psychology Compass, 1*(1), 115–128.

Black, D. W., Kehrberg, L. L., Flumerfelt, D. L., & Schlosser, S. S. (1997). Characteristics of 36 subjects reporting compulsive sexual behavior. *American Journal of Psychiatry, 154*(2), 243–249.

Bowlby, J. (1969). *Attachment and loss: Vol. 1. Attachment.* New York, NY: Basic Books.

Bowlby, J. (1973). *Attachment and loss: Vol. 2. Separation: Anxiety and anger.* New York, NY: Basic Books.

Bowlby, J. (1980). *Attachment and loss: Vol. 3. Loss: Sadness and depression.* New York, NY: Basic Books.

Bravo, I. M., & White Lumpkin, P. (2010). The complex case of marital infidelity: An explanatory model of contributory processes to facilitate psychotherapy. *American Journal of Family Therapy, 38*(5), 421–432.

Brennan, K. A., Clark, C. L., & Shaver, P. R. (1998). Self-report measurement of adult attachment: An integrative overview. In J. A. Simpson & W. S. Rholes (Eds.), *Attachment theory and close relationships* (pp. 46–76). New York, NY: Guilford Press.

Campbell, W. K., Foster, C. A., & Finkel, E. J. (2002). Does self-love lead to love for others?: A story of narcissistic game playing. *Journal of Personality and Social Psychology, 83*(2), 340.

Carpenter, B., Reid, R., Garos, S., & Najavits, L. (2013). Personality comorbidity in treatment-seeking men with hypersexual disorder. *Sexual Addiction & Compulsivity, 20,* 79–90.

Carver, C. S., & Scheier, M. F. (1981). *Attention and self-regulation.* New York, NY: Springer-Verlag.

Coleman, E. (1986, July). Sexual compulsion vs. sexual addiction: The debate continues. *SIECUS Report,* pp. 7–11.

Corcoran, K. O. C., & Mallinckrodt, B. (2000). Adult attachment, self-efficacy, perspective taking, and conflict resolution. *Journal of Counseling & Development, 78*(4), 473–483.

Crocker, M. (2013). *Looking for attachment solutions in all the wrong places: Out of control sexual behavior as a symptom of insecure attachment in men* (Doctoral dissertation). University of Pennsylvania, School of Social Policy and Practice; Philadelphia, PA.

Davis, D., Shaver, P. R., & Vernon, M. L. (2004). Attachment style and subjective motivations for sex. *Personality and Social Psychology Bullet, 39*, 1076–1090.

Davis, D., Shaver, P. R., Widaman, K. F., Vernon, M. L., Follette, W. C., & Beitz, K. (2006). "I can't get no satisfaction": Insecure attachment, inhibited sexual communication, and sexual dissatisfaction. *Personal Relationships, 13*(4), 465–483.

DeWall, C. N., Lambert, N. M., Slotter, E. B., Pond R. S., Jr., Deckman, T., Finkel, E. J., ... & Fincham, F. D. (2011). So far away from one's partner, yet so close to romantic alternatives: Avoidant attachment, interest in alternatives, and infidelity. *Journal of Personality and Social Psychology, 101*(6), 1302.

Dewitte, M. (2012). Different perspectives on the sex-attachment link: Towards an emotion-motivational account. *Journal of Sex Research, 49*(2–3), 105–124.

Diamond, L. (2013). Concepts of female sexual orientation. In C. J. Patterson & A. R. D'Augelli (Eds.), *Handbook of psychology and sexual orientation* (pp. 3–17). New York, NY: Oxford University Press.

Diamond, L. (2014). Gender and same-sex sexuality. In D. Tolman, L. Diamond, J. Bauermeister, W. George, J. Pfaus, & M. Ward (Eds.), *APA handbook of sexuality and psychology: Vol. 1. Person-based approaches* (pp. 629–652). Washington, DC: American Psychological Association.

Drigotas, S. M., Safstrom, C. A., & Gentilia, T. (1999). An investment model prediction of dating infidelity. *Journal of Personality and Social Psychology, 77*(3), 509.

Easton, D., & Liszt, K. (1997). *The ethical slut: A guide to infinite sexual possibilities.* Gardena, CA: Greenery Press.

Feeney, B. C., & Collins, N. L. (2001). Predictors of caregiving in adult intimate relationships: An attachment theoretical perspective. *Journal of Personality and Social Psychology, 80*(6), 972.

Fisher, H. (2004). *Why we love: The nature and chemistry of romantic love.* New York, NY: Owl Books.

Foster, J. D., Shrira, I., & Campbell, W. K. (2006). Theoretical models of narcissism, sexuality, and relationship commitment. *Journal of Social and Personal Relationships, 23*(3), 367–386.

Fraley, R. C., Heffernan, M. E., Vicary, A. M., & Brumbaugh, C. C. (2011). The experiences in close relationships—Relationship structures questionnaire: A method for assessing attachment orientations across relationships. *Psychological Assessment, 23*(3), 615.

Gailliot, M. T., Baumeister, R. F., DeWall, C. N., Maner, J. K., Plant, E. A., Tice, D. M., ... & Schmeichel, B. J. (2007). Self-control relies on glucose as a limited energy source: Willpower is more than a metaphor. *Journal of Personality and Social Psychology, 92*(2), 325.

Gask, L., Evans, M., & Kessler, D. (2013). Personality disorder. *British Medical Journal, 347*, f 5276.

Greenspan, S., & Greenspan, N. (1985). *First feelings: Milestones in the emotional development of your baby and child.* New York, NY: Penguin.

Hazan, C., & Shaver, P. (1987). Romantic love conceptualized as an attachment process. *Journal of Personality and Social Psychology, 52*(3), 511.

Hurlbert, D. F., Apt, C., Gasar, S., Wilson, N. E., & Murphy, Y. (1994). Sexual narcissism: A validation study. *Journal of Sex & Marital Therapy*, 20(1), 24–34.

Janssen, E., & Bancroft, J. (2007). The dual control model: The role of sexual inhibition & excitation in sexual arousal and behavior. In E. Janssen (Ed), *The psychophysiology of sex*. Bloomington, IN: Indiana University Press.

Joireman, J. A., Needham, T. L., & Cummings, A. L. (2002). Relationships between dimensions of attachment and empathy. *North American Journal of Psychology*, 3, 63–80.

Jones, D. N., & Weiser, D. A. (2014). Differential infidelity patterns among the Dark Triad. *Personality and Individual Differences*, 57, 20–24.

Katz-Wise, S., & Hyde, J. (2014). Sexuality and gender: The interplay. In D. Tolman, L. Diamond, J. Bauermeister, W. George, J. Pfaus, & M. Ward (Eds.), *APA handbook of sexuality and psychology: Vol. 1. Person-based approaches* (pp. 29–62). Washington, DC: American Psychological Association.

Kaufman, G., & Raphael, L. (1996). *Coming out of shame: Transforming gay and lesbian lives* (p. 7). New York, NY: Doubleday.

Kinsey, A. C., Pomeroy, W. B., & Martin, C. E. (1948). *Sexual behavior in the human male*. Philadelphia, PA: W.B. Saunders.

Krueger, R. F. (2005). Continuity of axes I and II: Toward a unified model of personality, personality disorders, and clinical disorders. *Journal of Personality Disorders*, 19(3), 233.

Lloyd, M., Raymond, N. C., Miner, M. H., & Coleman, E. (2007). Borderline personality traits in individuals with compulsive sexual behavior. *Sexual Addiction & Compulsivity*, 14(3), 187–206.

Loewenstein, G., & O'Donoghue, T. (2007). The heat of the moment: Modeling interactions between affect and deliberation. *Unpublished manuscript*. Retrieved from https://odonoghue.economics.cornell.edu/heat.pdf

McGonigal, K. (2011). *The willpower instinct: How self-control works, why it matters, and what you can do to get more of it*. New York, NY: Penguin.

McNulty, J. K., & Widman, L. (2013). The implications of sexual narcissism for sexual and marital satisfaction. *Archives of Sexual Behavior*, 42, 1021–1032.

McNulty, J. K., & Widman, L. (2014). Sexual narcissism and infidelity in early marriage. *Archives of Sexual Behavior*, 43, 1315–1325.

Mikulincer, M., & Shaver, P. R. (2007). Boosting attachment security to promote mental health, prosocial values, and inter-group tolerance. *Psychological Inquiry*, 18(3), 139–156.

Mikulincer, M., & Shaver, P. R. (2010). Attachment in adulthood; Structure, dynamics, and change. New York, NY: Guilford Press.

Miller, W. R., & Rollnick, S. (2002). *Motivational interviewing: Preparing people for change*. New York, NY: Guilford Press.

Moller, N. P., & Vossler, A. (2015). Defining infidelity in research and couple counseling: A qualitative study. *Journal of Sex & Marital Therapy*, 41(5), 487–497. doi:10.1080/0092623X.2014.931314

Money, J. (1988). *Gay, straight, and in-between: The sexology of erotic orientation*. Oxford, UK: Oxford University Press.

Money, J. (1999). *Principles of developmental sexology*. New York, NY: Continuum.

Morin, J. (1995). *The erotic mind: Unlocking the inner sources of sexual passion and fulfillment*. New York, NY: HarperCollins Publishers.

Muraven, M. (2010). Builidng self-control strengthen: Practicing self-control leads to improved self-control performance. *Journal of Experimental Social Psychology, 46,* 465–468.

Muraven, M., Baumeister, R. F., & Tice, D. M. (1999). Longitudinal improvement of self-regulation through practice: Building self-control strengthen through repeated exercise. *Journal of Social Psychology, 139,* 446–457.

Muraven, M. R., & Baumeister, R. F. (2000). Self-regulation and depletion of limited resources: Does self-control resemble a muscle? *Psychological Bulletin, 126,* 247–259.

O'Sullivan, L., & Thompson, A. (2014). Sexuality in adolescene. In D. Tolman, L. Diamond, J. Bauermeister, W. George, J. Pfaus, & M. Ward (Eds.), *APA handbook of sexuality and psychology: Vol. 1. Person-based approaches* (pp. 433–486). Washington, DC: American Psychological Association.

Péloquin, K., Brassard, A., Lafontaine, M. F., & Shaver, P. R. (2013). Sexuality examined through the lens of attachment theory: Attachment, caregiving, and sexual satisfaction. *Journal of Sex Research, 51,* 561–567.

Perel, E. (2006). *Mating in captivity: Unlocking erotic intelligence.* New York, NY: Harper.

Perelman, M. (2014). The history of sexual medicine. In D. Tolman, L. Diamond, J. Bauermeister, W. George, J. Pfaus, & M. Ward (Eds.), *APA handbook of sexuality and psychology: Vol. 2. Contextual approaches* (pp. 137–179). Washington, DC: American Psychological Association.

Pfaus, J. G., Kippin, T. E., Coria-Avila, G. A., Gelez, H., Afonso, V. M., Ismail, N., & Parada, M. (2012). Who, what, where, when (and maybe even why)? How the experience of sexual reward connects sexual desire, preference, and performance. *Archives of Sexual Behavior, 41*(1), 31–62.

Prochaska, J. O., & DiClemente, C. C. (2005). The transtheoretical approach. *Handbook of Psychotherapy Integration, 2,* 147–171.

Raymond, N. C., Coleman, E., & Miner, M. H. (2003). Psychiatric comorbidity and compulsive/impulsive traits in compulsive sexual behavior. *Comprehensive Psychiatry, 44*(5), 370–380.

Reid, R. C., & Carpenter, B. N. (2009). Exploring relationships of psychopathology in hypersexual patients using the MMPI-2. *Journal of Sex & Marital Therapy, 35*(4), 294–310.

Savin-Williams, R. C., & Ream, G. (2007). Prevalence and stability of sexual orientation components during adolescence and young adulthood. *Archives of Sexual Behavior, 36,* 385–394.

Schachner, D. A., & Shaver, P. R. (2004). Attachment dimensions and sexual motives. *Personal Relationships, 11,* 179–195.

Shore, A. (2003). *Affect regulation and the repair of the self.* New York, NY: W. W. Norton.

Siegel, D. J. (2011). *Mindsight: The new science of personal transformation.* New York , NY: Bantam Books.

Storms, M. D. (1979). Sexual orientation and self-perception. In P. Pliner, K. Blankstein, & I. Spiger (Eds.), *Perception of emotion in self and others* (pp. 165–180). New York, NY: Plenum.

Storms, M. D. (1980). Theories of sexual orientation. *Journal of Personality and Social Psychology, 38*(5), 783.

Storms, M. D. (1981). A theory of erotic orientation development. *Psychological Review, 88*(4), 340.

Tolman, D., & Diamond, L. (2014). Sexuality theory. In D. Tolman, L. Diamond, J. Bauermeister, W. George, J. Pfaus, & M. Ward (Eds.), *APA handbook of sexuality and psychology: Vol. 1. Person-based approaches* (pp. 3–27). Washington, DC: American Psychological Association.

Trusty, J., Ng, K. M., & Watts, R. E. (2005). Model of effects of adult attachment on emotional empathy of counseling students. *Journal of Counseling & Development, 83*(1), 66–77.

Vohs, K. D., & Heatherton, T. F. (2000). Self-regulatory failure: A resource-depletion approach. *Psychological Science, 11*, 249–254.

Wagner, D. D., Heatherton, T. F., & Todd, F. (2015). Self-regulation and its failure: The seven deadly threats to self-regulation. In M. Mikulincer, P. R. Shaver, E. Borgida, & J. A. Bargh (Eds.), *APA handbook of personality and social psychology, Vol. 1: Attitudes and social cognition* (pp. 805–845). Washington, DC: American Psychological Association.

Widiger, T. A., Simonsen, E., Krueger, R., Livesley, W. J., & Verheul, R. (2005). Personality disorder research agenda for the DSM–V. *Journal of Personality Disorders, 19*(3), 315.

Widman, L., & McNulty, J. K. (2010). Sexual narcissism and the perpetration of sexual aggression. *Archives of Sexual Behavior, 39*(4), 926–939.

Williamson, I. R. (2000). Internalized homophobia and health issues affecting lesbians and gay men. *Health Education Research, 15*(1), 97–107.

Wood, W., & Neal, D. T. (2007). A new look at habits and the habit–goal interface. *Psychological Review, 114*, 843–863.

Wryobeck, J. M., & Wiederman, M. W. (1999). Sexual narcissism: Measurement and correlates among college men. *Journal of Sex & Marital Therapy, 25*(4), 321–331.

OUT OF CONTROL SEXUAL BEHAVIOR ASSESSMENT

CHAPTER FIVE

SCREENING PROCEDURE

In this section, we describe how the dual-process model of human behavior (Loewenstein & O'Donoghue, 2007) and sexual health principles are operationalized within our clinical protocol. We call this operation the OCSB (Out of Control Sexual Behavior) Clinical Pathway. This pathway is a multistep process used to guide providers of OCSB assessment and treatment. The next four chapters describe each step in the pathway prior to offering OCSB individual and group therapy. The OCSB Clinical Pathway begins with an initial phone call, a screening appointment, followed by assessment, and then treatment preparation. Section 3 completes the pathway discussion and reviews OCSB group and individual psychotherapy practices, as well as the specific treatment intervention case examples for Jay, Hector, Frank, Peter, Will, and Anthony. In this section, we first look at the big picture of the Out of Control Sexual Behavior Model and introduce the OCSB Clinical Pathway. We describe each element of the treatment-preparation protocol and the therapist's clinical work for preparing men to change their sexual behavior.

OCSB CLINICAL PATHWAY

The OCSB Clinical Pathway is a sexual health-based outpatient clinical assessment and psychotherapy treatment protocol for men experiencing problematic or OCSB (Figure 5.1). The OCSB Screening Procedure is the first component of the multistage OCSB Clinical Pathway. It is an initial consultation appointment to determine whether to recommend an OCSB assessment. (This can be done with an OCSB professional or a non-OCSB specialist.) The screening procedure combines OCSB clinical

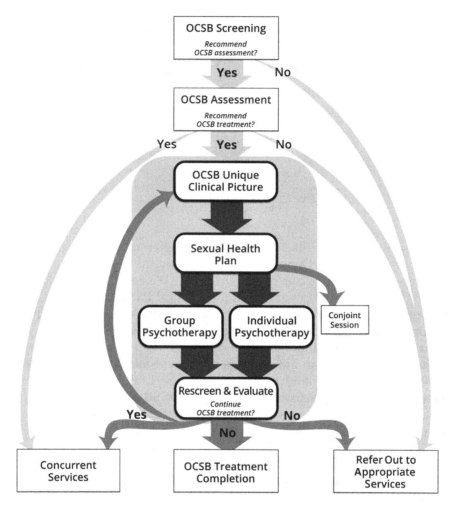

Figure 5.1 *The OCSB Clinical Pathway.*

distinctions and vulnerability factors to guide therapists' opinions about suggesting further assessment. The OCSB assessment gather's information about each man's competing motivations in the three clinical areas while engaging in motivation-enhancement processes for sexual health. The goal of the assessment is to establish a man's Unique Clinical Picture and determine whether to recommend combined individual and group OCSB treatment. The last OCSB assessment component establishes a sexual health plan and clarifies each client's vision of sexual health, which shapes the overall direction of OCSB treatment.

The Out of Control Sexual Behavior Model

The OCSB Model is based on the dual-process model of human behavior (Loewenstein & O'Donoghue, 2007). Figure 5.1 visually depicts how competing motivations contribute to dysregulated sexual behavior by influencing the affective–deliberative interaction. We identify three clinical areas (self-regulation, attachment patterns, and sexual/erotic conflicts) and examine how competing motivations within each of these areas can imbalance the affective–deliberative relationship leading to men feeling that their sexual behavior is out of control. The *competing motivations* box encircles the affective and deliberative systems to illustrate the central influence of these clinical areas on the affective–deliberative balance. The OCSB assessment is intended to identify and clarify how each of the four vulnerability factors influences a man's affective–deliberative interaction. Any combination of the vulnerability factors can induce imbalances that men experience as being out of control. OCSB treatment is based in the hypothesis that recalibrating a man's affective–deliberative interaction will improve his sexual health and reduce his out of control sexual experiences. Figure 5.2 illustrates the OCSB Model.

The OCSB screening criteria encircles the competing motivations and affective–deliberative systems. This schematically illustrates the screening criteria hierarchy as a treatment priority over the three OCSB clinical areas. The criteria are the treatment priority because of the significant negative impact on establishing the affective–deliberative balance necessary for overall wellness and improving sexual health.

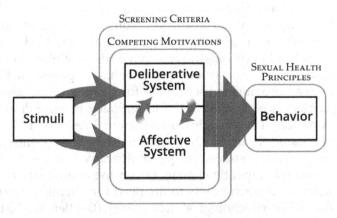

Figure 5.2 *The OCSB Model.*

The OCSB Model identifies six screening criteria that are assessed for each client. Two of the screening criteria are *motivation for change* and *sexual consent*. We label these criteria as clinical distinctions because of their role in ruling out further consideration for OCSB assessment or treatment. We call the remaining four screening criteria (i.e., *physical safety, physical health, mental health, relationship with drugs/alcohol*) OCSB vulnerability factors. All six screening criteria are clinically monitored throughout treatment because of their disruptive influence on the affective–deliberative interaction. Specifically, these vulnerability factors, left unaddressed, generate numerous behavioral and sexual health consequences. The initial OCSB screening interview identifies potential sources of imbalance and assists with generating preliminary plans for addressing men's physical safety, mental health, physical health, or his relationship with drugs or alcohol. The *Screening Criteria* box surrounds both the affective–deliberative interaction and the competing motivations to schematically convey their significance in the triaging of OCSB assessment and treatment (Figure 5.2).

A Psychotherapy Integration Model

Wolfe (2001) describes psychotherapy integration as a process of moving toward increasing assimilation and integration between a therapist's "home orientation" and "foreign techniques." "Different theories focus on different phenomena, which means that the existing specific theories of therapy leave out important phenomena regarding the nature of psychopathology and its modification" (Wolfe, 2001, p. 125). A pathway model is a useful approach for integrating both familiar and new OCSB psychotherapy practices that address a range of psychopathology as well as sexual behavior that has negative consequences. The pathway was designed to integrate a range of psychotherapy techniques and processes to address the diverse combination of factors that contribute to OCSB. Until such time that sexual and psychological research leads to etiological and diagnostic agreement about consensual sexual behavior problems, the OCSB Clinical Pathway provides a useful map for treating OCSB as a human behavior problem (see Bancroft, 2013; Steele, Staley, Fong, & Prause, 2013).

The American Psychological Association Presidential Task Force on Evidence-Based Practice (2006) strongly endorsed integrating a range of empirically established psychotherapy components associated with psychotherapeutic change. Given the complexity of change, current empirical research points to the need for scientific practitioners to focus on many psychological treatments (Beutler & Castonguay, 2006). The APA Task Force concluded that integration of independently established factors of change (client characteristics, therapy techniques, and clinical relationship) was most strongly associated with psychotherapy that leads to client change (Beutler & Castonguay, 2006). In other words, effective psychotherapy considers client characteristics, clinical technique, and the therapeutic alliance as essential elements of change rather than focusing on one empirically established factor as the primary mechanism of change.

Integrative psychotherapy models encourage flexible clinical approaches to address mental health and behavioral issues related to the client's intra- and interpersonal experiences. OCSB treatment relies on evidence-informed practices when providing treatment for the many ways OCSB can mask, mimic, or exacerbate the symptoms of another condition. OCSB assessment and treatment assimilates a range of empirically validated psychotherapy practices that correspond to the client's Unique Clinical Picture—a multidimensional understanding of the client that informs treatment decisions (adapted from unique client picture by Chadwick Center for Children and Families, 2009). OCSB treatment planning is incomplete without a comprehensive approach for clinically addressing each man's multiple clinical factors.

Change Processes

The primary objectives of the OCSB Screening Procedure and Assessment Plan (e.g., administering validated surveys, clinical interview, monitoring of behavior) are to identify men's motivations for change and facilitate the readiness process. The stages of readiness for change are imbedded within the OCSB Clinical Pathway. The transtheoretical model of health behavior change (TTM) is an integrative framework that encompasses a series of stages people repeatedly and incrementally pass through as they change (DiClemente & Prochaska, 1998). Change relies on sustained motivational energy. Like all energy supplies, it wanes and needs to be replenished. Expending a lot of energy for a difficult decision leaves little in the energy tank, hampering one's ability to maintain intentions for change. Sexual health behavior change is no different. It is rarely achieved through one-time expenditures of energy via catharsis or a moment of profound insight. Changing sexual behavior is more often a gradual upending of distorted beliefs, interpersonal relationship patterns, and developing new ways of relating to one's sensual and sexual desires. Change requires effort and no effort can be implemented without energy (DiClemente & Velasquez, 2002).

The primary objectives of the OCSB Screening Procedure and Assessment Plan (e.g., administering validated surveys, clinical interview, monitoring of behavior) are to identify men's motivations for change and facilitate the readiness process. The OCSB Screening Procedure and OCSB Assessment Plan are not merely information-gathering processes. OCSB screening and assessment integrate elements of treatment designed to enhance client motivation for sexual health change. Prochaska, Norcross, and DiClemente (1994) identify nine processes of health behavior change. Each process is applied during different stages of client readiness for change: consciousness-raising, social liberation, emotional arousal, self-reevaluation, commitment, countering, environmental control, reward, and helping relationships. Clients initiating therapy with an OCSB specialist are likely at the precontemplative or contemplative stages of change and the OCSB Assessment Plan integrates change strategies that research suggests are well matched with these early stages. Precontemplative and contemplative change strategies are consciousness-raising, emotional arousal, self-reevaluation, and social liberation (Prochaska et al., 1994).

OCSB Screening Procedure

The OCSB Screening Procedure closely examines six criteria that either rule out an OCSB assessment or identify factors for immediate clinical intervention. We separate the six screening criteria into two *clinical distinctions* that determine the appropriateness of OCSB treatment and four *vulnerability factors* that may mask, mimic, or exacerbate sexual problems. The clinical distinctions are client motivation and sexual consent. The remaining four vulnerability factors are commonly assessed in psychotherapy and are inextricably linked with human sexuality and biopsychosocial systems. These four factors—physical safety, physical health, mental health, and drug and alcohol use—will be familiar with most mental health professionals. OCSB treatment-seeking men are unlikely to change their sexual health behavior if one or more of the screening criteria remain unexplored or problematic. The screening explores these distinct and interconnected factors, which then determines the next step of the OCSB Pathway (Figure 5.3 illustrates the OCSB Screening Procedure).

Screening Ethics

In Chapter 2, we discuss the OCSB therapist's responsibilities to uphold the "freedom from/freedom to" ethical standard when providing sexual health-based psychotherapy. As a reminder, men have a right to be free from the sexual constraints imposed by interventions based on an unsubstantiated or inaccurate sexual-disorder diagnosis. This sexual right is

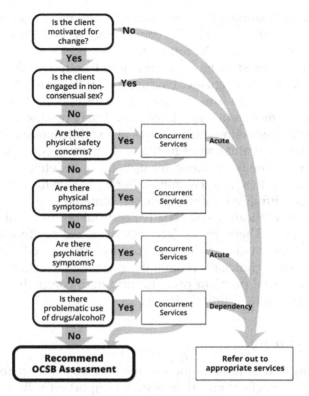

Figure 5.3 *OCSB Screening Procedure.*

honored alongside the client's right to personal sexual expression. The OCSB Screening Criteria provide a tool to relationally investigate client's sexual behavior concerns without utilizing labeling language. "What aspects of your sexual behavior concern you the most?" "What are you feeling as you are being so open and honest with me about your sexual activities?" What events led up to your decision to call a specialist in OCSB?" The client motivation criterion is best implemented by avoiding language that infers a clinical conclusion but rather explores the labels clients use to describe their behavior. Slowing the clinical conversation down and moving away from conclusory labels prevents premature characterization of the individual clinical picture.

In the screening interview, men may label their sexual behavior a sexual addiction or sexual compulsivity. Others may speak metaphorically, referring to their sexual behavior as "a drug." The client may be colloquially familiar with conclusory language and appear familiar with using these similes throughout the screening interview. Therapists may also adopt the client's language. "When did you first think you needed help for your sex addiction?" "How did your partner respond to your compulsive sexual behavior when he found out you paid for sex?" The motives for this dialogue need to be counterbalanced with avoiding premature evaluative diagnostic language. Finding a way to mirror, build rapport, and demonstrate active listening are important therapy tools when first establishing the therapeutic relationship and may need to be adjusted to avoid implicitly endorsing the diagnosis of an addiction or compulsion.

Focusing on evaluation of health and wellness issues in the OCSB Screening Procedure is a method for upholding the ethical obligation to protect client liberties. The screening criteria protects the client and therapist from unwittingly reinforcing an act-centered sexual value system as well as from replicating sex-negative cultural norms within the OCSB clinical interview. Therapist anxiety, lack of sexual health education, or low self-confidence with leading and guiding client sexual health conversations increases a clinician's premature movement to action that focuses on naming a sexual problem prior to forming a comprehensive understanding of the client's clinical picture.

Fostering Curiosity

The screening criteria are designed to quickly create a space for empathic curiosity between client and therapist. An important task for the therapist is to consistently implement empathic communication (Staemmler, 2012). Empathic communication "is a professional *act* and because of this, it can be undertaken or not, just as it can also succeed or fail" (p. 69). Commitment to the screening criteria process decreases both a rush to judgment by client and therapist and provides a consistent container for therapist empathic responses to client distress. When a client is highly distressed, having the screening criteria as a map for the initial interview may provide a source of confidence for the therapist. The OCSB screening interview structure helps decrease the threat of therapist countertransferential reactions from infecting the therapeutic space and limiting deeper, nuanced discussions (see Staemmler, 2012).

Miller and Rollnick (2013) consider the rush to issue diagnostic labels as indicative of a counselor asserting his or her expertise, which is similar to a family member conveying judgment, disapproval, or discomfort. This rush to judgment confines client and therapist to an expectation that one person in the clinical relationship will provide the right answers. Studies in motivating change identify this pattern as a hindrance to forming an active collaboration (Miller & Rollnick, 2013). The OCSB Screening

Process shelters the initial client–therapist space from a hasty movement to providing treatment based on the client's perceived emergency. The emergency situation to enter treatment may be motivated by a spouse's discovery of secretive and hurtful sexual behavior. The screening criteria vulnerability factors determine the level of care and prevent the clinical assessment from overly focusing on the client's immediate fear and shame. Applying the screening criteria protects against unsubstantiated conclusions by encouraging a sufficient level of curiosity and meaningful client dialogue before moving to any specific course of action.

The Consultation

Some therapists may choose to learn the screening and assessment protocol and only refer clients for OCSB treatment if their assessment indicates that the client may need that specialized care. If that is the case, the screening criteria are a useful checklist to apply whenever a client discloses his concerns about sexual behavior problems or dysregulation. Other professionals may be invested in adapting some of the OCSB Model into their current clinical work with OCSB. In this section, we shift the focus to our OCSB Screening Process and therapists who specialize in working with sexual behavior problems. In this circumstance, the initial screening determines whether an OCSB assessment is indicated and is agreed to by the client. Scheduling this one-time appointment is neither an agreement to enter therapy, nor does it include any commitment to change. It is a 50-minute confidential conversation for OCSB treatment-seeking men to discuss their sexual health concerns. Like all first appointments with a psychotherapist, counselors are also encouraged to observe their relational experience to determine whether they are a good fit for the prospective client.

Client Methods of First Contact

"I found you online." "My friends therapist suggested you." "Someone in AA said to call." OCSB specialists are familiar with e-mails, voicemails, text messages, or even men walking into the waiting room to schedule an appointment. When first talking about their sexual situations men will commonly say phrase like "sex addiction" or "compulsive sexual behavior." The content of the client's initial voicemail may indicate his familiarity with talking about sexual behavior. "Things just got out of hand, I need to finally treat this addiction." "I want to get into your group for sex addicts." "My therapist said I might have compulsive sexual behavior and that I needed to call you."

The therapist response to the client's initial inquiry sets the frame for the screening interview. The therapist explains that the initial screening appointment is not a conjoint session with their intimate partners, friends, or family members. The screening appointment is scheduled directly between the therapist and the prospective client. We have had intimate partners, parents, and administrative assistants try to schedule a screening appointment. Requests by a third party to schedule the OCSB screening appointment are declined. The OCSB approach places a high value on direct conversation between client and therapist to assess client motivation and begin the process of establishing a collaborative relationship for planning treatment.

E-mail requests

Given the pervasiveness of e-mail and text communication, we provide a few comments about how we handle e-mail or text requests to schedule an appointment. It is best to keep the electronic message brief given that there is not an established relationship with the potential client. After thanking the sender for the inquiry, we request the client schedule a phone call. That is the extent of the message. Because of confidentiality risks, no comment on what the e-mail said about the circumstances is mentioned in the return e-mail. Both Michael and Doug's e-mail addresses do not identify a psychotherapy specialization in OCSB (e.g., no e-mail addresses like @OCSBhelp.com or @sexadditiontherapy.com). To emphasize the relational aspect of OCSB treatment and to protect his health information, we schedule the OCSB screening appointment by directly speaking with the client over the phone.

Initial phone call

The focus of the phone conversation is to schedule an OCSB screening or referral. It is not a time to screen clinical content. Callers often find it reassuring to know there is a clear, step-by-step screening process before any commitment to an OCSB assessment or therapy. The only decision is whether to schedule a screening appointment. Some callers may be looking for or need nonconsensual sexual behavior treatment. Given that OCSB treatment is limited to consensual sexual behavior problems, listening on the phone for vague references to lawyers or court proceedings are cues for screening for this clinical distinction. Men usually appreciate the clarity of the OCSB treatment parameters even if the circumstance requires a referral to another professional.

OCSB SCREENING CRITERIA—CLINICAL DISTINCTIONS

The OCSB screening appointment determines whether an OCSB assessment is warranted and, if so, when to begin the process. After discussing confidentiality, the screening procedure focuses on the six screening criteria, building rapport, and coming to a decision regarding recommending an OCSB assessment.

Clinical Distinction: Motivation for Change

What is the client's motivation for change?

A common voicemail message received in our office sounds like: "Hello, my name is Kurt. I found your website and wanted to see whether we can schedule an appointment." Something motivated Kurt to go online, search for a variation of "sex addiction therapy" and make a phone call. Motivation is a subjective force that moves people toward action. Understanding motivation in the context of seeking OCSB treatment focuses the therapist and client to empathically examine what is driving clients toward change. If men had their way, they would likely not be talking with a health care professional about their embarrassing or frightening sexual dilemmas. Frank was motivated to talk about his workplace online sexual behavior with his psychiatrist, Beth, because he was scared. Frank's fear came from the self-discrepancy between what he was doing and how his behavior contradicted with his broader life goals. Seeing this contradiction activated enough distress to motivate him to reach out for help. The status quo now was disrupted because of the negative sexual consequences. "Scandinavians have a word for this for which there is no direct equivalent term in English: *lagom* in Swedish. It means just so, the right balance, just enough" (Miller & Rollnick, 2013, p. 244).

Does Frank see himself in conflict with the principles of sexual health? Probably not. Imagine men calling for help because their sexual behavior is out of alignment with sexual health standards. That would mean he had somehow internalized sexual health principles from external sources (e.g., society, schools, medical professionals), had the self-awareness to recognize that his behavior crossed these fundamental lines, and experienced *lagom* in his motivation to change his sexual behavior. This ideal is highly improbable with today's cultural lens of addictive sex.

Men will likely arrive at the screening appointment with a mental picture of their sexual problem. This client's pathology language is too narrow of a focus for an OCSB screening. Rather than structuring the first appointment solely on why clients think they cannot stop a specific sexual behavior, we want to know what they want to achieve. At some point in the screening, we ask a form of this question: "What is your vision for sexual health?" It is a variation of the solution-focused technique referred to as the "miracle question" (De Shazer & Dolan, 2012) that uncovers the client's goals for changing sexual behavior. If a man woke up tomorrow and everything in his life was the way he wanted it, how would his sexual behavior look? Constructive behavior change arises from connecting the behavior with something of intrinsic value, something cherished (Miller & Rollnick, 2002).

In his early OCSB treatment work, Michael learned an important lesson in client motivation. Jeremy, a self-diagnosed "sex addict," reported numerous extrarelational sexual encounters with women during the course of his 20-year marriage. A White, heterosexual-identified father of four, his wife recently discovered one of his many extramarital relationships. She confronted him and asked whether there were other affairs. His wife demanded Jeremy seek treatment after he revealed more, but not all, of his sexual behavior with other partners. In the screening appointment with Michael, Jeremy's wife's expectation that he seek treatment was unmistakably clear. However, Michael was more focused on Jeremy's motivation. As he listened to Jeremy say over and over how much he wanted to save his marriage, Michael assumed that Jeremy was conflicted about not being a good husband. Michael soon learned that actually Jeremy was more conflicted about who he was as a father. "When my children are older and they ask me if it is okay to cheat on their spouses, I want to be able to look them in the eye and say 'no' without hesitation or hypocrisy." Michael's reaction was a mixture of tenderness for Jeremy's parenting motivation and disappointment with his unmentioned motivation for being a good husband. Michael thought to himself, "What about his wife?" Jeremy did not keep his sexual agreements with his wife for 20 years. Did he love her? Jeremy did not seem to have an attachment-related fear about losing his wife. Jeremy's motivation, what he cherished, resided within a future image as a credible proponent of fidelity. This did not align with Michael's unconscious wish for Jeremy to be the remorseful husband. Michael felt disappointment and regulated his countertransference to maintain his focus on Jeremy's actual motivation for change. Michael's ability to suspend his judgment dissipated his countertransference and made space to empathize with his client's stated self-discrepancy. Establishing the client's motivation preserved the OCSB screening framework and Jeremy's decision to consider an OCSB assessment. Therapists risk activating precontemplative defenses if they attempt to develop a self-discrepancy that is not there.

Client internal discrepancies are the most enduring motivations that activate the change process (Miller & Rollnick, 2002). The intention of the OCSB screening is to verbalize self-discrepancy to spell out a man's current motivation for change. The OCSB Screening Procedure invites men to identify, label, and express the internal conflicts connected to their sexual urges, thoughts, and behaviors. The self-discrepancy provides energy for motivating sexual behavior change. "People are often more persuaded by what they hear themselves say than by what other people tell them" (Miller & Rollnick, 2002, p. 39).

Managing Psychological Reactance

Jay was in deep distress during the first moments of his couple therapy session. Jay's anguish and shame might have been interrupted had David interpreted his feelings as an indication of Jay's readiness to change his sexual behavior. After all, Jay was adamant about stopping his online sexual activity and delete all his explicit sexual video. In this moment, he sounded determined to change.

Jay did not delete all of his files because he was ready to change his sexual behavior. His actions stemmed more from wanting to quell a terrifying threat (losing his marriage) and relieving his guilt about his secret online sexual life. Jay's intense fear and insecurity were more likely his motivation to suddenly declare an end to his online sexual behavior. A stages-of-readiness perspective would predict a loss of motivation to restrict his sexual urges once Jay's immediate alarm and uncertainty lessens. In this moment of crisis, Jay intended to preserve his marriage before he had balanced this reactive decision with a clear understanding of the value he places on his now prohibited sexual activity. What will Jay do when his sexual desires return? What happens when his sexual excitation no longer has these temporary inhibitions?

Identifying client stage of readiness for change and one's sexual behavior self-discrepancies is a benchmark of OCSB screening and assessment. The OCSB assessment offers a methodical approach to investigate the benefits and costs of current and past sexual behavior. This process allows clients to formulate how and why they are motivated to improve their sexual health. The OCSB assessment process emphasizes men's subjective freedom to choose how they sexually behave once their behavior is more aligned within the sexual health principles.

How do people react when external factors destabilize this balance between sexual behavioral freedom and responsibility to sexual principles? Brehm (1966) developed a theory of "psychological reactance" to describe the aversive reactions that are set in motion when freedom and autonomy are threatened or reduced. According to Brehm, the emotional state ignited by a perceived diminution in freedom elicits behavior directed toward restoring the important lost freedoms. The affective motivation found within psychological reactance has direct relevance to understanding a client's diminished motivation for upholding restrictive sexual agreements.

Treatment methods that emphasize restricting aspects of the client's behavior will more likely activate psychological reactance. This tends to lead men to eventually reassert sexual freedom when faced with sexual behavior constraints. To be mindful of this possible reaction to the screening and assessment, therapists must look at the presence of moralizing, reinforcing culturally uninformed sexual information, replicating overly restrictive societal sexual rules, or by premature adherence to a narrow bandwidth of acceptable sexual behavior. It is also important for OCSB therapists not to prematurely expect men to align their sexual attitudes, values, and behaviors with sexual health principles. The theory of psychological reactance "predicts an *increase* in the rate and attractiveness of a 'problem' behavior if a person perceives that his or her personal freedom is being infringed or challenged" (Miller & Rollnick, 2002, p. 18). The vulnerability of the initial sexual behavior disclosure crisis leads many men to unquestionably agree to any sexual behavior change or comply with therapist suggestion or spousal demands. Crisis-moment sexual agreements will likely need to be contemplated and reconsidered as men begin to identify and understand the sexual health values and goals that emerge from OCSB treatment.

Dillard and Shen (2005) developed conceptual perspectives on the nature of reactance. Their studies demonstrated that reactance is a combination of cognitive and emotional processes similar to those described in the dual-process model of human behavior (Loewenstein & O'Donoghue, 2007). Their participants' perceptions of losing freedom combined with feeling angry led to actions that entrenched their problematic behavior (Dillard & Shen, 2005). Sexual problems might look more mysterious and pathological if therapists do not consider the forces of psychological reactance on freedom infringement within the OCSB screening and assessment process.

To minimize psychological reactance, the OCSB screening interview matches the clinical assessment process with the man's motivation to change his sexual behavior. Frequently lost in early evaluation of dysregulated sexual behavior is the men's sexual pleasure. Clinical models that focus extensively on the negative consequences will miss identifying vital sexual-pleasure motivations that compete with the men's motivation to change. Raising consciousness about both sexual pleasure and painful consequences activates curiosity and often mirrors the tension that men have been addressing secretly on their own. Raising consciousness is more than focusing on why one should stop a sexual behavior. It is also a space for men to honestly discuss why they want to continue their current sexual behavior, even though they experience it as out of control. What is so enticing about the sexual behavior that even their own foresight about negative consequences was not enough to cause a change? What does he miss about it?" Balancing the discussion between pleasure and consequences provides therapist and client with a clearer picture regarding men's conflicting motivations for considering change.

Managing Self-Manipulation

Cubitt, Starmer, and Sugden (2004) describe the self-manipulation of beliefs as "the situation in which a rational agent deliberately avoids free information that would reduce his uncertainty before acting" (p. 91). Self-manipulation defenses prohibit men from considering the consequences of their sexual behavior and transcend their immediate moment of sexual excitation. Self-manipulation defenses effectively block information that creates uncertainty prior to the sexual act and impedes the mind's deliberative system from asserting influence over the affective system's action tendencies. This obstruction of the deliberative system allows men to remain highly motivated to have sex. Self-discrepancy and uncertainty evaporate when sexual behavior consequences are self-manipulated away like unwelcomed intruders. The OCSB assessment provides multiple opportunities to implement consciousness-raising techniques to weaken self-manipulation defenses and enhance client motivation for change.

Self-manipulation theory explains how some men with OCSB have avoided developing and internalizing an ethical sexual map that would conflict with their immediate sexual urges. OCSB treatment-seeking men benefit from having an intentional discussion that raises their awareness about the self-manipulation patterns that enable sexual behavior. Sexual self-manipulation significantly decreases when the negative consequences of men's sexual behavior become unavoidable and are juxtaposed with the man's increasing internalization of the sexual health principles. As these defenses decrease, the short-term sexual interests that are not aligned with men's sexual health plan generate a greater self-discrepancy.

Clinical Distinction: Consensual Sexual Behavior

The OCSB Screening Procedure distinguishes between two sets of sexual behavior problems that warrant separate treatment approaches: consensual sex and nonconsensual sex. The OCSB Clinical Pathway is a treatment model for men whose consensual sexual urges, thoughts, or behaviors feel out of control. For OCSB screening, consultation shifts to determining whether a referral to a nonconsensual specialist is warranted when men report a history of engaging in nonconsensual sex or have nonconsensual fantasies and urges. As such, the OCSB Screening Procedure evaluates the consent dynamics for every client. In most situations, men who report nonconsensual sexual behaviors in the screening interview or at any time during the assessment or treatment are referred to a nonconsensual specialist for further evaluation.

We advocate screening for nonconsensual sexual urges, thoughts, and behaviors with all men presenting for problematic sexual behavior or OCSB treatment. The OCSB Clinical Pathway reflects our clinical judgment about separating populations based on nonconsent. Nonconsensual sex is such an emotionally laden topic that we have dedicated space to discuss the various parameters that define nonconsensual sex and informed our recommendation.

What is nonconsensual sexual behavior?

Defining *nonconsensual sex* is complicated by the various attitudes, priorities, and values associated with this behavior (Meuhlenhard & Peterson, 2004). The essence of nonconsensual sex is seen when one's behavior violates another person's freedom from sexual contact. It resides at the friction point between the sexual autonomy of two (or more) people. Wertheimer (2003) developed a moral and legal theory of consent grounded in the psychology of perpetrators and victims. He includes philosophical, legal, and social science perspectives in his examination of nonconsensual sex. Wertheimer (2003) suggests that the central dynamic of consent is not the stereotypical "no means no," but rather the clear responsibility of all sexual partners to determine that "yes really does mean yes." A man must balance the moral dimension of consent with the woman's autonomy to render permission for him to engage in sex with her in circumstances in which she is competent, informed, and voluntarily consenting (Wertheimer, 2003). [Note: Wertheimer uses the female pronoun throughout his book to discuss the role of the person who gives valid consent and uses the male pronoun for the person responsible for obtaining valid consent from a sexual partner prior to sexual relations.] Wertheimer articulates consent as a balance between one's autonomy to give clear unambiguous consent for sex in combination with everyone's right to engage in sex with whomever he or she chooses. Sexual consent is most likely maintained when men best approximate this balance between autonomy and freedom. Sexual violence and nonconsensual sex increase in probability when the potential violator bases his threshold for consensual sex on the certainty of the partner's permission ("yes"; Wertheimer, 2003).

Consent Spectrum

It is useful to organize nonconsensual sexual behaviors along a continuum to better define this behavior and discern clinical distinctions. Rasmussen and Miccio-Fonseca (2007) describe nonconsent as sexual permission that is elicited through coercive behavior that exploits power differences to gain access to sexual contact. Although there are no universally accepted standards that determine sexually coercive conditions, "the type of influence used to obtain sex and the circumstances of the individuals involved are all likely to affect people's judgments" (Meuhlenhard & Peterson, 2004, p. 247). Coercion and exploitation must be absent for valid consent to be given.

Miccio-Fonseca and Rasmussen (2011) developed a nomenclature for describing two distinct categories of sexually abusive youth. Of particular focus in their work is the focus on distinguishing between the vast majority of sexually abusive youth who engage in coarse sexual improprieties (sexually vulgar comments, expressions, and behaviors; crude, indecent, behavior outside societal norms of propriety; examples include: crude sexual gestures, sexually suggestive comments, mooning, looking up skirts, a young child rubbing his or her genitals in public or trying to grab another's genitals, a child looking over a stall in a public restroom) and adjudicated or nonadjudicated youth whose violent sexually abusive behaviors and improprieties reside within a continuum of low, moderate, high, or very high (i.e., lethal) risk (Miccio-Fonsecca & Rasmussen, 2011).

Bancroft (2009) proposes a nonconsent continuum from the most harmful to least intrusive: rape by penile penetration; rape with other body parts (finger, tongue) or object; variety of sexual acts with children and one's own children or family relations; sexual threats; exposing genitals to strangers and becoming aroused; sexual arousal by spying on sexual activity of others; sexual touching on the continuum of naked genitalia to touching genitals, breasts, bottom; or kissing in such a manner that the person feels fear, alarm, or distress. Bancroft delineates nonconsent as an individual's sexual expression overriding the right of another person to be free from unwanted sexual behavior and gestures.

Nonconsent as Illegal Sex

Sexual consent laws are in place to protect people by defining and forbidding forms of unwanted sexual contact between individuals (Bancroft, 2009). In addition, vulnerable classes of people have specific provisions protecting them from sexual violations, such as minors, people with disabilities, and seniors. The nature of legal and public safety laws and regulations are act-centered prohibitions of specific nonconsensual sexual activities. Although consent laws are present across the country, the legal details change over time (e.g., marital rape laws) and vary by jurisdiction (e.g., ages of consent). This means relying on legal definitions to guide clinical conceptualization and treatment has significant limitations.

Furthermore, illegal sex is not necessarily nonconsensual sex. Laws can also restrict adult consensual sexual behaviors considered repugnant by many segments of society (see Klein, 2012). Such laws include regulations prohibiting paying for sex, obscenity, incest, and sex-toy sales. Laws governing sexual relations between consenting adults often use criminal statutes under the guise of public safety to enforce act-centered sexual values.

Sex offense laws are intended to promote consent as a fundamental principle of sexual rights (World Association for Sexual Health, 2008) despite contradictions among sex offense laws and the overreach of many regulations of consensual sex. The threat of legal sanctions is considered one of the most effective methods for regulating potential sex offenses (Bancroft, 2009). We clearly endorse the sexual health principle of consent as a human right and essential parameter for societal membership (see Cossman, 2009). Our intention with advancing nonconsent as an OCSB clinical distinction is to help therapists navigate the clinical space in which public safety and mental health treatment priorities coexist.

Nonconsent as a Psychiatric Symptom

Nonconsensual sexual urges, thoughts, and behaviors are psychiatricly explained as either psychosexual paraphiliic disorders or subsumed within current sexual addiction, impulsive/compulsive sexual behavior, and hypersexual behavior disorder diagnostic models. Paraphilic psychosexual disorders include both consensual and nonconsensual sexual activities. However, psychiatric diagnostic preoccupation with nonconsensual sex crimes has left consensual paraphilic disorders within mental health care invisible. The most frequently diagnosed of the paraphilias are those that involve illegal sex offenses; those that describe legal sexual behavior generally go undiagnosed or misdiagnosed (Money, 1999). Moser (2011) cautions the profession that including nonconsensual sex as a paraphilic criterion has confused a criminal act with a mental disorder. This risks an "inappropriate medicalization of criminal behavior to serve a practical public safety purpose" (Frances & First, 2011, p. 560). Medicalizing public safety may obscure and compete with the health care-providing role of the psychotherapist, leaving the therapist vulnerable to omitting the current body of sexual science and emphasizing legal formulations of diverse sexual interests (Ortmann & Sprott, 2013).

Nonconsensual sexual experiences have also been subsumed into the proposed diagnostic criteria of sexual dysregulation disorders. For instance, the methods used to diagnose a sexual addiction have historically included a focus on the content of a person's sexual fantasies. Sexual fantasies that are far afield of relational, sociocultural, and gender-normative scripts have been included within addictive sexual behavior treatment. "Healthy sexuality for most sexually addicted individuals involves not only a change in behavior, but also an avoidance of fantasizing about behaviors that are unhealthy" (Carnes, 2007, p. 360). Healthy sexuality is framed within a relational dynamic in which increased sexual excitement leads to increased closeness. Unhealthy sexual imagery that is deemed disrespectful, increases objectification, involves hostility-based bonding, and depersonalizing is not considered sober or consistent with recovery from sexual addiction (Carnes, 2007).

Sexual addiction as a disease is conflated with long-standing beliefs in degeneracy. This fusion of the disease progression with the corruption of sexual self-discipline implies an inevitable fall into human depravity when the disease is not adequately treated. Degeneracy involves the movement from conventional, consensual sex to unconventional or nonconsensual sex. Rather than differentiating between consensual and nonconsensual as qualitatively distinct, addictive sexual behavior is organized around ideological norms about orgasm frequency and nonrelational sex that are an unhealthy deviation from the norm and will degenerate without intervention. Understandably, nonconsensual sex acts generate disapproval and intense feelings of fear, disgust, and revulsion. If one adheres to the slippery slope of the degeneracy conceptualization, the logical progression of sexual addiction is toward nonconsensual sex acts. For instance, a spouse may generalize a partner's disease as a menacing threat that could progress (degenerate) into molesting their children or grandchildren, expose family members to violent sexual imagery, or violate sound judgment of basic parental safety if children are left alone with the sexually addicted parent. Unfortunately, sexual degeneracy theory obscures the critical evaluation of combined clinical treatment methods for consensual and nonconsensual sexual behavior.

Coleman has written about the current gap in a clear clinical understanding of nonparaphilic impulsive/compulsive sexual behavior (2007): "A challenge remains to understand non-paraphilic compulsive sexual behavior, find where this clinical syndrome fits in our classification of sexual disorders, determine clear diagnostic criteria, and find effective treatment approaches" (p. 356). Clinical formulations of hypersexual behavior focus on distinguishing paraphilic psychosexual disorders from hypersexuality. Kafka proposed that hypersexual disorder and paraphilic disorders are distinct from each other and can be simultaneously present within the same patient (Kafka, 2010). Impulsive/compulsive sexual behavior and hypersexual disorder conceptualizations expect clinicians to discern criminal acts, mental disorders, sexual variation, and culturally embedded notions of sexual degeneracy while not directly commenting on differentiating consent and nonconsent independent from the medicalization lens of paraphilias.

Excluding Nonconsensual Sexual Behavior From OCSB Treatment

Sex is nonconsensual when someone has sexual contact with a person who is unable to consent or when consent is obtained through coercion or force. Relational dynamics, situational contexts, personal motives, and the law complicate the specific forces at work within each individual engaging in nonconsensual sexual activity. Consent is now a universal component of all internationally endorsed definitions of sexual health. Consent is also a clinical distinction in the OCSB Model. OCSB assessment and treatment are limited to men who feel that their consensual sexual activity is out of control and who do not use force or coercive behavior to engage in sexual activity with another person. We propose the factors that influence the affective–deliberative interaction that produce nonconsensual sexual behaviors are different than those that produce consensual sexual problems. Therefore, prospective clients who engage in nonconsensual sex should be assessed and treated by trained specialists. We find support for our distinction from studies on sexual offending youth and adults and the Standards of Care for the Treatment of Adult Sex Offenders (Coleman et al., 2000). These standards and practice guidelines concur with the need for specialized training and programming for assessing and treating nonconsensual sexual practices. Nonconsensual sexual treatment training is currently not required to provide sexual addiction, impulsive/compulsive sexual behavior, or hypersexual behavior therapy. In this section, we describe our rationale for excluding most of the nonconsensual spectrum of sexual behavior from OCSB treatment.

Nonconsensual sexual behavior includes a wide breadth of human psychpathology. The Sexual Attitudes and Behavior Inventory (SABI), developed by San Diego forensic psychologist Clark Clipson, is a self-report instrument that provides "a standardized way to assess an individual's sexuality in relation to a community sample as well as to know sex offender populations" (Clipson, 2009, p. 1). To comprehensively measure sex offender populations, measures, such as the SABI, include scales to assess antisocial attitudes and behaviors; hostility toward women; sexual interest in prepubescent and pubescent children; various motivations for rape, voyeurism, exhibitionism; cognitive distortion scales for child molesters; and a separate scale for rapists. Although the SABI has additional scales for relationships, sexual functioning, attachment, and other various sexual behavioral and historical themes, to comprehensively measure nonconsent is well beyond relevant measures for consensual OCSB. Given that this additional range in psychopathology is more frequently present within men who are compelled to engage in nonconsensual sex, this population would benefit from different treatment inventions to regulate their sexual behavior than clients seeking treatment for consensual sexual problems.

Differences between erotic arousal in consensual and nonconsensual situations lend themselves to different sexual behavior treatment approaches. For some OCSB clients, their consensual sexual problems stem from an obstructed erotic-identity development involving an unconventional turn-on. The goal is to integrate their erotic orientations into their self-concept and intimate relationships. The ultimate objective is to create congruence among their sexual behavior, orientation, and identity. This "coming out" process usually involves changing shame-based attitudes and beliefs about the turn-on within the larger sexual health goal of accepting and integrating their turn-ons into their sexual expression. Men with rigid, narrow, or highly unconventional turn-ons may feel conflicted and ambivalent about accepting their more fixed arousal capacity. Expanding a fixed sexual repertoire is complicated by the gap between the fixed erotic template and their idealized and more desired erotic orientation. The personal journey of erotic orientation integration is complicated further by the level of partner disinterest, disgust, or even revulsion in participating with their partner in his erotic turn-on. As is typical with any coming-out process, grieving the sexual ideal and accepting the reality of one's immutable sexual self is a significant journey toward sexual health. For clients with an unconventional erotic orientation with nonconsensual themes, the goals are different. Treatment is not directed toward helping men integrate nonconsensual behavior with partners. The therapist has a duty to maintain public safety as a primary goal rather than to guard a man's freedom for violent, coercive, or forced nonconsensual sexual autonomy. Thus, we recommend referring OCSB treatment-seeking clients who are concerned about nonconsensual sexual experiences to specialists trained to navigate the public safety concerns along with the clinical needs of this population.

The final reason for excluding nonconsent from OCSB treatment is specific to our clinical approach. OCSB treatment is an outpatient, combined group, and individual psychotherapy model. Our style of group psychotherapy is a semi-structured, process-oriented approach incorporating here-and-now interactions for understanding defenses, interpersonal patterns, and regulation skills. Through treatment, clients become aware of the mental tricks performed by their defenses, which contribute to gaining more control over their process of change (Prochaska et al., 1994). The defenses of clients engaged in nonconsensual sex, especially those well beyond coarse sexual impropriety, rely on defenses that are more likely to create aggression and injure another group member. The defenses often found among many nonconsent actors, combined with their more complex psychopathology, leads to relational patterns and limitations that are not compatible in a group of out of control, consensual sexual behaviors. We propose that a process-oriented psychotherapy group with a combined membership of consensual and nonconsensual presenting problems poses a formidable challenge for maintaining an adequate treatment frame for group cohesion.

Identifying Nonconsensual Sexual Behavior as a Sexual Health Intervention

Anthony's peak sexual excitement is masturbating in places where he might be discovered. His encounter with Amy presents an important opportunity for a sexual health intervention. Since his early teens, Anthonly has engaged in potentially exhibitionistic solo sex. The onset of his nonconsensual behavior occurred long before it came to the attention of professionals or law enforcement. Sex-offending research uses the terms "actual onset" and "official onset" to mark the years a person spends engaging in nonconsensual sex without legal consequences. The time between the historical first crossing into nonconsensual behavior and a man's first conviction for sexual offense is called "cost avoidance" (Mathesius & Lussier, 2013). Anthony's cost-avoidance story from actual onset to official onset is not unusual. He began nonconsensual sexual behavior as a teen. It continued unabated and remained hidden within his adult sexual life. For some, the actual onset of nonconsensual sexual behavior is explained by the dawning awareness, especially when hormonal puberty commences, of a nonconsensual sexual arousal and fantasy. Many juveniles whose nonconsensual behaviors involve a range of reoccurring sexually abusive behaviors will persist in their offending into adulthood (Lussier & Blokland, 2013). Most adolescents and adults are identified and labeled "sex offenders" as part of their transition from cost avoidance and official onset and a criminal prosecution and sentencing. Thus, men who engage in nonconsensual sexual behaviors—from coarse sexual improprieties to sexually abusive and violent behavior—follow a developmental trajectory and time period in which they are "haunted by the unspeakability of what one has done" (Money, 1999, p. 3). It is during this *cost-avoidance* period that the individual lives a "damned if you do—damned if you don't" dilemma. Money (1999) describes the bind of this predicament as either a secret isolated chamber of silence or a confinement resulting from the wrath of retribution and derision. This is a time when individuals hide the nonconsensual behavior as well as maintain the necessary psychological defenses and behavior to ensure their nonconsensual sex life remains an unspeakable act. The coping strategies used to maintain nonconsensual behavior and maintain the coping strategies for keeping unspeakable acts invisible leads to an array of behavioral problems, mental illnesses, medical problems, and distorted or delusional thinking. Most important is the development of defenses that significantly disable their ability to make accurate cause-and-effect associations between their nonconsensual behavior and their escalating distress and suffering. As the time gets closer and closer to official onset, their avoidant coping strategies falter and a crisis ensues. This was Anthony's story.

Nonconsent ranges on a continuum from various degrees of coarse sexual improprieties to low, medium, high, and lethal levels of sexual abuse and violence. The current relationship a person has with his nonconsensual behavior at any one time resides within one of these three categories:

1. Unobserved/undocumented
2. Observed/undocumented
3. Observed/documented

Prior to his hospital-room discovery, Anthony lived with an unobserved and undocumented exhibitionistic arousal. He was avoiding consequences of discovery while enduring the consequences and distress of hiding a fundament component of his sexuality. The discovery in the hospital was a change in his relationship with his sexual turn-on. It became observed but undocumented. It is undocumented because psychological treatment or diagnosis had not been given; law enforcement was not involved; and employment, divorce, or child-custody proceedings involving his sexual conduct had not commenced. Anthony, and other clients in his situation, may schedule an initial OCSB assessment in response to this change from unobserved to observed, but it is an undocumented transition. Men might engage in sexually harassing behavior in the workplace, or distribute digital sexual images of a former girlfriend, or look through their neighbor's window while masturbating, or press against subway passengers with an erect penis, or masturbate in a men's public bathroom, all behaviors that have remained unobserved and undocumented for years. The client may be invested in a sex addiction (SA), impulsive–compulsive sexual behavior (ICSB), or hypersexual disorder (HD) diagnosis as a way to document the condition in response to the onset of legal consequences. This is where the utility of a sexual-disorder diagnosis can emerge in the life of someone engaged in nonconsensual sex. Self-identifying as a sex addict provides a process to access appropriate treatment services and remain observed while a medical, legal, employment, or court document can be established and lead to appropriate treatment.

OCSB treatment screens for unobserved and observed as well as undocumented and documented coarse or abusive sexual behavior. Referring for treatment with a nonconsensual specialist becomes the priority once the nonconsensual sexual activity is disclosed and identified in the screening interview. We have existing professional relationships with respected nonconsensual specialists who assess undocumented men who are interested in leaving their cost-avoidant prison. We recommend therapists consult with a nonconsensual specialist to determine the course of treatment if a client reveals undocumented low-level, coarse sexual behavior. If the behavior clearly involves nonconsensual sex with minors and other forms of sexual coercion and violence, the OCSB screening shifts course to become a dialogue that facilitates a referral to a nonconsensual specialist. We recommend educating the client so he understands that he can seek treatment prior to being arrested, and that he should be seen only by nonconsensual specialists until the nonconsensual issue has been professionally assessed. Lussier and Cale (2013) warn of the risks of a therapist either underestimating or overestimating the reoffending risk of a documented sex offender when he or she lacks highly specialized training in working with men who have ended the cost-avoidance stage of their nonconsensual sexual activity. Preventing premature recommendations for SA, ICSB, or HD treatment is essential for an individual's sexual health and public safety. The clear clinical distinction of nonconsent as a part of the screening interview is an OCSB Pathway component to prevent an underresponse by the therapist when a client discloses nonconsensual activity. There are licensed professionals, trained in both sexual-offender treatment and OCSB, who are qualified to develop their own processes to manage public and client safety. The vast majority of licensed mental health professionals do not have this level of training.

For example, a man reveals in an OCSB screening or assessment that he is aroused by images of sex with 13-year-old early-pubescent boys and lives with long-hidden fears that he will someday actually have sex with a minor. His long history of looking at images is combined with a haunted pride of having "never touched a boy." He is both tormented by the fear of crossing this line and comforted by the fact that he never has. It is a disservice to these men and the safety of communities that the only avenue available to move from the shadow of undocumented cost-avoidant nonconsensual sex is with an arrest or incarceration. The sexual health consequence for each man and his victims is tragic. The vast majority of these men gain access to treatment only *after* they have engaged in nonconsensual sex and are arrested for a sex crime. The mental health field is contributing to this societal problem by not adequately screening for nonconsensual sex with all their clients or providing treatment for nonconsensual sex without advanced training and ongoing supervision. Under- or overresponding to clients' distress or uncertainty about their propensity or risk for acting on their nonconsensual sex urges will likely impede their ability to change out of control sexual behavior and live their personal vision for sexual health. It is our responsibility to connect treatment-seeking men to the most capable professional in the community who can assess their current undocumented nonconsensual sexual behavior and identify risk factors for nonconsensual sex.

OCSB SCREENING CRITERIA: VULNERABILITY FACTORS

Motivation and consent are the two clinical distinctions that differentiate between who is recommended for an OCSB assessment and who is referred to alternative resources for further assessment. There are four remaining criteria that must be explored as part of the the OCSB Screening Process within the OCSB Clinical Pathway: (a) physical safety, (b) physical health, (c) mental health, and (d) relationship with drugs and alcohol. In the OCSB Model, these factors influence and mediate the relational balance between the affective and deliberative processes. Their potential to disrupt the dual process requires that they be considered before drawing conclusions about a client's sexual behavior control. The criteria are familiar components of responsible mental health psychosocial assessments. Screening for these four vulnerability factors ensures that the conditions for sexual health behavior change are in place. Before addressing the vulnerability factors, we introduce the concept of allostasis and its role in health-behavior change.

Sexual Health and Allostasis

Allostasis refers to balancing one's physiology to retain homeostasis in various circumstances of change (McEwen & Seeman, 2009). Higher levels of overall health and well-being exist when the body is able to have a well-coordinated physiological response to one's lifestyle and environment as well as physical, mental, and social circumstances (McEwen & Seeman, 2009). Researchers at the MacArthur Research Network on Socioeconomic Status and Health at the University of California, San Francisco (UCSF), developed environmental and psychosocial pathway models to understand how socioeconomic and biological systems interact, not within groups of people, but within each person, leading to disease risk, disease progression, and, ultimately, mortality.

"The widespread use of the term 'stress' in popular culture has made this word a very ambiguous term to describe the ways in which the body copes with psychosocial, environmental and physical challenges" (McEwen, 2000, p. 108). Researchers at UCSF adopted the term "allostasis," which looks beyond the word "stress" to encompass a process of health that allows a person to maintain internal viability amid changing conditions (Sterling & Eyer, 1988). The UCSF team is composed of a psychologist, sociologists, psychoneuroimmunologists, physicians, epidemiologists, neuroscientists, biostatisticians, and economists who studied how well individuals maintain homeostasis when going through change (McEwen & Seeman, 2009). Their research explores the health consequences that arise from the expenditure of physiological resources to maintain balance in response to chronic stress. Every biophysiological mechanism requires energy expenditure. A person must gather his or her body's resources to adapt (attempt to maintain homeostasis) in response to changes in his or her environment. The cumulative negative effects of "allostatic load" are determined by genetic makeup, how many challenges individuals face, when in their lives these challenges were they faced, and their brain's efficiency in managing its resources (McEwen, 2000). Allostatic health is measured by a person's mental abilities expended to maintain stability during change. Screening for OCSB vulnerability factors is designed to identify and address current factors that are associated with allostatic load. Sexual behavior regulation will improve when distressing or disruptive circumstances that require a physiological allostatic response become less and less frequent over the course of OCSB treatment.

Allostatic mechanisms for regulating the dual-process affective–deliberative interaction is reflected in a person's ability to maintain adequate levels of stability when faced with stressful stimuli or life events. The affective system becomes activated proportional to the degree of stress (Metcalfe & Mischel, 1999). The stress levels depend on both the stress induced by the appraisal of the specific situation and the evolving lifelong chronic stress levels specific to the history of each person. The degree of allostatic load contributes to the energy available to access the deliberative system processes that balance the affective activation. A man may be able to enhance his deliberative activation in low to moderate levels of stress, but higher stress may foretell poor deliberative processing or even a shutting-off response. Treating the OCSB vulnerability factors will significantly reduce the allostatic load that diverts much needed energy for self and attachment regulation and positive sexual- and erotic-identity development.

A childhood spent adapting to chronically stressful conditions has long-term, adult consequences on health, emotional regulation, and behavior (Repetti, 2011). Adult OCSB may reflect a child's (mal)adaptation in response to physical, environmental, or psychosocial challenges. A boy may stroke his penis while listening to his drunken father threaten to harm his mother and learn that the self-soothing sensations calm his body's anxiety and fears. However, he may rely on this sexual mechanism for self-soothing to achieve multiple consecutive orgasms that also lead to skin irritation, bleeding, and soreness. We incorporate these perspectives during the OCSB assessment to explore and understand the developmental allostatic adaptions that contribute to OCSB. The OCSB screening focuses on identifying vulnerability factors that may require separate clinical interventions to reduce the client's allostatic load.

Vulnerability Factor: Physical Safety

Current risks of violence or self-harm are important health conditions to screen when clients present for OCSB treatment. The probability of succeeding in the difficult work of changing sexual behavior patterns decreases if the client is not free from bodily harm or the threat thereof. One of the primary roles of the affective system is to protect against physical harm. When faced with a threatening stimulus, the affective system prioritizes immediate action and the deliberative system is less engaged. Persistent affective activation used to manage threats to physical safety can obscure other factors that contribute to OCSB or contribute to the allostatic load clients manage.

Distress in response to OCSB may lead clients and intimate partners to react with harmful or violent behavior. Men may attempt to reassure themselves that their partners are not leaving them by snooping through their e-mail, following them after work, or leveraging their partner's financial dependency. Some men may feel so hopeless about their futures that they regulate their emotional pain with self-injurious behaviors or become suicidal. A highly reactive partner may resort to verbal attacks or physical assault after discovering details of the partner's sexual infidelity.

The physical safety screening criterion is divided into two risk areas:

1. Self-harm
2. Relationship violence

Self-Harm

Suicide
Nine percent of the world's population has seriously considered suicide at some point in their lives, making suicide a leading cause of death worldwide (Borges et al., 2010). Approximately 3% of the world's population attempts to kill themselves. Suicide research has helped therapists to identify suicide risk factors. Clinician knowledge of suicide risk factors is crucial for differentiating between clients who may attempt suicide in the next few hours, days, or months (Borges et al., 2010). Men with co-occurring mood disorders and drug and alcohol problems are at an increased risk for suicide. OCSB treatment-seeking clients may exhibit symptoms similar to these at-risk populations. Their suicidal preoccupation may increase in response to a discovery of secretive sexual behavior, rejection by an intimate partner, or may be related to a chronic or ongoing concern linked with an untreated psychiatric disorder.

Men who keep suicide as a problem-solving option are highly unlikely to succeed at OCSB treatment. There is an inherent conflict between keeping an "emergency exit" of suicide as a viable treatment option while moving forward and facing significant life fears. Some clients may be so accustomed to their suicidal thinking that they remain unaware of the influence that this defense of hopelessness has on their day-to-day lives and sexual behaviors. Because an OCSB assessment raises emotional activation ending suicide as an individual's conscious or unconscious self-soothing strategy establishes the safety boundaries necessary for taking the first steps toward sexual health.

Self-injury
Not all self-harming behaviors involve suicidal ideation; clients may engage in intentional bodily injury without suicidal intent. Self-injury ranges from cutting, burning, and scratching of skin to grander actions like hitting one's body, banging one's head, preventing wounds from healing, pulling out hair follicles, or swallowing objects (Sutton, 2007). Self-injury provides another "emergency exit" from emotional distress. Clients utilize self-injury to disrupt their unregulated activation states. The injury process is frequently experienced as an effective means for controlling and calming emotions. Sutton describes this as an exchange of one pain for another. Turning an invisible psychological pain into a visible physical wound transforms the circumstance to a concrete physical manifestation (a wound) that organizes emotional and cognitive distress (Sutton, 2007). The treatment objective for self-injurious clients is to expand their affect tolerance and reduce their reliance on problematic coping behaviors; an objective that is similar to that of OCSB clients. Treatment becomes the opportunity for clients to develop safer coping strategies.

Relationship Violence

In their lifetimes, about 25% of women and 14% of men will experience severe physical violence. Nearly half of all women and men have experienced psychological aggression from an intimate partner. Similar to the varying degrees of nonconsensual sex, violence within relationships can vary by form, intensity, and intention. There is no consensus on what to label this phenomenon as the field continues to debate conceptualization and ideology (McHugh, Livington, & Ford, 2005). The U.S. Department of Justice defines domestic violence as:

a pattern of abusive behavior in any relationship that is used by one partner to gain or maintain power and control over another intimate partner. Domestic violence can be physical, sexual, emotional, economic, or psychological actions or threats of actions that influence another person. This includes any behaviors that intimidate, manipulate, humiliate, isolate, frighten, terrorize, coerce, threaten, blame, hurt, injure, or wound someone. (Office on Violence Against Women, 2014, p. 1)

McHugh and Frieze (2006) distinguish between intimate partner violence (IPV) and abuse. They define *intimate partner violence* (IPV) as "physical injury to one's partner in the context of intimate (romantic/sexual) relationships; *intimate partner abuse* refers to physical, psychological, and/or sexual coercion perpetrated in the context of an intimate relationship" (p. 122). We screen for acute violence between clients and their intimate partners to determine the best course of treatment. Most acute expressions of IPV require immediate intervention in order to address both partner's safety. This may involve a referral to specialized IPV services rather than beginning an OCSB assessment. Clinicians should consult an IPV specialist when men report a history of IPV that predates the discovery of their sexual behavior, have immediate access to firearms as well as a history of drug and alcohol abuse, obsessive possessiveness, homicidal/suicidal threats, or recent estrangement (Websdale, 2000).

Despite the prevalence rates of male perpetrators of IPV (M. C. Black et al., 2011), the most common form of IPV we have seen with clients presenting for OCSB treatment involved male clients being hit by their female partners after the discovery of extrarelational sex. Men describe struggling with asserting a safety boundary because they believe they deserve the assault and minimize the consequences of violence in the relationship. For OCSB treatment-seeking clients with current IPV, a safety plan and no-harm contract are recommended prior to initiating the assessment. A referral to an IPV specialist is recommended if the acuity of IPV is beyond the scope of OCSB treatment.

Stalking

Meloy (1998) defines *stalking* as the "willful, malicious and repeated following and harassing of another person" (p. 2). Mullen, Pathe, Purcell, and Stuart (1999) delineated five categories of stalkers based on motivations and context: rejected, intimacy seekers, incompetent, resentful, and predatory. Defenses of denial, minimization, devaluation, and projection of blame play a significant role when someone is engaged in obsessional following of another person (Meloy & Gothard, 1995; Skoler, 1998). Given the nature of insecure or pathological attachment patterns, and the disturbingly high frequency of violence directed toward their victims, these men require a trained stalking specialist to assess levels of lethality, context, and motivations for the behavior (Meloy & Fisher, 2005). Three specific elements elevate a man's stalking behavior to an extreme risk that requires assessment with a stalking specialist: (1) Is the stalking behavior intentional? (2) How credible are the client's verbal threats? (3) Are the threats inducing fear in the victim? When stalking behaviors are clearly intentional with credible threats that provoke fear in the victim, stopping the stalking behavior is the priority and an OCSB assessment is postponed until a stalking-treatment specialist has assessed the client.

If IPV or stalking behavior is discovered or emerges after entering OCSB treatment, continued participation in outpatient individual or group psychotherapy should be reevaluated. Given the potential psychopathology present in men who engage in these violent behaviors, combined with the potential for significant psychological, physical, and legal consequences for the OCSB client and his victims, an outpatient OCSB treatment setting is not the appropriate venue to effectively address stalking and IPV perpetration. Furthermore, managing group member fear and terror elicited by hearing group members terrorize others may be harmful to the other OCSB group members. It is the group leader's responsibility to protect the whole group from coming up against a member's unwillingness to address the fear and terror evoked by his stalking or IPV.

Homicidal threat
Current risk of homicide may also be relevant for some men seeking treatment for OCSB. Are death threats a spoken response to a man's disclosure of OCSB? Is the client currently living with a mentally ill family member who is unpredictably violent? The homicidal threat may come from an intimate partner, adult sibling, child, or others involved in family life. Although a low-frequency occurrence, it is important to listen for men's language, innuendo, or gallows humor that alludes to current threats of homicide. We have encountered a small subset of OCSB treatment-seeking men who, as children or young adults, lived in chronic fear that someone in their household would commit a homicide. This fear developed from being the target of direct verbal homicidal threats and physical assaults or witnessing homicidal threats to others in the household. Recent threats of homicide may activate historical wounds of family violence as well as contribute to an individual's current allostatic load. It is difficult for men to realistically move toward improving their sexual health if they continue to live with homicidal threats in their homes, workplaces, or other environments. Therapists whose OCSB clients are currently navigating

homicidal threats should seek case consultation with supervisors or specialists in this form of family violence. It is crucial to determine the acuity level of current homicidal threats prior to any further movement in OCSB evaluation or treatment.

Vulnerability Factor: Physical Health

Physical health plays an important role in all behavior health treatment, and OCSB treatment is no exception. Physical health problems can contribute to sexual behavior problems. Medical conditions can damage or impair parts of the brain that alter the deliberative–affective interaction. As a result, we recommend a physical health screening criterion to identity issues that may undermine the client's biological foundations of health.

Medical Conditions

Neurobiological impairment may undermine or overwhelm men's sexual inhibition leading to an imbalance with their levels of sexual excitation that could contribute to OCSB. For instance, hypersexual behavior is a symptom linked with neuropsychiatric conditions, brain injury, and medication side effects (Kafka, 2010). Hypersexual behavior is symptomatic of underlying disease states, such as frontal and temporal lobe lesions, temporal lobe epilepsy, dementia, Klüver–Bucy syndrome, multiple lesions in multiple sclerosis, and dopaminergic agents used for treatment of Parkinson's disease, each of which requires slightly different therapy (Chughtai et al., 2010). Some brain injuries may cause sexual disinhibition, impaired sexual decision making, sexual impulse control problems, and impair the ability to empathize with or care about others (Dombrowski, Petrick, & Strauss, 2000; Elliot & Biever, 1996).

It is important to not underestimate the significance of overall physical health as an OCSB vulnerability factor. How is the client currently sleeping, eating, and exercising? Having a body that is capable of providing a full range of sexual functioning, behavior, and pleasure is necessary for sexual health and overall sexual satisfaction. Sleep, for instance, is particularly important considering how sleep loss impairs high-level cognitive functioning and the ability to regulate sexual behavior. Having one's mental and physical energy depleted by treating a medical condition or physical problem limits the available reservoir of energy for regulating behavior, interpersonal relationship patterns, as well as one's sexual desires and interests (see Wolverton, 2013). A basic physical health screening is recommended for all OCSB treatment-seeking men.

It is also important to consider how the interplay between physical health and sexual behavioral symptoms may contribute to OCSB. For example, we have treated men whose sexual behavior symptoms functioned as ill-informed or unconscious solutions to address an undiagnosed erectile disorder or problems with rapid ejaculation. Men may attempt to build confidence in their ability to achieve and sustain an erection through a self-prescribed sexual imagery masturbation regimen. They may have experienced difficulties achieving a firm enough erection to vaginally or anally enter a partner and find the solo sex a welcome reprieve from the performance threat that intrudes partnered sex. They may feel tremendous shame for their erectile problems and seek OCSB treatment with a narrative that blames erection dysfunction on "porn addiction." Other men manage their sexual shame and anxiety from erectile dysfunction or rapid ejaculation through paid sex. They hire a professional sex worker as an unofficial sexual surrogate to build confidence or avoid an intimate partner's reactions to his sexual functioning. In these situations, screening for biogenic erectile dysfunction is an important first step before exploring the systemic or psychogenic contributors associated with erectile dysfunction. Biogenic causes of impaired erectile functioning (i.e., hormonal imbalances, low penile blood flow, or physical trauma) risk being obscurred by a "sex addiction" narrative.

HIV/STIs

The stress of untreated, newly diagnosed, or chronic medical conditions add to men's allostatic load. Addressing a co-occurring medical health condition competes with the energy, focus, and time it take for changing sexual health. A serious unexpected health crisis can usurp men's prioritization of their sexual behavior concerns, particularly when the health crisis is also a life-threatening diagnosis. One significant risk among OCSB treatment-seeking men is a newly diagnosed HIV infection. Studies have demonstrated positive correlations between high scores on sex addiction, sexual compulsivity, and hypersexual disorder measures and HIV risk behaviors, such as receptive anal intercourse without condoms, high frequency of sexual partners, paying for sex, and sex under the influence of drugs and alcohol (Parsons, Grov, & Golub, 2012; Yeagley, Hickok, & Bauermeister, 2014). Clarifying HIV status among OCSB treatment-seeking clients is also important considering that approximately 15.8% of people living with HIV do not know their status (Centers for Disease Control and Prevention [CDC], 2013).

The first sexual health treatment goal for OCSB treatment-seeking men is taking an HIV and sexually transmitted infection (STI) test. It is important for overall health and, in particular, OCSB treatment for men to know their HIV/STI status. In particular, HIV infection is associated with mental health problems such as neurocognitive impairment (Clifford & Ances, 2013) and depression (Rabkin, 2008). People with undiagnosed HIV infections pose a greater risk for infecting their sexual partners because they are not taking virus-suppressing medications (CDC, 2009). Not knowing one's HIV status may be a source of allostatic load because of the stress associated with engaging in behavior that is clearly linked with HIV transmission. Equally important is the reduction in allostatic load when men change their sexual behaviors in a manner that allows them to have a completely accurate negative HIV test result. Concretely knowing that they are HIV negative once and for all (which may be first time since they became sexually active) may be an opportunity to motivate sexual health behavior change and provide the impetus to remain HIV negative.

One's relationship with HIV expands beyond knowing one's status. The sexual practices and erotic interests of some men place them at little to no risk for infection, whereas the sexual desires and activities of other men place them in a closer, ongoing relationship with HIV. A triad model of HIV transmission risk is a helpful means for gauging an individual client's risk of HIV infection. This model organizes transmission risk using three areas: (a) infectivity per sex act, (b) rate of partner change, and (c) prevalence of disease among potential partners (Rotello, 1997).

Men living with HIV have a significantly different relationship with the virus. How an HIV-positive man lives is greatly influenced by the degree to which he integrated his HIV status into his self-concept. As with any identity formation process, psychological dis-ease is often generated when a person defends against accepting an immutable element of oneself. These defenses are frequently linked with problematic coping strategies. Dysregulated solo or partnered sexual behavior, for instance, may function to disconnect clients from their relentless self-talk narratives of being "damaged goods" or "undesirable." Men in OCSB group therapy have described the allure of certain sexual contexts or activities as a cognitive "HIV-free zone" that acts as a respite from the persistent stress surrounding all the complexity of living with HIV. These discussions provide insights into the motivations that HIV-positive men experience that compete with their overall sexual health goals.

Vulnerability Factor: Mental Health

Counselors should address psychiatric conditions at the outset of treatment given that mental health factors are one of the largest barriers to sexual health (Edwards, Delmonico, & Griffin, 2011; Reid, 2013).

Individuals with elevated scores of compulsive sexual behavior and hypersexual behavior have a high prevalence rate of comorbity with mood disorders, anxiety, substance addiction, and attention deficit hyperactivity disorder (ADHD; Bancroft, 2009; D. W. Black, Kehrberg, Flumerfelt, & Schlosser, 1997; Kafka & Prentky, 1994; Kaplan & Krueger, 2010; Raymond, Coleman, & Miner, 2003; Reid, 2007; Reid, Carpenter, Gilliland, & Karim, 2011). A meta-analysis of the literature found a positive correlation between nonparaphilic hypersexual behavior and depressive symptoms (Schultz, Hook, Davis, Penberthy, & Reid, 2014). Psychiatric disorders commonly found among men with hypersexual disorder include a range of Axis I mood disorders, anxiety disorders, substance abuse disorders, and ADHD (Kafka, 2010). Carpenter, Reid, Garos, and Najavits (2013) suggest that men seeking treatment for hypersexual disorder are at modestly higher risks for comorbid personality disorder (PD). These outcomes are juxtaposed with studies that found a relatively small proportion of PD in a hypersexual treatment-seeking population (Lloyd, Raymond, Miner, & Coleman, 2007; Reid & Carpenter, 2009) and those that found substantially more comorbid PD among their samples (D. W. Black et al., 1997; Raymond et al., 2003). ADHD (inattentive type), major depressive disorder, bipolar disorder, and anxiety disorders are most frequently associated with Internet sexual compulsivity (Edwards et al., 2011).

It should be noted that comorbidity commonly refers to the occurrence of two or more psychiatric disorders existing simultaneously in the same person, currently or over a lifetime (Kaplan & Krueger, 2010). Studies have found positive correlations with various psychiatric disorders with people who score highly on SA, ICSB, or HD measures. Although we do not consider OCSB a sexual disorder, but rather, a human behavior sexual health problem, we use the term *comorbidity* to acknowledge that OCSB treatment-seeking men frequently meet criteria for other psychiatric disorders. We do not mean to imply that they meet criteria for a sexual disorder *and* another psychiatric disorder. In addition, it is important to remember that the association between clinical disorders and the scores on sexual dysregulation measures are correlational and do not reveal the direction of that relationship.

It is clear that comorbid mental illness is a common aspect of the overall clinical picture of clients seeking treatment for OCSB. Men and women seeking consultation for sexual behavior problems represent a highly diverse clinical population with a wide range of co-occurring mental health issues (Reid et al., 2009). Our clinical application of the comorbidity literature on SA, ICSB, and HD is to treat men's difficulty with regulating their sexual behavior as a symptom of an underlying psychiatric disorder. The psychiatric disorder may be disrupting the affective–deliberative interaction, resulting in unsuccessful sexual regulation and problematic decision making. The hyperactivation associated with an untreated clinical disorder may result in uncharacteristically high levels of sexual behavior. Or the OCSB may function as a distraction from unaddressed issues that induce a negative mood (Bancroft, 2009). Screening for the potential influence of psychiatric disorders on sexual behavior problems is a vital step.

Occasionally, OCSB symptoms resolve because treatment is introduced or improved for an untreated or mistreated psychiatric disorder. In other circumstances, the mental health issue is essential to diagnose and treat while the client works on improving their sexual health. A new diagnosis and treatment plan for the clinical disorder will need to be integrated within a man's vision of his sexual health. For someone newly diagnosed with generalized anxiety disorder, for instance, the integration question for the client becomes, "What is your vision of sexual health living with anxiety?" His anxiety treatment may also shift his sexual expression. Will his anxiety medications inhibit his typical levels of sexual excitement? Will an improvement in anxiety treatment reveal underdeveloped sexual and relational abilities? Will a diagnosis of an untreated lifelong anxiety illuminate and alter the shame-based narratives he developed about sexual developmental milestones? (e.g., "Oh, I get it, my inability to control my ejaculation during intercourse was connected with untreated anxiety, not that I'm hopeless, a bad lover.")

As with all of the screening criteria vulnerability factors, we educate clients that it is unlikely that they can achieve their sexual health goals if they do not address this vulnerability factor. Psychiatric disorders must be addressed in order to create the psychotherapy conditions necessary for the client to achieve his sexual health goals. Although clients request treatment from us to change their sexual behavior, we frequently provide traditional mental health disorder treatment and case management. There may also be a stage discrepancy in client readiness to explore psychiatric symptoms concurrent with their OCSB. A client may be determined to change his OCSB, yet have no curiosity about his symptoms of anxiety. Some clients may have adapted to their untreated mood disorder over several decades and are completely unaware that the levels of depression that they experience are treatable. Men may believe that they will "feel better" once their sexual behavior is under control, especially if they assume their moods are the result of their OCSB. Motivational interviewing strategies, in tandem with understanding common client defenses, are helpful in working with discrepant motivational stages (see Miller & Rollnick, 2013).

Vulnerability Factor: Relationship With Drugs and Alcohol

Everyone has a relationship with drugs and alcohol. Having a clear understanding of one's relationship with drugs and alcohol is essential for effective treatment. Drug and alcohol use has great potential to disrupt the affective–deliberative interaction and undermine conditions necessary for health. These substances are inescapable. Over the life span, women and men form many opinions and make an enormous array of decisions about their use of drugs and alcohol. They directly experience benefits and unwanted consequences from their consumption or indirectly experience the negative consequences when someone in their life abuses drugs and alcohol. We use the phrase "relationship with drugs and alcohol" to emphasize the complex connections people have with substances. Relationships vary among substances, change over time, and shift depending on circumstances. For the purposes of the OCSB screening, we recommend focusing on the client's current and direct relationship with alcohol and drugs (including medications) and where it falls on the continuum of nonuse, use, misuse, abuse, and dependence. The presence of drug and alcohol dependency has obvious sexual health implications, but an addiction is only one relationship a client may have with drugs and alcohol. Clients may rely too much on alcohol as a social lubricant when meeting potential dating partners. When attending circuit parties, gay or bisexual men may abuse recreational drugs that influence their decisions about condomless sex. Therapists shape their understanding of the clients relationship to drugs and alcohol with the use continuum to assist with determining a man's readiness for OCSB assessment.

We frame this vulnerability factor as the client's relationship with drugs and alcohol as opposed to simply screening for a more binary threshold of dependent/nondependent use. A relationship with drugs and alcohol is lifelong and can be in flux depending on the man's stage of life. A relationship-centered discussion may decrease the probably of provoking client defensiveness. This approach is less threatening for clients who have a problematic relationship with drugs and alcohol, but who have not come to that conclusion yet. Asking the client to discuss his relationship with drugs and alcohol is more inviting than a focus on determining criteria for dependency. This is an important position to consider because we are asking this screening question at the first session when rapport is limited and we want to welcome the possibility that the client is not ready to change his problematic relationship with drugs and alcohol. Clients may be aware of the risks, costs, and harm of both their substance abuse and their sexual behavior, but only feel ready to change their sexual behavior (Miller & Rollnick, 2013). Clients describing high levels of substance use may perceive the therapist inquiries about drinking as judgmental. Any premature movement to action will likely evoke precontemplative defenses against changing their drug and alcohol use. Screening a client's relationship with drugs and alcohol takes time and is an important process for rapport building and treatment planning. Discussing this issue at the initial consultation also establishes the language and purpose for discussing a man's relationship with drugs and alcohol as it relates to his sexual behavior.

Clients who are substance dependent and are actively using at the time of the screening appointment are not recommended for OCSB assessment. Outpatient OCSB assessment and treatment is not an adequate milieu to fully address an abusive or addictive relationship with drugs and alcohol. For clients at the acute end of the dependency continuum, referrals to medically monitored detox and inpatient treatment are prioritized over an OCSB assessment. If the sexual behavior symptoms persist after chemical dependency treatment, the client can be rescreened for an OCSB assessment. If the level of acuity resides somewhere between nonuse and abuse, we recommend proceeding with the OCSB assessment and looking more closely at this OCSB vulnerability factor. The OCSB assessment can also widen the scope to current or historical indirect consequences from drugs and alcohol (e.g., being raised by an alcoholic parent or having a current partner who abuses prescription drugs).

We may recommend an OCSB assessment or treatment for clients who are substance dependent, are not actively using, and who agree that they maintain their recovery boundaries while in OCSB treatment. Some men who are in recovery for their drug and alcohol addiction seek out an OCSB screening because their sexual behavior continues to be a concern. For these men, maintaining recovery is a necessary component of their health. Some men's problematic relationship with drugs and alcohol reemerge over time in the assessment or during ongoing OCSB treatment. This vulnerability factor, like all of the screening criteria, must be continually monitored throughout the assessment.

The OCSB assessment considers a man's range of affect tolerance when he is using drugs and alcohol or is in early recovery. The OCSB assessment is an in-depth and emotionally evocative process. If it is the clinical judgment of the therapist that the client's recovery is not sufficiently established, the therapist should collaborate with the client to discern whether adding additional stress will risk maintaining his recovery. The OCSB assessment can be postponed until the client's recovery and emotional regulation capacity are more stable. This is the most commonly occurring vulnerability factor: We frequently disappoint clients by either delaying or, ultimately, not recommending outpatient OCSB assessment when they initially request it.

The relationship between men's substance use or abuse and their sexual behavior may have little connection with each other. Others may show a very strong link between their substance use and sexual behavior. This screening vulnerability factor not only questions the amount of a man's substance use, but also the association between substance use and sexual behavior. Cocaine, marijuana, crystal methamphetamine, and alcohol are associated with triggering hypersexuality, either by reducing sexual inhibitions or by altering the level of dopamine in the brain, which, in turn, affects the user's perception of sexual arousal and pleasure (Finlayson, Stealy, & Martin, 2001). As a screening process, the goal is to clarify the client's current use of drugs and alcohol and educate the client about the role drugs and alcohol in sexual behavior.

Sex/Drug-Linked Patterns

Sex/drug-linked behavior is "the merging of drug- and/or alcohol-dependent behavior and sexual activity" (Braun-Harvey, 2011, p. 4). Some people's relationship with drugs and alcohol is indistinguishable from their sexual lives. Clients may access services in a variety of health care settings: chemical dependency treatment, STI/HIV clinics, and mental health offices. An unfortunate consequence of compartmentalized health care is the lack of comprehensive care for clients whose relationship with drugs and alcohol is undifferentiated from their sex lives. Clients may avoid discussing their sexual behavior problems in chemical dependency and mental health settings. They may openly discuss their sexual behavior with an STI/HIV counselor, but the focus of that session will likely remain on reducing sexual risk behaviors, not how to develop a satisfying and pleasurable sex life in recovery.

In many substance addiction treatment programs, the primary message about sex and recovery is to avoid sex during the first year of sobriety unless you are partnered or married. Often sexual behavior problems are framed as another addiction from which the client should abstain. Unlike using drugs and alcohol, however, sexuality is an integral part of human life and abstaining from sex is not an effective long-term solution to sex/drug-linked patterns. Newly sober clients may be unaccustomed to sex without drugs and alcohol and unprepared to manage the triggers associated with sexual urges, thoughts, or behavior. Without adequate treatment that integrates sexual health into their recovery and prepares them to reintegrate sexuality without substance abuse, clients with sex/drug-linked behaviors are vulnerable to drug and alcohol relapse. These men frequently view OCSB treatment as a necessary adjunctive service needed to introduce a sexual health component into their substance abuse treatment.

Recommending an OCSB Assessment

Similar to the way in which the consultation started, we end the consultation with a query about the client's motivation for sexual health. After the screening is complete and it is clear that a client would benefit from an OCSB assessment, we focus on the client's commitment for change. If he is not certain about proceeding with an assessment, we suggest that he go home to think about it, schedule another appointment to further evaluate his readiness, go back to his referring therapist and talk it over or decide not to go any farther or schedule an appointment for the assessment process. We advise him that agreeing to an assessment is not a commitment to change his sexual behavior, but rather an agreement to explore the factors that are contributing to the out of control sexual experiences. We want to avoid the situation in which the client does not feel accountable or invested in this decision. The final moments of the consultation hold the space in which the client determines his readiness to commit to the assessment process.

There are a couple issues to consider when recommending a formal OCSB assessment. For non-OCSB specialists who have conducted an OCSB screening, if the sexual symptoms persist, a formal OCSB assessment is recommended when the potential contributing factors have been identified and a management plan to address them is created. For the OCSB specialist conducting the screening during the initial consultation, a few additional considerations are important. First, an outpatient OCSB assessment is recommended if a higher level of care is not needed to address a co-occurring issue. Second, an assessment is recommended when the client is motivated to change his consensual sexual behavior and there is a plan to address any co-occurring issues that are present.

In the preceding chapters, we have discussed key elements of our model for assessment and treatment of OCSB. We have outlined a sexual health theory in combination with a model of human behavior as the map for understanding problems in regulating sexual behavior. We provided the historical context for the OCSB protocol by discussing the evolving conceptualizations of OCSB and sexual health. We described the dual-process theory of human behavior to contextualize sexual behavior problems. We proposed that the primary objective for OCSB treatment is to align sexual behavior with the six sexual health principles and the client's personal sexual health vision. A person's competing motivations (captured in the metaphorical relationship between elephant and rider) in which he struggles to maintain a balance between the affective and deliberative systems of the mind, are at the heart of OCSB. We organized the assessment of competing motivations into three clinical areas: self-regulation, attachment regulation, and sexual/erotic conflicts, which form the core of our OCSB assessment and treatment protocol. We have now added the last piece of new information to the OCSB protocol: screening criteria—a list of significant clinical distinctions and established biopsychosocial factors that may contribute to out of control sexual experiences.

REFERENCES

APA Presidential Task Force on Evidence-Based Practice. (2006). Evidence-based practice in psychology. *American Psychologist, 61*, 271–285.

Bancroft, J. (2009). *Human sexuality and its problems* (3rd ed.). London, UK: Churchill Livingstone.

Bancroft, J. (2013). Sexual addiction. In P. M. Miller (Ed.), *Principles of addiction: Comprehensive addictive behaviors and disorders* (Vol. 1, pp. 855–861). San Diego, CA: Academic Press.

Beutler, L. E., & Castonguay, L. G. (2006). The task force on empirically based principles of therapeutic change. In L. G. Castonguay & L. E. Beutler (Eds.), *Principles of therapeutic change that work: Integrating relationship, treatment, client, and therapist factors* (pp. 3–11). New York, NY: Oxford University Press.

Black, D. W., Kehrberg, L. D., Flumerfelt, D. L., & Schlosser, S. S. (1997). Characteristics of 36 subjects reporting compulsive sexual behavior. *American Journal of Psychiatry, 154*, 243–249.

Black, M. C., Basile, K. C., Breiding, M. J., Smith, S. G., Walters, M. L., Merrick, M. T., ... & Stevens, M. R. (2011). *The National Intimate Partner and Sexual Violence Survey (NISVS): 2010 summary report*. Atlanta, GA: National Center for Injury Prevention and Control, Centers for Disease Control and Prevention.

Borges, G., Nock, M., Haro Abad, J., Hwang, I., Sampson, N., Alonso, J., ... & Kessler, R. (2010). Twelve-month prevalence of and risk factors for suicide attempts in the World Health Organization World Mental Health Surveys. *Journal of Clinical Psychiatry, 71*(12), 1617–1628.

Braun-Harvey, D. (2011). *Sexual health in recovery: A professional counselor's manual.* New York, NY: Springer Publishing Company.

Brehm, J. W. (1966). *A theory of psychological reactance.* New York, NY: Academic Press.

Carnes, P. (2007). Understanding sexual addiction. In M. S. Tepper & A. F. Owens (Eds.), *Sexual health, volume 2: Physical foundations. Sex, love, and psychology* (pp. 356–363). Westport, CT: Praeger.

Carpenter, B., Reid, R., Garos, S., & Najavits, L. (2013). Personality comorbidity in treatment-seeking men with hypersexual disorder. *Sexual Addiction and Compulsivity, 20*, 79–90.

Centers for Disease Control and Prevention. (2009). *Effect of antiretroviral therapy on risk of sexual transmission of HIV infection and superinfection.* Retrieved from http://www.cdc.gov/hiv/pdf/prevention_art_factsheet.pdf

Centers for Disease Control and Prevention. (2013). Monitoring selected national HIV prevention and care objectives by using HIV surveillance data—United States and 6 U.S. dependent areas—2011. *HIV Surveillance Supplemental Report, 18*(5), 1–47. Retrieved from http://www.cdc.gov/hiv/pdf/2011_monitoring_hiv_indicators_hssr_final.pdf.

Chadwick Center for Children and Families. (2009). *Assessment-based treatment for traumatized children: A trauma assessment pathway (TAP)*. San Diego, CA. Retrieved from http://www.taptraining.net/documents/Master%20TAP-12-09.pdf.

Chughtai, Â. B., Sciullo, D. Khan, S. A., Rehman, H., Mohan, E., & Rehman, J. (2010). Etiology, diagnosis & management of hypersexuality: A review. *Internet Journal of Urology, 6*(2). doi:10.5580/1231

Clifford, D. B., & Ances, B. M. (2013). HIV-associated neurocognitive disorder. *The Lancet, 13*, 976–986.

Clipson, C. (2009). *Sexual attitudes and behavior inventory: Manual*. Unpublished manuscript.

Coleman, E. (2007). Sexual health: Definitions and construct development. In M. S. Tepper & A. F. Ownes (Eds.), *Sexual health volume 1: Psychological foundations* (pp. 1–15). Westport, CT: Praeger.

Coleman, E., Dwyer, S. M., Abel, G., Berner, W., Breiling, J., Eher, R., ... & Weiss, P. (2000). Standards of care for the treatment of adult sex offenders. *Journal of Psychology & Human Sexuality, 11*(3), 11–17.

Cossman, B. (2009). Sexual citizens: Freedom, vibrators, and belonging. In L. C. McClain, & J. L. Grossman (Eds.), *Gender equality: Dimensions of women's equal citizenship* (pp. 289–306). New York, NY: Cambridge University Press.

Cubitt, R., Starmer, C., & Sugden, R. (2004). Dynamic decisions under uncertainty: Some recent evidence from economics and psychology. In I. Brocas & J. D. Carrillo (Eds.), *The psychology of economic decisions. Vol 2: Reasons and choices* (pp. 81–107). Oxford, UK: Oxford University Press.

De Shazer, S., & Dolan, Y. (2012). *More than miracles: The state of the art of solution-focused brief therapy*. Binghamton, NY: Hawthorne Press.

DiClemente, C. C., & Prochaska, J. O. (1998). Toward a comprehensive, transtheoretical model of change: Stages of change and addictive behaviors. In W. R. Miller & N. Heather (Eds.), *Treating addictive behaviors* (2nd ed.). New York, NY: Plenum Press.

DiClemente, C. C., & Velasquez, M. M. (2002). Motivational interviewing and the stages of change. In W. R. Miller & Rollnick S. (Eds.), *Motivational interviewing: Preparing people for change* (Vol. 2, pp. 201–216). New York, NY: Guilford Press.

Dillard, J., & Shen, L. (2005). On the nature of reactance and its role in persuasive health communication. *Communication Monographs, 72*(2) , 144–168.

Dombrowski, L., Petrick, J., & Strauss, D. (2000). Rehabilitation treatment of sexuality issues due to acquired brain injury. *Rehabilitation Psychology, 45*, 299–309.

Edwards, W. M., Delmonico, D., & Griffin, E. (2011). *Cybersex unplugged: Finding sexual health in an electronic world*. CreateSpace Independent Publishing Platform.

Elliot, M., & Biever, L. (1996). Head injury and sexual dysfunction. *Brain Injury, 10*, 703–717.

Finlayson, A., Stealy, J., & Martin, P. (2001). The differential diagnosis of problematic hypersexuality. *Sexual Addiciton & Compulsivity, 8*, 241–251.

Frances A., & First, M. B. (2011). Paraphilia NOS, nonconsent: Not ready for the court-room. *Journal of American Academy of Psychiatry Law, 39*, 555–561.

Hilton, D. L. (2013). Pornography addiction—A supranormal stimulus considered in the context of neuroplasticity. *Socioaffective Neuroscience & Psychology, 3*, 197–211.

Kafka, M. (2010). Hypersexual disorder: A proposed diagnosis for *DSM-V*. *Archives of Sexual Behavior, 39*(2), 377–400.

Kafka, M. P., & Prentky, R. A. (1994). Preliminary observations of *DSM-III–R* Axis I comorbidity in men with paraphilias and paraphilia-related disorders. *Journal of Clinical Psychiatry, 55*, 481–487.

Kaplan, M. S., & Krueger, R. B. (2010). Diagnosis, assessment, and treatment of hyper-sexuality. *Journal of Sex Research, 47*(2–3), 181–198.

Klein, M. (2012). *America's war on sex: The continuing attack on law, lust and liberty* (2nd ed.). Santa Barbara, CA: Praeger.

Lloyd, M., Raymond, N. C., Miner, M. H., & Coleman, E. (2007). Borderline person-ality traits in individuals with compulsive sexual behavior. *Sexual Addiction & Compulsivity, 14*(3), 187–206.

Loewenstein, G., & O'Donoghue, T. (2007). *The heat of the moment: Modeling interac-tions between affect and deliberation.* Unpublished manuscript. Retrieved from http://www.academia.edu/2840116/The_heat_of_the_moment_Modeling_interactions_between_affect_and_deliberation.

Lussier, P., & Blokland, A. (2013). The adolescence-adulthood transition and Robin's continuity paradox: Criminal career patterns of juvenile and adult sex offenders in a prospective longitudinal birth cohort study. *Journal of Criminal Justice, 42*(2), 153–163.

Lussier, P., & Cale, J. (2013). Beyond sexual recidivism: A review of the sexual criminal career parameters of adult sex offenders, *Aggression and Violent Behavior, 18*(5), 445–457.

Mathesius, J., & Lussier, P. (2013). The successful onset of sex offending: Determining the correlates of actual and official onset of sex offending, *Journal of Criminal Justice, 42*(2), 134–144.

McEwen, B. (2000). Allostasis and allostatic load: Implications for neuropsychophar-macology. *Neuropsychopharmacology, 22*(2), 108–124.

McEwen, B., & Seeman, T. (2009). *Allostatic load and allostasis.* Retrieved September 10, 2014, from http://www.macses.ucsf.edu/research/allostatic/allostatic.php.

McHugh, M. C., & Frieze, I. H. (2006). Intimate partner violence: New Directions. *Annals of the New York Academy of Sciences, 1087*, 121–141.

McHugh, M. C., Livingston, N. A., & Ford, A. (2005). A postmodern approach to women's use of violence: Developing multiple and complex conceptualizations. *Psychology of Women Quarterly, 29*, 323–336.

Meloy, J. R. (1998). *The psychology of stalking: Clinical and forensic perspectives.* New York, NY: Academic Press.

Meloy, J. R., & Fisher, H. (2005). Some thoughts on the neurobiology of stalking. *Journal of Forensic Sciences, 50*(6), 1472–1480.

Meloy, J. R., & Gothard, S. (1995). Demographic and clinical comparison of obsessional followers and offenders with mental disorders. *American Journal of Psychiatry, 152*(2), 258–263.

Metcalfe, J., & Mischel, W. (1999). A hot/cool system analysis of delay of gratification: Dynamics of willpower. *Psychological Review, 106*, 3–19.

Meuhlenhard, C., & Peterson, Z. (2004). Conceptualizing sexual violence: Socially acceptable coercion and other controversies. In A. Miller (Ed.), *The social psychology of good and evil* (pp. 240–268). New York, NY: Guilford Press.

Miccio-Fonseca, L. C., & Rasmussen, L. (2011). A concise review on validated risk assessment tools for sexually abusive youth. *Sexual Offender Treatment, 6, 2.*

Miller, W. R., & Rollnick, S. (2002). *Motivational interviewing: Preparing people for change.* New York, NY: Guilford Press.

Miller, W. R., & Rollnick, S. (2013). *Motivational interviewing: Helping people change* (3rd ed.). New York, NY: Guilford Press.

Money, J. (1999). *The lovemap guidebook: A definitive statement.* New York, NY: Continuum.

Moser, C. (2011). Yet another paraphilia definitions fails. *Archives of Sexual Behavior, 40,* 483–485.

Mullen, P. E., Pathe, M., Purcell, R., & Stuart, G. W. (1999). A study of stalkers. *American Journal of Psychiatry, 156,* 1244–1249.

Ortmann, D. M., & Sprott, R. (2013). *Sexual outsiders: Understanding BDSM and communities.* Plymouth, MA: Rowman & Littlefield.

Parson, J., Grov, C., & Golub, S. A. (2012). Sexual compulsivity, co-occurring psychosocial health problems, and HIV risk among gay and bisexual men: Further evidence of a syndemic. *American Journal of Public Health, 102*(1), 156–162.

Prochaska, J. O., Norcross, J. C., & DiClemente, C. C. (1994). *Changing for good.* New York, NY: William Morrow.

Rabkin, J. G. (2008). HIV and depression: 2008 review and update. *Current HIV/AIDS Report, 5,* 163–171.

Rasmussen, L. A., & Miccio-Fonseca, L. C. (2007). Paradigm shift: Implementing MEGA, a new tool proposed to define and assess sexually abusive dynamics in youth ages 19 and under. *Journal of Child Sexual Abuse, 16*(1), 85–106.

Raymond, N. C., Coleman, E., & Miner, M. H. (2003). Psychiatric comorbidity and compulsive/impulsive traits in compulsive sexual behavior. *Comprehensive Psychiatry, 44*(5), 370–380.

Reid, R. C. (2007). Assessing reading to change among clients seeking help for hypersexual behavior. *Sexual Addiction & Compulsivity, 14,* 167–186.

Reid, R. C. (2013). Management perspective: Perspectives on the assessment and treatment of adult ADHD in hypersexual men. *Neuropsychiatry, 3*(3), 295–308.

Reid, R. C., & Carpenter, B. N. (2009). Exploring relationships of psychopathology in hypersexual patients using the MMPI-2. *Journal of Sex & Marital Therapy, 35*(4), 294–310.

Reid, R. C., Carpenter, B. N., Gilliland, R., & Karim, R. (2011). Problems of self-concept in a patient sample of hypersexual men with attention-deficit disorder. *Journal of Addiction Medicine, 5*(2), 134–140.

Reid, R. C., Carpenter, B. N., & Lloyd, T. Q. (2009). Assessing psychological symptom patterns of patients seeking help for hypersexual behavior. *Sexual and Relationship Therapy, 24*(1), 47–64.

Repetti, R. L. (2011). Allostatic processes in the family. *Development and Psychopathology, 23,* 921–938.

Rotello, G. (1997). *Sexual ecology: The birth of AIDS and the destiny of gay men.* New York, NY: E. P. Dutton.

Schultz, K., Hook, J. N., Davis, D. E., Penberthy, J. K., & Reid, R. C. (2014). Non-paraphilic hypersexual behavior and depressive symptoms: A meta-analytic review of the literature. *Journal of Sex and Marital Therapy, 40*(6), 477–487.

Skoler, G. (1998). The archetypes and psychodynamics of stalking. In J. R. Meloy (Ed.), *The psychology of stalking: Clinical and forensic perspectives.* New York, NY: Academic Press.

Staemmler, F. (2012). *Empathy in psychotherapy: How therapists and clients understand each other.* New York, NY: Springer Publishing Company.

Steele, V., Staley, C., Fong, T., & Prause, N. (2013). Sexual desire, not hypersexuality, is related to neurophysiological responses elicited by sexual images. *Socioaffective Neuroscience & Psychology, 3,* 20770.

Sterling, P., & Eyer, J. (1988). Allostasis: A new paradigm to explain arousal pathology. In S. Fisher & J. Reason (Eds.), *Handbook of life stress, cognition and health.* New York, NY: John Wiley.

Sutton, J. (2007). *Healing the hurt within: Understand self-injury and self-harm, and heal the emotional wounds.* Oxford, UK: How to Books, Ltd.

Websdale, N. (2000). *Lethality assessment tools: A critical analysis.* Harrisburg, PA: VAWnet, a project of the National Resource Center on Domestic Violence/ Pennsylvania Coalition Against Domestic Violence. Retrieved February 18, 2014, from http://www.vawnet.org

Wertheimer, A. (2003). *Consent in sexual relations.* Cambridge, UK: Cambridge University Press.

Wolfe, B. E. (2001). A message to assimilative integrationists: It's time to become accommodative integrationists: A commentary. *Journal of Psychotherapy Integration, 11*(1), 123–131.

Wolverton, M. (2013, September/October). Chasing slumber. *Psychology Today,* pp. 68–77.

World Association for Sexual Health. (2008). *Sexual health for the millennium. A declaration and technical document.* Minneapolis, MN: World Association for Sexual Health.

Yeagley, E., Hickok, A., & Bauermeister, J. A. (2014). Hypersexual behavior and HIV sex risk among young gay and bisexual men. *Journal of Sex Research, 51*(8), 1–11.

CHAPTER SIX

ASSESSMENT—INFORMATION GATHERING

The first step in fostering intentional change is to become conscious of the self-defeating defenses that get in our way.
—Prochaska, Norcross, and DiClemente

The OCSB (Out of Control Sexual Behavior) Assessment Plan provides an opportunity to deliberately and comprehensively examine the worries and fears surrounding a client's sexual world. We hope reading about the Assessment Plan presents also an opportunity for you to consider your reactions and thoughts about facilitating a detailed OCSB sexual health conversation. Some readers may be looking for an alternative to their existing methods for responding to clients concerned about their out of control sexual experiences. Others may read this description of the OCSB assessment process looking for specific elements to integrate into their current OCSB assessment practices. We invite you to reflect on your experiences as we move from describing OCSB theory to outlining specific clinical application of the OCSB sexual health model. An OCSB assessment offers a unique situation for both therapist and client to have a sexual health conversation. How often do we, not to mention our clients, take the time to consider and articulate our own personal visions of sexual health? Most therapists have experienced their own psychotherapy or completed a range of psychological or personality tests in their personal mental health care or throughout their professional training and career. But the percentage of readers who have had another professional lead them through an intentional process for assessing their own sexual health is likely significantly smaller. As such, we have suggestions for you that are not dissimilar to what we would recommend for OCSB clients beginning their assessment. Delay conclusions about the OCSB assessment protocol conventions until you have completed the section. Similarly, we ask you to read the assessment chapters with an open mind that is not limited by a predetermined opinion or perspective. Approach this chapter as a part of a larger process of determining whether our sexual health approach interests you. Notice how we apply our OCSB Model and introduce sexual health principles to our clients. Just as we inform our clients that the assessment is designed to help them envision how to align their sexual behavior with their values, perhaps you can approach these chapters as an opportunity to evaluate interest in implementing a sexual health assessment approach that is consistent with your overall theory and psychotherapy methods.

OCSB ASSESSMENT PREPARATION

Current psychotherapy education, clinical training, and sexual behavior treatment methods poorly integrate sexual health knowledge into their clinical conceptualizations and psychotherapy. The OCSB assessment relies on therapists who are prepared to enter into an intentional sexual health conversation to discuss and confidently explore how men balance deliberation about their sexual behavior with their sexual activation. The assessment requires more of therapists than just collecting information; it necessitates an ability to move between historical events and the processing of here-and-now emotions that surface in the conversation. This process presents not only a rich opportunity for therapeutic dialogue that explores client activations, it also prepares clients for OCSB treatment, which relies on the therapeutic relationship. J. K. Edwards and Bess (1998) argue that applying what therapists have learned through their psychotherapy education and training has limited usefulness unless they are aware of who they are "as a person in the room with the client" (p. 89). Slade (2000) advocates that therapists should be aware of their attachment style to better understand their patient interactions so as to facilitate therapeutic alliance. Because of the use-of-self techniques that are recommended in the OCSB assessment, we encourage counselors to establish a self-reflection process to manage countertransference that may arise during sexual health conversations. Therapists who choose to walk their clients through an OCSB assessment and want to integrate this use-of-self style will need to identify their personal qualities, life events, and sexual standards that enhance rapport building and, most important, unknowingly hinder their ability to suspend judgmental responses and sustain objective listening and responding. In the OCSB assessment, therapists gather detailed information about men's sexual activities and situations that may generate negative emotional reactions. Much like a trauma specialist must prepare to manage emotions that surface when listening to clients disclose painful events, OCSB therapists must develop skills to manage their activated emotions and thoughts while listening to men disclose their sexual activities, values, motivations, and injurious actions. Sexual activities that men discuss in OCSB assessment may be unfamiliar or include unconventional elements for arousal, pleasure, and meaning. The unfamiliar and unconventional may challenge therapists' beliefs about healthy or normative sex. Some sexual interests or turn-ons may generate feelings of disgust, arousal, or envy. Supervision, sex therapy training, and one's own therapy prepare therapists to become familiar with these aspects of themselves and develop a plan to manage their countertransference when it inevitably arises. Therapists are not fully aware of all the areas of themselves that may undermine objectivity, damage rapport, or reinforce the client's negative self-concept. Psychotherapists can improve sexual health conversation skills by attending ongoing case consultation and sex therapy continuing education that focuses on the therapist's attitudes and values and addresses unrealistic expectations of oneself in doing work with men and OCSB.

Not unlike the early years of drug and alcohol addiction treatment, many pioneers in sexual addiction treatment were inspired to become treatment professionals after their own recovery from their OCSB. These professionals could establish and maintain rapport through a shared personal experience in sexual behavior recovery. An OCSB assessment does not share the same recovery parallel for fostering rapport between therapist and client. However, a parallel can exist when therapists realize that their own personal vision for sexual health faces similar societal values and pressures that influence their client's sexual health. Therapists can find a deep well of empathy for clients in an OCSB assessment if they access their own experiences in discussing, developing, and asserting their sexual health vision.

The multisession OCSB assessment determines whether to recommend treatment and, if so, to prepare men to enter into combined individual and group OCSB therapy. The assessment process constructs a unique clinical picture for discerning clinical judgments, diagnostic distinctions, behavioral patterns, and treatment recommendations. The OCSB Unique

Clinical Picture presents a multidimensional understanding of the client's case that informs treatment decisions (Chadwick Center for Child and Families, 2009). It comprises the details of the client's sexual symptoms and the factors that influence the deliberative/affective interaction, including the screening criteria and the competing motivations.

The OCSB Assessment Plan (Figure 6.1) visually represents both the information gathering and treatment elements of the OCSB assessment. The information-gathering portion is a semistructured interview conducted in tandem with standardized measures that provide both subjective and objective clinical information. The OCSB assessment is not a hierarchical system in which the therapist collects symptom information and relevant personal history to identify the problem and prescribe a remedy to the client. Integrating the stages of readiness for change and motivational enhancement techniques places the therapist in a role that is more like a guide, someone who is a skillful listener who offers

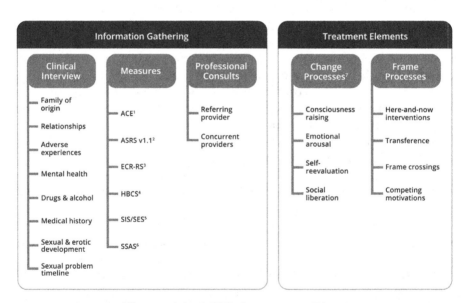

Figure 6.1 *OCSB Assessment Plan.*

[1] Adverse Childhood Experiences Study questionnaire (Felitti et al., 1998).
[2] Adult ADHD Self-Report Scale (Reid, Garos, & Fong, 2012).
[3] The Relationship Structures Questionnaire (Fraley, Niederthal, Marks, Brumbaugh, & Vicary, 2006).
[4] Hypersexual Behavior Consequences Scale (Reid et al., 2012).
[5] The Sexual Inhibition and Sexual Excitation Scales (Janssen, Vorst, Finn, & Bancroft, 2002).
[6] Sexual Symptom Assessment Scale (Raymond, Lloyd, Miner, & Kim, 2007).
[7] Prochaska, Norcross, and DiClemente (2006).

expertise when needed (Miller & Rollnick, 2013). A strength of motivational interviewing (MI) is the collaborative and conversational spirit it fosters, which strengthens motivation and commitment to change (Miller & Rollnick, 2013). Accordingly, we designed our assessment as a structured collaboration that infuses the essence of MI's underlying principles. How we gather information develops the OCSB Unique Clinical Picture *and* motivates behavioral change. The assessment helps clients begin to understand their contradictory sexual urges, thoughts, and behaviors within an in-session structure that elicits motivation to change sexual health. The therapist moves between gathering clinical information and in-the-moment interventions that raise self-awareness, process emotional activation, and develop client self-discrepancies. Men's affective–deliberative interaction is revealed during the assessment sessions as they recount their sexual stories and complete the measures. Similar to MI teachings, "the interview seeks to create a positive interpersonal atmosphere that is conducive to change but not coercive" (Miller & Rollnick, 2013, p. 15). The assessment is an interactive space for clients to honestly consider the costs and benefits of sexual behavior change within a clinical relationship that minimizes the external pressure for immediate change (e.g., social norms, partner expectations, religious values) while looking closely at the consequences of the clients' sexual behaviors.

For example, at the first assessment appointment, a client may open the meeting by saying, "I paid for sex right after our first appointment." "I went online and hooked up with someone last night." When a client reports engaging in problematic sexual behavior, the therapist may utilize a person-centered here-and-now intervention, such as asking about the client's choice to be transparent: "What was it like for you to come here today and tell me about this?" "How did you make the decision to mention this in our assessment today?" "How often do you tell people about this sexual behavior, like you just told me?" The focus for this moment is to set the stage for a semistructured interview, which lets the client know we are interested in obtaining information as well as talking about what is happening right now. The therapist may follow up this exchange by reaffirming that the OCSB assessment is not a time for making commitments to change, but is rather a space to be curious about all the factors related to his OCSB and his experience in the assessment process.

The assessment meetings are a time for men to honestly discuss their sexual values and relational commitment discrepancies as they learn to talk openly about their sexual pleasures. We frame the assessment as a rare opportunity to explore all motivations that influenced their sexual behaviors and choices without fear of an act-centered values system steering the conversation. In this way, the client gradually becomes a specialist in his sexuality, which empowers him to formulate answers to his sexual health problems. Together, in a structured collaboration, men find the solutions to their sexual health problems.

In this section, we outline specific therapist interaction strategies to gather information designed to enhance client motivation and resources for change. Each assessment component discerns an aspect of the client's internal experience to clarify the underlying competing motivations affecting his sexual health. After reviewing the various measures in conjunction with the clinical interview, we discuss the format, structure, and treatment elements of the OCSB assessment. The clinical questions outlined in Chapter 4 guide the assessment content and process.

Self-Regulation:
1. How are OCSB symptoms related to self-regulation ingredients?
2. How are sexual urges, thoughts, or behaviors solutions to regulating uncomfortable activation?
3. Are the OCSB symptoms an outcome of hyper/hypoactivated states?
4. How does the client regulate sexual activation?

Attachment Regulation:
1. How do the OCSB symptoms reflect the client's attachment style?
2. How does the client maintain relationship agreements?
3. Does the client have traits of sexual narcissism?

Sexual and Erotic Conflicts:
1. Are the OCSB symptoms related to sexual or erotic conflicts that clients have with themselves?
2. Are the OCSB symptoms related to sexual or erotic conflicts that clients have with others?
3. Does the client exhibit fixed or unconventional arousal patterns?

INFORMATION GATHERING: MEASURES

Adverse Childhood Experiences Scale

The Adverse Childhood Experiences (ACE) study is groundbreaking research that investigated the association between childhood maltreatment and adult health and well-being (Felitti et al., 1998). The ACE study, sometimes referred to as the most important public health study you never heard of (Stevens, 2012), is composed of a health score based on five areas of personal abuse and neglect and five areas of adverse household experiences that occur prior to a child's 18th birthday. The original ACE study sample comprised about 17,000 mostly middle-class, working adults who were Kaiser Permanente enrollees in San Diego, California. An ACE score (from 0 to 10) is used to tally childhood abuse, neglect, and exposure to other traumatic stressors during childhood. The higher the ACE score, the greater the risk for a wide range of health problems that increase in strength and frequency. In the original research, only one in three had a zero or "no ACE." One in 10 had a score of four or more. Since 1998, the ACE study has progressively uncovered a stunningly high correlation between adverse childhood experiences and chronic adult diseases and social and emotional problems (Anda et al., 2006). An ACE score of 4 or more is where serious health, social, and mental health consequences emerge. Dr. Jeffrey Brenner, the 2013 MacArthur Foundation "Genius Grant" winner, believes ACE scores should become as important a vital sign as blood pressure, height, and weight (Brenner, 2014). All clients who participate in an OCSB assessment determine their ACE score.

ACE Health Problems and the OCSB Model

The ACE study lists 17 different health problems that research has correlated with ACE scores greater than or equal to 4. We organized the 17 ACE-related health problems within our screening criteria, excluding the clinical distinctions of client motivation and nonconsensual sex and added a sexual health domain.

Physical Safety:
- Risk for intimate partner violence
- Suicide attempts

Physical Health:
- Health-related quality of life
- Chronic obstructive pulmonary disease (COPD)
- Liver disease
- Ischemic heart disease (IHD)

Mental Health:
- Depression

Relationship With Drugs and Alcohol:
- Alcoholism and alcohol abuse
- Illicit drug use

- Early initiation of smoking
- Smoking

Sexual Health:
- Multiple sexual partners
- Sexually transmitted diseases (STDs)
- Early initiation of sexual activity
- Adolescent pregnancy
- Fetal death

Two thirds of ACE study participants had at least one adverse experience, which brings into focus just how common these events may be among America's children. The ACE study linked many common social problems and major chronic illnesses with adverse childhood experiences. The correlation between multiple early-life stressors with adult onset of disease, mental illness, and persistent social ills suggests a contextual perspective that the risk for diseases increases when a person spends the first 18 years of life coping with a mixture of early life adverse experiences.

Research on childhood brain development suggests that during exposure to severe and chronic adverse events, the brain releases hormones in response to intense fear or danger. Prolonged exposure to these hormones may physically damage the brain. These neurobiological mechanisms are activated to respond to immediate and serious threats. Once the threat is resolved, these mechanisms usually return to a restful state. This is the allostatic process for returning the brain to the equilibrium of homeostasis. When this allostatic process is called on early and often, it wears out and harms the developing child's brain. The evidence suggests that children's brains are overtaxed when they must constantly rely on their emergency response system (Repetti, Robles, & Reynolds, 2011).

Brain development research and the ACE study support the concept that allostatic load may lead to a fatigued and impaired neurological mechanism. Framing observable maladaptive coping behaviors as a fatigued neurological system stemming from persistently taxed and insufficient allostatic resources provides an alternative narrative for understanding physical and mental health problems. Behavioral coping strategies, such as overeating, drinking, smoking, drug abuse, sexual activity, high-risk activities/sports, and excessive work and overachievement, are found among men and women in every aspect of health care (Stevens, 2012). Perhaps these behavioral patterns are the problematic solutions of a tired brain seeking solace and homeostasis. Repeated adverse childhood experiences may impair reliable homeostasis processes and lead to problematic, but effective, behavioral solutions to restore the affective–deliberative balance. Specific to OCSB, sexual behavior can be a short-term fix for a distressed body and fuel-deprived brain that can decrease persistent and chronic states of anxiety, fear, shame, demoralization, despair, and isolation. Therefore, we propose out of control sexual thoughts, urges, and behaviors may be linked to early-life coping strategies against real and frequent adverse childhood experiences that shaped their deliberative/affective interaction. Beginning the OCSB assessment with the ACE measure sets the stage for a systematic assessment of sexual behavior functionality.

Administering the ACE Study Questionnaire

Clients are requested to complete the ACE measure at the end of the screening interview before returning for their first assessment appointment. We provide a brief synopsis of the ACE measure and indicate that we believe everyone should know his or her score as part of his or her basic health information. We instruct clients to download the form from our websites or ACEStudy.org. This is the first of many interventions in the assessment process that help us understand how clients meet their agreements and the extent of their motivations for change. The spirit of the OCSB assessment is focused less on whether the client completes the ACE measure and more on making sense of the mental states and affective experiences involved in approaching the task. Not meeting this initial assessment agreement introduces an opportunity to explore the client's thinking process and defenses against self-observation and uncomfortable activation. Curiosity allows us to uncover the motivations that compete against change and result in patterns of avoidance or dissociative defenses. As this is an assessment, we maintain a curious stance to avoid premature interpretations and conclusions.

If the client has either not completed the ACE or left it at home, provide a copy and complete each item together in the session. Clients read each item out loud one at a time and choose "yes" or "no." The reasoning behind reading each item aloud is to give the clients a more embodied experience with their thoughts than completing the form silently would provide. Pacing the exercise is important to prevent the clients from emotional flooding, avoiding thoughtful examination of their history, or misattunement to nuanced facial expressions. Empower the clients to control the pace and depth of the interview by letting them know that they can pause after any item to clarify meaning, to discuss something in more detail, or to regulate their affect. The therapist can also slow the discussion to clarify meaning, examine thresholds that determined a *yes* or *no*, as well as process the emotions experienced while describing these events. It is not necessary to get through all items in one appointment. We use the ACE as a process to learn about the impact of adverse childhood experiences and identify important historic events relevant to childhood development. The ACE questions ascertain information about significant childhood events and chronically stressful family environments described with specific behavioral frequency, consequences, feelings, and thoughts.

The client reads aloud:

Did a parent or other adult in the household often or very often...
Swear at you, insult you, put you down, or humiliate you? or
Act in a way that made you afraid that you might be physically hurt?
If yes to either or both, enter 1 _____

Some clients may have few experiences speaking about abusive behaviors out loud without pejorative, judgmental, or vague language. "They beat the shit out of me"; "He was so mean, he hit me with anything he could get his hands on"; "I just lay there and took it" may be more familiar than the dry, clear, measured detail of the ACE. Reading each sentence aloud familiarizes clients to new words and perspectives that suspend judgment but clearly describes painful experiences in the context of a supportive OCSB assessment relationship.

If the answer is *no* to the first item, consider asking if the question were worded differently, would the answer be *yes*? For example, "Did these behaviors happen sometimes or even just once?" For the purposes of the ACE, score the answer as a *no*, but for the purpose of the assessment, this nuanced inquiry is useful for establishing the structured informality of going between rating a specific item on a measure to a conversation about the client's history. If he answered *yes*, inquire as to which items/words allowed him to answer *yes*. Have him identify which frequency dimension *often* or *very often* and the specific behaviors he endorses. "I was always afraid of my dad" or "My mom used to humiliate me, calling me her girly boy when I cried." When men immediately say *yes*, then return to discussing the dimension of *often* or *very often*. Use the exact language of the item to ascertain the perspective of the client as to what *often* or *very often* means to him.

Men are asked to explore their perceptions about the frequency of specific behavior throughout OCSB assessment and treatment. Taking the time to explore their calculations (deliberative system) during highly activated states is important for developing this integral OCSB treatment skill. Going through each item in the same routine provides excellent early exposure to this learning skill. Each ACE item works well for discussing basic psychosocial history details in a conversational manner and can be easily integrated into a therapist's current psychosocial assessment process. An ACE score conversation can be easily integrated into a therapist's current psychosocial assessment process.

Over the years we have seen ACE scores range from 0 to 9. We also find that clients access a greater degree of empathy for their childhood circumstances and their individual coping responses to adverse childhood events in a discussion format rather than an unprocessed reporting of the total score. The lack of the labels like "trauma," "abuse," "neglect," and "dysfunction" within the ACE items is consistent with our OCSB assessment approach to sexual health dialogue. Words like "trauma," "abuse," and "neglect" are conclusions and judgments with unclear thresholds that can be easily dismissed by clients who are not ready to face the harmful realities of their childhood. Instead, each ACE item offers a behavioral description. The situations and feelings are described solely from the clients' perspective. Additionally, clients may be defended against thinking of their parents as abusers or themselves as victims. Using clear behavioral descriptions without conclusive language or colloquial phrases pertaining to family violence, mental illness, or parental neglect creates a constructive space for reflection on these adverse childhood experiences.

It is important for the therapist to use the exact ACE phrases and words. This is not the time to insert different labels that summarize information rather than simply describe events. For example, the therapist is advised to inquire, "Who used street drugs in your home when you were a child?" "What kind of street drugs were you aware they were using?" rather than asking, "Which household member was addicted to drugs?" Repeating the language the client endorsed from the ACE can prevent a stage-discrepant intervention.

This conversational ACE discussion integrates the therapist's clinical style and theory of practice while relying on the ACE protocol to expose clients to the therapist's relational style for establishing rapport. The ACE interview is also an early glimpse into a client's self-regulation and attachment style. When clients describe their childhood adverse events, therapists can make note of the clients' observable defenses that regulate their emotions. Is there a detached, disengaged, minimizing, and even dismissive tone to some discussion? "My mother put up with a lot of crap, what else is new?" "My dad was an imbecile, he still is." "I got outta there as soon as I could." "I am not just another whiney adult who had it so bad." "My wife thinks you're going to feel sorry for me and just excuse what I did to her."

Some clients may feel guilt and shame when discussing parental behaviors that they think betray family privacy. Others might hold a great deal of self-blame and have a distorted perception of their culpability for their family dynamics. "I had sex with my dad so he would leave my other sisters alone." "One time I took a Christmas present and threw it at him [stepfather] so he would stop hitting my mom." Therapists will need to be prepared to guide men to regulate their activated emotions in response to each item. Here-and-now interactions that invite the clients to name their feelings, identify their thoughts, and describe their process while discussing their ACE score is well within the frame of the assessment agreement.

When all 10 areas have been reviewed, we ask the clients to total their score and to say the number. It may seem like a trivial detail, but announcing the ACE score is important. Much like speaking the precise degree of your fever, the actual number matters. Clients sometime stare at the sheet of paper and go back to specific memories, mentally leaving the room. In their minds, they often return to a place they have not revisited for quite a while. When the client comes back to the present moment, the therapist can gently ask, "Where did you just go?" This is an opportunity for the client to learn how the therapist responds to a break in contact. For some men this may be an uncomfortable moment to receive caring attention exemplified by a curious question or gentle inquiry without a demand for detail. This may be an unfamiliar experience for some men. This brief process inquiry is an early example of examining a client's attachment capacity through here-and-now moments in the assessment.

The ACE score of 0 to 10 presents an opportunity for psychoeducation feedback. A low ACE score, below 3, is less common among the men in our OCSB treatment program. We let them know that this is only one health measure and that men with low ACE scores may have other dimensions that significantly contribute to their OCSB. We discuss the ACE research outcomes and recommend considering preventative measures to reduce the risk of adult health consequences for men who score above 3.

Sexual Symptom Assessment Scale

The Sexual Symptom Assessment Scale (SSAS) is a useful tool and an excellent fit for the OCSB assessment process. It is a 12-item, self-report scale developed to measure the changes in compulsive sexual behavior symptoms over time (Raymond et al., 2007). Men complete the SSAS weekly throughout the assessment in a manner that is analogous to having one's blood pressure checked prior to each visit to the doctor. The SSAS measures the client's perception of his current sexual urges, thoughts, behaviors, and consequences and focuses on recent experiences without listing specific sexual acts (e.g., attending strip clubs, viewing online sexual imagery, paying for sex, masturbation practices). We prefer that clients identify the sexual behaviors that they would like to change based on their motivation or what they determine as problematic, not based on a list of sexual behaviors that are presumed to be problematic.

SSAS items ask men to specifically rate differentiated components of their OCSB. Each week men rate their perceptions of intensity, frequency, regulation, and cumulative time spent on "problematic sexual behaviors" (Raymond et al., 2007, p. 27). The SSAS is distinctive because it measures both subjective and objective symptoms of problematic sexual behavior (Hook, Hook, Davis, Worthington, & Penberthy, 2010). The SSAS is most strongly correlated with scales that measure current ability to control sexual impulses (Raymond et al., 2007). In a review of 17 measures pertaining to sexual addiction, Hook et al. (2010) found promise among several measures, including the SSAS. (They did caution, however, that a clinician's ability to determine diagnosis and prognosis with standardized measures is hampered by "weak theory" that does not precisely identify sexual addiction [p. 256].)

The SSAS combines the intensity and severity of the client's emotional experiences with observable frequency and duration of sexual urges, thoughts, and behaviors associated with each man's specific sexual concerns. Additionally, the weekly practice of deconstructing OCSB into sexual urges, thoughts, and behaviors strengthens observational skills so men can better understand their sexual behavior in a manner congruent with the dual-process model. It's helpful for men to repeatedly answer clinical questions that ask them to rate changes in self-regulation and willpower capacities through the practice of self-monitoring. The weekly ratings of urges, thoughts, and behavior, over time, reveal the competing motivations that negatively impact their sexual regulation.

Administering the SSAS

Clients download the measure from our websites and bring the completed form to each weekly assessment appointment. We review the four sub-scales of the measure along with the total score. As with the ACE survey, the client process for completing or not completing the SSAS offers important information about motivation and ability to honor commitments.

Clients first define the SSAS phrase *problematic sexual behaviors* based on the sexual behaviors that they believe are creating negative consequences in their lives. As the therapist introduces the sexual health principles, the men begin to identify and evaluate their sexual health behavior in terms of exploitation, dishonesty, behavior incongruent with emerging values, sexual pleasure, as well as placing themselves at risk for a range of health-related consequences. The SSAS offers a weekly opportunity to increase sexual health self-observation capacity in tandem with building a capacity for discussing the various components of OCSB.

In the following section, we discuss how we work with each sub-scale in the measure. Figure 6.2 is the OCSB-adapted version of the SSAS.

THE SEXUAL SYMPTOM ASSESSMENT SCALE

The following questionnaire is aimed at evaluating problematic sexual behaviors **DURING THE PAST SEVEN DAYS**. Please read the questions carefully before you answer.

1. **If you had urges to engage in problematic sexual behaviors, on average, how strong were your urges? Please circle the most appropriate number:**

None	Mild	Moderate	Severe	Extreme
0	1	2	3	4

2. **How many times did you experience urges to engage in problematic sexual behaviors? Please circle the most appropriate number:**

None	Once	2 to 3 times	Several to many	Constant to near constant
0	1	2	3	4

3. **How many hours (add up hours) were you preoccupied with your urges to engage in problematic sexual behaviors? Please circle the most appropriate number:**

None	1 hr or less	1 to 7 hrs	7 to 21 hrs	+21 hrs
0	1	2	3	4

4. **How much were you able to control your urges? Please circle the most appropriate number:**

Completely	Much	Moderate	Minimal	No control
0	1	2	3	4

5. **How often did thoughts about engaging in problematic sexual behaviors come up? Please circle the most appropriate number:**

None	Once	2 to 3 times	Several to many	Constant to near constant
0	1	2	3	4

6. **Approximately how many hours (add up hours) did you spend thinking about engaging in problematic sexual behaviors? Please circle the most appropriate number:**

None	1 hr or less	1 to 7 hrs	7 to 21 hrs	+21 hrs
0	1	2	3	4

Figure 6.2 *Sexual Symptom Assessment Scale.*
OCSB-adapted version.

7. How much were you able to control your thoughts of problematic sexual behaviors? Please circle the most appropriate number:

Completely	Much	Moderate	Minimal	No control
0	1	2	3	4

8. Approximately how much total time did you spend engaging in problematic sexual behaviors? Please circle the most appropriate number:

None	1 hr or less	1 to 7 hrs	7 to 21 hrs	+21 hrs
0	1	2	3	4

9. On average, how much anticipatory tension and/or excitement did you have *shortly before* you engaged in problematic sexual behaviors? If you did not actually engage in such behaviors, please estimate how much tension and/or excitement you believe you would have experienced if you had engaged in problematic sexual behaviors. Please circle the most appropriate number:

None	Mild	Moderate	Severe	Extreme
0	1	2	3	4

10. On average, how much excitement and pleasure did you feel when you engaged in problematic sexual behaviors? If you did not actually engage in such behaviors, please estimate how much excitement and pleasure you would have experienced if you had. Please circle the most appropriate number:

None	Mild	Moderate	Severe	Extreme
0	1	2	3	4

11. How much emotional distress (mental pain or anguish, shame, guilt, embarrassment) has your problematic sexual behavior caused you? Please circle the most appropriate number:

None	Mild	Moderate	Severe	Extreme
0	1	2	3	4

12. How much personal trouble (relationship, financial, legal, job, medical, or health) has your problematic sexual behavior caused you? Please circle the most appropriate number:

None	Mild	Moderate	Severe	Extreme
0	1	2	3	4

Figure 6.2 *(continued)*

SSAS Subscale: Sexual Urges

---

1. **If you had urges to engage in problematic sexual behaviors, on average, how strong were your urges? Please circle the most appropriate number:**

None	Mild	Moderate	Severe	Extreme
0	1	2	3	4

2. **How many times did you experience urges to engage in problematic sexual behaviors? Please circle the most appropriate number:**

None	Once	2 to 3 times	Several to many	Constant to near constant
0	1	2	3	4

3. **How many hours (add up hours) were you preoccupied with your urges to engage in problematic sexual behaviors? Please circle the most appropriate number:**

None	1 hr or less	1 to 7 hrs	7 to 21 hrs	+21 hrs
0	1	2	3	4

4. **How much were you able to control your urges? Please circle the most appropriate number:**

Completely	Much	Moderate	Minimal	No control
0	1	2	3	4

Sexual Urges, the first of the four subscales, are understood as the physiological activation referred to as sexual impulse, drive, or excitation. It is an embodied sense of action, movement, and, at times, is an intrusive drive to take an action. Monitoring and rating urges connected to each problematic sexual behavior are important for changing the felt sense of "being out of control." Even with this description of an urge, we still do not know what each client feels when he endorses these SSAS items, nor how an urge motivates sexual behavior. Are the sexual urges related to their sex drive, a response from an erotic stimulus, or desire for sexual connection? Did the urge precede a sexual behavior and thought or did it follow them? Were the sexual urges connected or unrelated to the immediate moment in which the urge was most intensely felt? The urge subscale items clarify these distinctions by combining the client self-rating with his in-session discussion.

The sexual urge subscale asks clients to subjectively rate the strength of their recent urges and to separately rate their ability to control these urges. The subscale measures the frequency of urges (of various intensities) and the time spent managing various urge-state intensities. In the first review of each SSAS item, it is important to ask clients to describe their urges, no matter how low they score all four items. Take time to slowly unpack the clients' reflective understanding of their embodied senses associated with urge states. Allow clients to carefully contemplate each question. They may be less confident when asked to describe their own activation (affective system) than they are with talking about sexual situations or offering a judgment (deliberative system). If they are unsure about how to discuss an urge, direct them to observe the sensations in their bodies such as heart rate, breath, muscle tension, or energy states. Orient the clients to the bodily experience associated with the urge. Men with OCSB rarely examine or name the internal reflexive processes associated with sexual urges. It is important for the therapist to allow ample time for men to struggle with their language. The therapist's patience and nonjudgmental stance gives men permission not to do this well at first. Building reflective capacities of body sensations improves self-monitoring and prepares men for OCSB individual and group psychotherapy.

Clients often confuse an urge state with a judgment about how they feel or an opinion about the situation. "I felt bad." "I felt like jerking off." "I had to do it." "There was no turning back." Gently clarify that these statements described their thoughts or judgments of their embodied feelings. They did not describe the urge or the activation in their bodies. Accurate bodily descriptions of urges include the aforementioned heart rate, temperature (i.e., hot), muscle tension, and breathing. Urges also include feeling words like *anxious, excited,* or *shame*. Clients commonly report lack of awareness of an urge state and describe a sense of increasing engulfment and sensations of intensity, as if a wave is coming in on the shore and they don't believe it will recede back to sea. It can be helpful to educate clients that all feelings are temporary and will recede with or without direct intervention. A helpful homework assignment to illustrate this point is to suggest the client perform an experiment. Recommend that the next time the client has an urge he observe how long the urge state lasts without him having solo or partnered sex. He may be surprised that it stopped over time.

Clients react with a variety of defenses to avoid directly investigating their urge states. Precontemplative defenses may surface as dismissive or demeaning attitudes, especially when the client perceives he is not identifying his feelings perfectly. Other clients may describe a sense of relief at having new words for urge states other than "my addiction" or "my compulsion." Our intention is to slowly build men's capacity for nuanced self-awareness and to develop curiosity about their internal worlds through weekly completion of the SSAS. Affective self-awareness gradually increases through repetition in both the assessment and treatment.

When urge scores change from one week to the next, ask clients to discuss any behavior or thought modifications that they think may account for the rating. Clients may say, "I took a breath and remembered what we talked about in the assessment." "I told myself this is only an urge, it doesn't mean I have to have sex now." "I put my hand on my heart and pictured my family." "I imagined that my body was trying to say something to me, and I focused on what it was trying to say rather than planning what to do sexually." Or "I prayed." The specific urge-reduction technique is not the main focus of the SSAS urge-rating discussion, rather, the focus is highlighting the client's budding realization that observing and recording urges has a regulation function.

SSAS Subscale: Thoughts About Sexual Behavior

---

5. **How often did thoughts about engaging in problematic sexual behaviors come up? Please circle the most appropriate number:**

   None   Once   2 to 3 times   Several to many   Constant to near constant
   0   1   2   3   4

6. **Approximately how many hours (add up hours) did you spend thinking about engaging in problematic sexual behaviors? Please circle the most appropriate number:**

   None   1 hr or less   1 to 7 hrs   7 to 21 hrs   +21 hrs
   0   1   2   3   4

7. **How much were you able to control your thoughts of problematic sexual behaviors? Please circle the most appropriate number:**

   Completely   Much   Moderate   Minimal   No control
   0   1   2   3   4

This subscale moves the focus from the affective to the deliberative system of the mind. Most OCSB treatment-seeking men have clearer recollections and better vocabulary to describe their sexual thoughts than their feelings. As Haidt (2006) points out, people tend to overly focus on the conscious, verbal process and are less aware of the nonverbal activations in their mind. Their mind may think about planning the next sexual experience, fantasize about a desired sexual partner, remember a previous encounter, or vividly recall images from explicit sexual media. An essential self-monitoring skill for improving sexual health is to distinguish sexual thoughts from sexual urges and behaviors. It is hoped that discussing these three items in the assessment will evoke more detailed content of their thoughts and increase their ability to identify which thoughts generate concern for dysregulation; escalate activation; cause values conflicts; or evoke feelings of pleasure, guilt, or shame. For example, therapists can ask how the client interprets "thoughts about engaging in problematic sexual behavior" from question 5. What thoughts are the clients reporting? How intrusive or intentional are these thoughts? Do they occur in response to or precede specific stimuli, urges, or behaviors? Do they generate conflict, confusion, or contradictions with their sense of self? Are any of the thoughts old, perhaps dating back to childhood or adolescence? Are there thoughts they only have in sexual situations (like masturbation or partnered sex)?

A common self-discrepant motivation for OCSB treatment-seeking men is the loss of time spent thinking about or engaging in sexual behavior. Men often sound exasperated or look chagrinned when they say, "I am so sick of all the time I waste on this!" Typically, the time spent thinking about sex is far greater than time spent having sex. Because the SSAS is a weekly measure, at some point the therapist should ask about time spent over the past months, years, or even decades to establish a baseline. Does the time spent fluctuate, determined by certain periods of life, situations, moods, or relationship status? When in the midst of sexual preoccupation, can they describe what they are experiencing? The less conscious nonverbal components can be explored by the therapist, inviting the client to become an observer. "If I were in the office and able to observe you when you're preoccupied by these thoughts, what would you look like? What would you be doing? If your thoughts were audible, what would I hear?" This is an opportunity to gauge ability to self-monitor when men experience intensely activating sexual thoughts. The client may say, "I lock my office door. I am afraid someone will walk in and I will be so distracted that it will look like I was just daydreaming at work." Or "I sit and stare off into space. I'm thinking about getting online but I don't move much. Time sort of goes by, sometimes I realize 20 minutes has gone by and I am shocked!" Or "My mind begins racing, I can hardly think straight. I get really edgy. I will probably leave to go get a sexual massage."

Clinical dialogue that evaluates a client's ability to conceive of his own behavior or that of others as a reflection of a mental state has been defined as reflective functioning (Fonagy, 2008). Berry and Berry (2013) highlight how "deficient understanding of the *intentional* roots of behaviour is often a symptom of impaired reflective function" (p. 7). The SSAS item-response dialogue asks men to articulate their urges and thoughts as part of assessing current ability to see how they are distinct but interrelated. Some clients describe a coaching voice that acts as an observer to tell them how to cope with the intensity of their sexual urges and thoughts. Other clients excel at describing feeling states, mood, even body sensations and have great difficulty organizing these observations into a cognitive thought. Those who are better at describing the affective component will need help in articulating their thoughts. The therapist might say, "You described your reaction to time going by and the kind of state of mind you were in. Are there any specific thoughts or ideas or images that go through your mind when you're sitting there unaware that time is going by?" When redirected, clients may be able to report specific thoughts or ideas that go through their minds. They may be unaware or have little retainable cognition at this time and experience a quasialtered state of mind somewhere between daydreaming and dissociation. Clients who have difficulty describing specific thoughts when exploring their rating of this subscale may need an explanation from the therapist about how beneficial it can be to become aware of their thinking to create a more balanced relationship with the affective system. The contrast between clear language and ability to reflect on affective states is an important clinical assessment within the SSAS dialogue.

Other men are flooded with racing thoughts. They may be less articulate about the first four urge items, have underdeveloped affective reflection capacity, and become engulfed by their mental activity. Men may experience such rapid engulfment of their escalating thoughts that the verbal statements end up being a report of their defensive coping rather than an articulation of their state of mind. "I just feel like giving up." "This is too much, I can't take it anymore." "I just don't know what to do." These helplessness or hopelessness defenses are the words without the observation of the mental process that got them here. The SSAS subscales provide early practice for reflective functioning capacity that is an essential building block to improving sexual health and sexual behavior regulation.

Item 7 on the SSAS, "How much were you able to control your thoughts?" is another reflective-function question of the SSAS; this is a central question in OCSB treatment. We are most interested in the question "how much" because it illustrates a strength-based perspective of the client's current ability to exercise control. He may have been disappointed by the eventual outcome of his sexual behavior but disappointment is not the same as being "out of control." This item shifts client focus away from his perceived failure in sexual behavior so he notices the moments of control, no matter how small. Clients often overgeneralize their degree of control within a binary frame between success and failure. This is usually where they rely on the language of addiction. "My addict just took over." "I get to the point where my addiction overwhelmed me." "Nothing will stop me." The client whose "addict took over" is conflating his sexual behavior disappointment with an objective evaluation of his self-regulation. Question 7 invites men to contemplate how much control they exerted over their thoughts, not whether they completely controlled their thoughts. Therapists will need to listen closely for an inaccurate read of this item because men are engaged in all/none thinking after performing the unwanted sexual behavior. The therapist might say, "Yes, I understand, but this item is looking at *how much* (with emphasis) you were able to regulate your thoughts. I wonder whether we can slow this down a bit, and think about what thoughts you did control before the sex-seeking behavior started. It may be for only a few seconds, but I am interested in going back to that time to see whether you can describe your attempts to control your thoughts." Whether the client can do this well is not the main focus. This item reminds each client that observing thoughts is a skill required for change. When clients recall the times they asserted some control over their sexual thoughts, they are incrementally building their self-efficacy and confidence. It is important for the therapist to use the SSAS items to develop language that leads to accurate reflective descriptions of their deliberative processes.

SSAS Subscale: Observing Sexual Behavior

8. Approximately how much total time did you spend engaging in problematic sexual behaviors? Please circle the most appropriate number:

None	1 hr or less	1 to 7 hrs	7 to 21 hrs	+21 hrs
0	1	2	3	4

9. On average, how much anticipatory tension and/or excitement did you have *shortly before* you engaged in problematic sexual behaviors? If you did not actually engage in such behaviors, please estimate how much tension and/or excitement you believe you would have experienced if you had engaged in problematic sexual behaviors. Please circle the most appropriate number:

None	Mild	Moderate	Severe	Extreme
0	1	2	3	4

10. On average, how much excitement and pleasure did you feel when you engaged in problematic sexual behaviors? If you did not actually engage in such behaviors, please estimate how much excitement and pleasure you would have experienced if you had. Please circle the most appropriate number:

None	Mild	Moderate	Severe	Extreme
0	1	2	3	4

The SSAS subscale: Observing Sexual Behavior focuses on three areas of sexual behavior self-report. Question 8 quantifies the aggregate time spent engaging in problematic sexual behaviors over the last 7 days. Time spent is a fairly observable variable that men are typically motivated to monitor and accurately report. This may be reflected in the high correlation between time spent in sexual behavior and client motivation for treatment. Focusing on the hours spent engaging in problematic sexual behavior places emphasis on the opportunity costs of the behavior rather than moral disproval of a specific sex act. Opportunity costs are the benefits the client would have received if he engaged in different behaviors (e.g., investing that time in work, relationships, or hobbies).

The details of their sexual behavior are important. A distinct advantage of the SSAS is that it does not list specific sexual activities. This avoids implying moral disapproval of certain sexual behaviors or desires that are deemed de facto unhealthy because of their inclusion in a sexual dysregulation measure. It is important, however, that clients complete the SSAS after having identified which sexual behaviors are problematic for them. In other words, each client defines the specific sexual behaviors he will monitor and measure when completing the SSAS. Once they settle on what those behaviors are, we need to know too! No matter how the client answers question 8, we ask him to describe sexual behaviors that he identified as problematic as a touchstone used to calculate the time spent.

Ask for detailed descriptions of how he spent his time, what sexual activities are the most important, the most frustrating, and yield the most highly prized sexual experiences. Listen for competing motivations. "I know I should get to bed and then I end up staying up 2 more hours." Observe whether clients emphasize their thinking process or their emotional activated state. "I like to edge as long as I can. I keep searching for the next great scene, masturbate until I'm about to get off and then I stop. I try to hold off as much as I can." Here the therapist can ask process questions that may be less conscious and are rarely discussed by men. What were you thinking that kept you from having an orgasm? What made you finally choose to have an orgasm? Clients improve their reflective functioning capacity when they can suspend their judgmental thinking as they verbalize their process for regulating sexual release. Invitations for men to discuss their sexual excitation and inhibition establish familiarity with developing sexual self-observation capacity.

Question 9 returns to rating affective activation. This item connects thoughts with feelings in the time just before clients engage in their consequential unwanted behavior. The affective focus described as "anticipatory tension and/or excitement" is an opportunity to assess the details and intensity of the internal struggle before a client acts on his urge. This item also develops the client's potential to self-observe the pleasure or tension surrounding unwanted behavior, whether he engages in problematic sexual behavior or not. This item creates opportunities for men to articulate the motivations that propel them toward sex as well as the motivations that regulate behavior. To what degree is the client hyperfocused on his anticipated gratification? Is his ambivalence an outcome of his ability to transcend the moment and think about distal consequences that will negatively impact someone or something else in which he is invested? For instance, when a client is motivated to change his online masturbation patterns, the therapist may ask him to describe the specific images he was most excited about viewing. Was it the orgasm? Or was it returning to a highly specific sexual turn-on that needed to be recharged for ongoing masturbation pleasure? Was it a fantasy relationship with a particular person? Perhaps in thinking about finding a new video that excited him, he felt anticipatory excitement. What imagery or social media did he look forward to watching? Where did he focus his attention when he anticipated engaging in sexual behavior? Was it on particular body parts, facial expressions, sex acts, or erotic themes? Additionally, what created tension? What consequences worried him just when he was getting ready to engage in the problematic sexual behavior? Was he worried about losing sleep? Did the consequences of multiple solo-sex orgasms lead him to worry about sexual functioning with a partner later in the day? The anticipatory tension and excitement focus of item 9 provides ample clinical dialogue for client and therapist to collaborate with men to assist them in verbalizing "being of two minds."

Clients may be unfamiliar with deconstructing detailed thoughts and feelings before or during their problematic sexual behavior. This reflective-functioning process is an important component of increasing awareness of OCSB competing motivations. The particular thought and feeling states that follow a poorly regulated sexual activity are too often lost in the emotional turmoil and recriminating thoughts associated with betrayal and violation.

SSAS Subscale: Consequences of Sexual Behavior

The final two items focus on men's perceived emotional and situational consequences caused by their problematic sexual behavior over the last 7 days.

11. How much emotional distress (mental pain or anguish, shame, guilt, embarrassment) has your problematic sexual behavior caused you? Please circle the most appropriate number:

None	Mild	Moderate	Severe	Extreme
0	1	2	3	4

12. How much personal trouble (relationship, financial, legal, job, medical, or health) has your problematic sexual behavior caused you? Please circle the most appropriate number:

None	Mild	Moderate	Severe	Extreme
0	1	2	3	4

Scaling levels of emotional distress and personal troubles as a consequence of sexual behavior is the last subcategory of the SSAS. Rating emotional distress and personal trouble leads to a dialogue between client and therapist to identify relevant proximal consequences and the level of concern the client associates with each consequence. Identifying consequences that are not self-discrepant will clarify which consequences will not be a source for motivating change. Whatever levels of distress the client reports are discussed in a similar manner as earlier items. "What feelings listed in this item are you identifying as sources of distress?" "Can you identify what feelings concern you the most?" "What sexual behaviors most commonly trigger this distress?"

Question 12 measures the client's consequences with his relationship partner, job, physical health, financial health, and the law. Once again, clinicians can work with the client to articulate the consequences that are most concerning and link this with developing his self-discrepancy. With enough practice, men will increase their ability to focus on sexual symptoms that have the most self-discrepant consequences and link the outcomes with following and not following their sexual health boundaries. Clients' capacity for regulation increases as they learn to transcend the moment of immediate sexual gratification and remain aware of the lessons learned from examining previous boundary crossings.

Hypersexual Behavior Consequences Scale

The Hypersexual Behavior Consequences Scale (HBCS) is an important follow up to the SSAS. The HBCS is the more detailed review of the explicit linkages between sexual behavior and the many potential negative consequences the behavior causes. The HBCS is also the component of the assessment that is designed to further develop self-discrepancies that are essential for eliciting change talk. Reid et al. (2012) developed the HBCS partly because the existing measures identified more global overall patterns of OCSB rather than specific negative outcomes. The developers believed current measures relied on ambiguous sources of injury and distress that rated consequences like "harm" and "problems" without making clear distinctions whether consequences stemmed from either solo or partnered sex. "Higher HBCS scores were positively correlated with higher levels of emotional dysregulation, impulsivity, and stress proneness and lower levels of satisfaction with life and happiness" (Reid et al., 2012, p. 115).

Benefits of HBCS in OCSB Assessment

Specific sexual behaviors are not listed in the HBCS items. By not focusing on specific sex acts, the HBCS provides therapist and client an excellent debriefing dialogue that places the focus on consequences without the measure predetermining which consequence goes with which sex act. For example, item 10 asks, "I have betrayed trust in a significant relationship because of my sexual activities" (Figure 6.3). If the client endorsed this question with a 4 (Has happened once or twice), a follow-up question might be to ask the client to clarify what specific sexual activity happened once or twice that betrayed the trust in a significant relationship. The client also defines what he means by betrayal of a partner's trust. It is important that the client does the work of linking his sexual behavior to the consequence. This allows for the clinician to learn what the client perceives as betrayal; what he considers a "significant relationship"; what relationship agreements he betrayed; and what feelings, thoughts, and behaviors he links with this item. The quality of the assessment is enhanced when men find the language to describe consequential details linked with their sexual behavior.

   Reid et al. (2012) were motivated to develop a measure that improved on existing measures by better distinguishing between consequences attributable to masturbation and consequences resulting from partnered sex. Existing consequence measures exclude solo-sex activity because items are written to identify only partnered sexual activity, causing men with out of control masturbation practices to have inaccurate scores. Item 13, "I have been humiliated or disgraced because of my sexual activities" for instance, could be measured by a man's exclusively solo-sex activities, exclusively partnered sexual behavior, or both. Perhaps the

HYPERSEXUAL BEHAVIOR CONSEQUENCES SCALE

Below are a number of statements that describe various consequences people experience because of their sexual behavior and activities. As you respond to each statement, indicate the extent to which each item applies to you. If you haven't experienced a particular item, indicate the likelihood that you will in the future. Use the scale below to guide your responses and write a number to the left of each statement.

For the purposes of this survey: *Sex* is defined as any activity or behavior that stimulates or arouses a person with the intent to produce an orgasm or sexual pleasure. Sexual behaviors may or may not involve a partner (e.g., self-masturbation or solo sex, using pornography, intercourse with a partner, oral sex, anal sex, etc.).

Hasn't happened and is unlikely to happen:	*ONE*
Hasn't happened but might happen:	*TWO*
Hasn't happened but will very likely happen:	*THREE*
Has happened once or twice:	*FOUR*
Has happened several times:	*FIVE*

1. _____ I have lost a job because of my sexual activities.

2. _____ I have failed to keep an important commitment because of my sexual activities.

3. _____ A romantic relationship has ended because of my sexual activities.

4. _____ I have gotten a sexually transmitted disease or infection because of my sexual activities.

5. _____ I have had legal problems because of my sexual activities.

6. _____ I have been arrested because of my sexual activities.

7. _____ Important goals have been sacrificed because of my sexual activities.

8. _____ I have experienced unwanted financial losses because of my sexual activities.

9. _____ I have emotionally hurt someone I care about because of my sexual activities.

10. _____ I have betrayed trust in a significant relationship because of my sexual activities.

Figure 6.3 *Hypersexual Behavior Consequences Scale.*

Courtesy of Rory C. Reid. © 2012

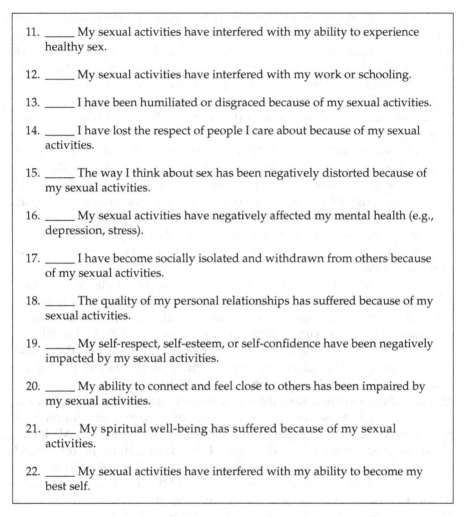

11. _____ My sexual activities have interfered with my ability to experience healthy sex.

12. _____ My sexual activities have interfered with my work or schooling.

13. _____ I have been humiliated or disgraced because of my sexual activities.

14. _____ I have lost the respect of people I care about because of my sexual activities.

15. _____ The way I think about sex has been negatively distorted because of my sexual activities.

16. _____ My sexual activities have negatively affected my mental health (e.g., depression, stress).

17. _____ I have become socially isolated and withdrawn from others because of my sexual activities.

18. _____ The quality of my personal relationships has suffered because of my sexual activities.

19. _____ My self-respect, self-esteem, or self-confidence have been negatively impacted by my sexual activities.

20. _____ My ability to connect and feel close to others has been impaired by my sexual activities.

21. _____ My spiritual well-being has suffered because of my sexual activities.

22. _____ My sexual activities have interfered with my ability to become my best self.

Figure 6.3 *(continued)*

client's humiliation resulted from masturbating online at work, but not from partnered sex. The item rating, when reviewed in a semistructured format, explains exactly what sexual behaviors had humiliating consequences. Clients may say, "I was disgusted that I felt excited by watching someone pee in his jeans in a video, I couldn't believe it excited me. And then I found out my assistant at the office found those images on the company laptop! I felt so humiliated. What is wrong with me?" Clients can feel pleasure during their exploration of an unconventional sexual interest as well as delayed disgust and humiliation in response to an unintentional exposure. Other clients may endorse this item not because of their sexual behavior but rather because their humiliation was the consequence of being confronted by the rage, hurt, and demeaning statements of an intimate partner after dishonoring the relationship agreement. The HBSC provides space for men to define the behaviors linked with the consequence.

The semistructured HBCS review follows the same procedure as the ACE Study questionnaire and SSAS. Clients complete the form in advance of the assessment appointment, read each item aloud, and discuss the range of sexual behaviors linked with the emotional, social, interpersonal, legal, and medical consequences. Slowly deconstructing the consequences is another change process that helps clients identify their motivations for defining and moving toward their personal vision of sexual health.

At this point in the assessment, the therapist builds on the clinical conversation of the ACE and SSAS to illustrate how specific sexual behaviors also have consequences linked with crossing sexual health principles. Linking sexual health consequences with HBCS clinical dialogue is essential for expanding men's capacity for future sexual decision making to align their sexual behaviors with the sexual health principles. Clients can develop their personal sexual ethics by evaluating the congruence of their current sexual activity with sexual health principles. For example, item 18 asks whether "The quality of my personal relationships has suffered because of my sexual activities" (see Figure 6.3). Michael's client Steve endorsed a 4 on this item. The sexual activity he referenced was having oral and vaginal sex with paid massage therapists. This activity violated his relationship agreement. When Michael explored his motivation to stop paying for sex, Steve reported that he wanted to honor his agreement with his wife. When Michael included the sexual health principles as another consequence to reflect on, Steve quickly saw that his behavior was not consistent with the principles of nonexploitation, honesty, protection from HIV/STIs, and unwanted pregnancy. He revealed to Michael that he was conflicted about paying for sex with Asian women at massage parlors who were vulnerable to exploitation because of their immigration status and may have been victims of sex trafficking. He felt sickened at times when he lied to his wife in response to her direct questions about where he goes after work, how he spent money that was removed from the bank account, or his self-disgust that he was putting her at risk for sexually transmitted infections. (Steve reported inconsistent condom use during paid penile–vaginal intercourse.) Evaluating his behaviors against the sexual health principles expanded his internal conflicts beyond his initial distress about violating his romantic relational agreements.

The Sexual Inhibition Scales/Sexual Excitation Scales

Assessing a man's individual sexual response is an essential component in developing the client's OCSB Unique Clinical Picture. In the same way that the OCSB Clinical Pathway underscores individual differences among clients, the dual control model of sexual response focuses on individual variability in human sexual response (Janssen & Bancroft, 2007). The dual control model of sexual response postulates that sexual arousal and associated behaviors rely on the balance between sexual excitation and inhibition (Janssen & Bancroft, 2007). "The model proposes that the weighing of excitatory and inhibitory processes determines whether or not a sexual response occurs within an individual in a given situation, and at the same time it assumes individual variability in the propensity for these processes" (p. 1). The dual control model of sexual response moves the focus of sexual response beyond existing one-dimensional sexual response models that conceptualize arousal as the outcome of only excitatory processes. In less than 10 years, the dual control model of sexual response has been widely accepted as a significant expansion of previous models by identifying the role of both excitatory *and* inhibitory processes within each person's sexual response (Janssen & Bancroft, 2007). It was this hypothesis that led to the survey that separately measures a person's sexual excitation and inhibition propensities understand this two-dimensional model. Sex-specific measures called the Sexual Inhibition/Sexual Excitation Scales (SIS/SES) were originally developed for use with men (Janssen et al., 2002). Because of several differences found in inhibition mechanisms in early research studies with women, a separate instrument was developed for women: Sexual Excitation/Inhibition Inventory for Women (SESII-W; Graham, Sanders, & Milhausen, 2006). As we only treat men with OCSB, we only discuss how to implement the SIS/SES. (For a review of both measures, see Bancroft, Graham, Janssen, & Sanders, 2009.)

The SIS/SES measures two male sexual inhibition factors and one excitation factor. The two inhibition scales measure threats due to performance failure (SIS1) and threats due to performance consequences (SIS2). The SIS/SES questionnaire has been used in OCSB research only once with a small sample of self-identified "sex addicts" ($N = 31$; Bancroft & Vukadinovic, 2004). In the OCSB group, they found no difference between

SIS1 and SIS2 scores but significantly higher SES scores. When divided between men who identified as "compulsive masturbators" and those whose behavior involved partnered sex, the partnered-sex group scored significantly lower on the threats due to performance consequences (SIS2) than did the control and masturbation groups. Another study looked at high-risk sexual behaviors among heterosexual and gay men (study did not differentiate between bisexual or not-exclusively heterosexual; Bancroft et al., 2009). Among the study participants, a high propensity for sexual excitation (SES) predicted men's number of casual partners. This was contrasted with an association between high-risk sexual activity (in particular, unprotected anal intercourse [UAI]) and a low propensity for sexual inhibition (SIS2) in sexually risky sexual encounters (Bancroft et al., 2009). To reduce risk of negative consequences, men who are capable of high levels of sexual excitation may need assistance in creating sexual health behavior inhibitors that adequately balance their high-excitation propensity.

Completing the SIS/SES allows clients to evaluate how their excitation and inhibition levels contribute to OCSB. We frequently find two profiles among men completing this measure as part of their OCSB assessment. The first profile, which reflects the research, is a client with high sexual excitation scores or low–moderate inhibition scores (SIS2). The second and less frequent profile involves clients with high sexual inhibition scores (SIS1) who disinhibit in problematic ways as a means to balance their inhibition and their average to low levels of sexual excitation.

Benefits of SIS/SES in OCSB Assessment

The SIS/SES measure provides an empathic, well-informed, and less pathological narrative that each client can use to learn about the connection between his sexual excitation/inhibition level and his sexual behavior. The dual control model of sexual response challenges client narratives that blame their high sexual excitement propensity for feeling out of control in their sexual behavior and offers an alternative, sexologically relevant model for understanding sexual response. Frequently, clients misattribute their OCSB symptoms to a one-dimensional perspective of an "overactive" excitation system. "I want sex too much," "I'm just a hound dog," and other narratives that ascribe sexual excitement capacity as the explanation for sexual behavior. This is understandable given the long history of the one-dimensional perspective of sexual response. When men see their sexual excitation scores (SES) in comparison to the general population, we often hear responses like, "Oh, my capacity for sexual excitement is high" that challenge their shame-based notion that "I'm a sex fiend." Men's shame and negative self-judgments about their sexual excitation capacity may lessen when excitation is viewed as a relatively stable dimension of a dynamic balance that determines his overall sexual response.

Combining the complete picture of a man's inhibitors with his level of excitation has great potential to decrease his sexual shame and redirect him toward an effective sexual health strategy. Clients often feel relieved to learn that their excitation levels are not disordered but rather are above or below average when compared to the general population. Insufficient or overwhelming inhibitors are the real focus for change. The goal of OCSB treatment is to develop men's inhibition capacity to balance their excitation propensity. This balance is necessary for men to have an enjoyable and pleasurable level of sexual response. Similar to other discredited mental health techniques aimed at changing people's sexual pleasure and orientation, psychotherapy treatment for compulsive, hypersexual, or sexual addiction is ineffective and harmful when deployed to change someone's capacity for consensual sexual excitation.

Men who have low–moderate excitation scores (SES) and high inhibition (SIS1) may report fearing erectile or ejaculation control problems during sexual activity. This configuration may be reflected in OCSB behaviors that are motivated by coping with low confidence in sexual functioning. Clients suffering from biogenic (e.g., low testosterone) or psychogenic (e.g., anxiety) sexual dysfunction may engage in problematic strategies to work around their high inhibition levels. They may hire a sex worker as a form of sexual surrogacy. They may engage in high rates of masturbation to practice maintaining an erection or delaying orgasm. Clients may use sexual novelty seeking to boost their sexual excitation. They use alcohol, illicit drugs, and medications without prescriptions to regulate their sexual anxieties.

Administering the SIS/SES

The 45-item SIS/SES questionnaire and dual control model of sexual response references are available free online at the Kinsey Institute website (www.kinseyinstitute.org/research/inhibition_excitation.html). Complete the measure yourself, and have your spouse, partner, and colleagues complete the measure. The more confident and familiar you are with the questionnaire and the model, the better you are able to integrate a client's score into his Unique Clinical Picture. The ability to obtain instant results is what makes online access to the questionnaire so convenient. After men complete the online survey, the three individual SES, SIS1, and SIS2 scores are immediately summarized in separate bar graphs that compare their answers within the distribution of scores among over 8,000 male participants. Before seeing each score, we frequently ask clients to predict where on the graph they expect to see their score. This is an interesting moment used to gauge their judgments about their levels of sexual excitation and inhibition capacities. After they view their scores and read the explanations, we debrief the experience of completing the questionnaire as well as their reactions to their scores. The SIS/SES process presents another opportunity to clinically discuss important elements of men's OCSB symptoms in a less defended situation. The intermediary role of the measure allows men an alternative for self-understanding of their sexual thoughts, feelings, and urges without having to answer direct questions that are expected in a standard sex history or clinical interview.

OCSB Sexual Symptom Measures

The three sexual symptoms measures (SSAS, HBCI, and SIS/SES) contribute to the reasonable and collaborative approximation to determine whether OCSB treatment is recommended or whether the assessment should move in a different direction. For some men, the measures do not reveal a sexual regulation problem. The primary cause for the client's sexual concerns may be an unresolved values conflict. Men with overly rigid or unreasonable sexual values become highly activated when their intrapersonal or interpersonal sexual activities are not fully aligned with their values. Values conflicts may be evident when the client has a low frequency of problematic sexual behavior, thoughts, and urges but a high degree of consequences. Consequences likely range from relational, spiritual, and psychological distress linked with threats of losing a primary partner, acceptance in his religious community, or a threat to a person's self-concept or identity. In these cases, the client or couple's sexual standards may be the originating source for deeply felt hurt and injury. Clients with significant sexual values conflicts may feel as if their sexuality or situation is out of control. They may be correct. If a highly religious man feels sexually excited when he sniffs women's panties, his intense orgasmic pleasure is not under his control and neither is the possible rejecting reaction from his wife or religious community. The pain from internal, relational, or institutional values conflicts and rejection is real. However, a values conflict is not a clinical profile we recommend resolving with specialized OCSB treatment. Couple therapy or non-OCSB individual therapy is usually the recommended course of treatment.

Experiences in Close Relationships—Relationship Structures Questionnaire

The Experiences in Close Relationships—Relationship Structures Questionnaire (ECR-RS) measures client attachment styles. The online attachment instrument we recommend assesses the dimensions of attachment-related anxiety and attachment-related avoidance in multiple relationship contexts (i.e., mother, father, romantic partners, and friends) and configures the client's global attachment style. (Fraley, Heffernan, Vicary, & Brumbaugh, 2011).

High levels of attachment-related anxiety are reflected in attachments in which a person tends to "worry whether their partner is available, responsive, attentive, etc. People who score on the low end of this variable are more secure in the perceived responsiveness of their partners" (Fraley, 2010, p. 5). People who score high on attachment-related avoidance "prefer not to rely on others or open up to others. People on the low end of the avoidance dimension are more comfortable being intimate with others and are more secure depending upon and having others depend upon them. A prototypical secure adult is low on both of the anxiety and avoidance attachment dimensions" (p. 5). The ECR-RS is free and available online at: www.yourpersonality.net/relstructures/.

Administering the ECR-RS

Similar to the OCSB measure, we provide psychoeducation information about attachment patterns, administer the ECR-RS, and debrief with a clinical dialogue to expand on the process. We ask clients to complete the online measure during an assessment session; administering, scoring, and discussing the measure may take an entire session. The ECR-RS consists of the same nine attachment questions in the context of the client's relationship with his mother (or mother figure), father (or father figure), close friend, and romantic partner. After completing the measure, the client's scores are immediately plotted on axes that represent dimensions of attachment-related anxiety and attachment-related avoidance. This four-quadrant graph provides a visual representation of each relationship attachment style. The four quadrants represent each attachment style: Secure, Fearful, Preoccupied, and Dismissive. Each dot on the chart represents the specific score on both attachment-related dimensions for one of the cleint's close relationships (see Figure 4.1).

Because attachment styles vary by degree and are not fixed by defined boundaries, these patterns are best thought of as styles rather than distinct categories (Fraley & Shaver, 2000). The OCSB Unique Clinical Picture summarizes the range and intensity of multiple factors that contribute to feeling sexually out of control. The textured relational contexts assessed by the ECR-RS questionnaire complement the overall OCSB assessment objective. Examining adult attachment styles within an OCSB assessment prepares men to consider their attachment-related anxiety and avoidance patterns throughout OCSB combined treatment. We remind men that this attachment survey does not determine whether something is wrong with the way they manage or how they feel in relationships. Attachment styles are a way to learn about relationship patterns and their possible links with OCSB. Clinical discussions may investigate how men negotiate and regulate attachment fears through dismissiveness, abandonment preoccupation, and reservations about depending on others. OCSB may function as a (deliberate or unintended) client strategy to defend against these attachment worries.

Attachment Measure Discussion

Attachment assessment presents an opportunity for important clinical dialogue. How does the assessment score reflect or not reflect the client's sense of relational connection? How does a man feel when people close to him want to depend on him? Do the attachment scores reflect his experience with opening up in his relationships with his mother, father, or intimate partners? How was his sexual desire expressed in romantic relationships when attachment-related anxieties arose? Some men experience relational closeness as a smothering feeling and rely on sexual behavior to create emotional space (e.g., solo sex or extrarelational sexual behavior). Some men experience higher levels of sexual excitement when they feel emotionally distant from their partners. Do they use sex to bridge this gap?

The dialogues that occur when administering the ACE, SSAS, and HCBI questionnaires have relational components. Noticing the feel, the pace, and nuances for connection enriches the attachment assessment, whereas the attachment measure is a useful tool for corroborating earlier OCSB clinical observations about how the client is relating to the therapist. Therapists may find the ECR-RS attachment styles clearly evident in these earlier interactions. A benefit of the measure is the potential to reveal unseen strengths as well. Perhaps the client's friendships are a source of secure attachment. This would clearly appear in the graph, but may have remained less visible in a standard psychosocial assessment interview.

Therapists may observe other patterns of in-session interaction consistent with the attachment measure results. For example, a dismissive attachment pattern is consistent with men who, in OCSB assessments, effortlessly provide summary statements, opinions, or conclusions about themselves and their sexual lives. They may find it difficult to contextualize their summations with specific memories, details, or events. The dismissive clients may discuss their sexual behavior in banal language and terms arising from common knowledge. "I know it's wrong to lie about my sexual behavior," "I should know by now that I was going to eventually get caught," or "I wasn't hurting anyone." But when asked for more detail or behavioral specifics like "How did you come to believe that paying for sex and hiding it from your spouse would not hurt her?" The conversation often meanders in a manner that is devoid of strong emotions or specific personal experience: "I don't know, it just seemed to make sense at the time." Or the client may become vague, blank, or unwittingly change the subject to another focus. "She never gave me a blow job, not once, it was humiliating. I finally gave up. What was I supposed to do, live the rest of my life never getting head?"

Preoccupied attachment styles appear in assessment discussions as well. They often involve an emotional story with many connected components but lack a coherent narrative that holds the intensely emotional memories together. The interaction eventually creates a disconnection between therapist and client in which one or both has difficulty remembering how the discussion got started. The therapist notices that she or he is the only one tracking the context of reviewing the assessment measure while the client is increasingly consumed in his emotionally activated state. The client's preoccupied attachment style is evidenced by this disorganized emotional response to evocative attachment-measure dialogue.

Fearful relational adult attachment style emerges in the scattered and confused discourse that occurs when the attachment-assessment discussion is related to ruptures, injuries, traumas, or losses. Clients who are otherwise quite skilled in verbalizing clear and coherent thoughts, ideas, and details about their lives may shift to surprisingly inarticulate, disjointed, disorganized expressions. "I don't know, you know, it was tough, and, uh, they really weren't around much. I was pretty out there on my own, you know, it was, well . . . , anyway, I was just glad to be out of there." The attachment style emerges if his unconscious fear of returning to these experiences comingles with his severely underdeveloped deliberative mind to verbalize these highly activating experiences within language. The client may have little experience discussing his memories or reexperiencing fearful early life events without activating the same embodied sensed of fear or fright that was intensely constant in the attached relationship.

The OCSB attachment-assessment discussion plants the seeds for future insights into the client's sexual behavior patterns, erotic conflict dynamics, long-standing marital or relationship patterns, as well as his shame and biting personal judgments about his relationship patterns. When the client learns that his attachments are often activated by high levels of anxiety and fear, he comes to understand how his current sexual behaviors have been an attempt to cope with his dependency fears, abandonment anxiety, or insecurities about being a man on whom others can depend.

Attention-Deficit/Hyperactivity Disorder Self-Report Scale—V1.1 Symptom Checklist

Clinicians treating sexual dysregulation may assume that attention deficit hyperactivity disorder (ADHD) prevalence among men concerned with controlling sexual behavior derives from their predisposition toward the hyperactive and impulsive behavior associated with ADHD. Reid, Davtian, Lenartowicz, Torrevillas, and Fong (2013) found an unexpected association between elevated adult ADHD in hypersexual men. Their research suggests a different correlation between untreated ADHD and painful interpersonal consequences. Reid and his team found a range of salient factors most likely to predict hypersexual disorder (HD), such as low self-esteem, lack of self-confidence, feeling unsure of oneself, and a belief that goal attainment will be obstructed by a diminished sense of self. They conclude from their study that some men may be vulnerable to using sexual behavior to escape or avoid the emotional discomfort of living with peer rejection, romantic relationship problems, and employment problems, issues commonly found among men with ADHD (Reid et al., 2013).

When examining the link between adult ADHD and OCSB, Reid et al. (2013) advise clinicians to avoid jumping to conclusions by ruling out comorbid medical and psychiatric conditions, as well as carefully considering the context in which a man's ADHD symptom emerges. OCSB clinical cases need thorough and informed evaluation to discern whether a man is vulnerable to OCSB symptoms because of his inattentive or hyperactive traits or as a consequence of living with ADHD. Reid and his colleagues propose an attention model for hypersexual behavior focused on the relationship between a "target" and a "distraction." They framed the attention deficit as inability to sufficiently inhibit when the sexual stimuli captures (i.e., distracts) the client's focus away from the present task, leading to difficulty staying on task. Reid's explanation conceptualizes sexual behavior dysregulation associated with the ADHD mind's inability to effectively regulate the tension between the immediate sexual stimuli and the longer term completion of a job.

Their work on ADHD and HD is an important reminder for therapists to be open to new research to change existing yet not fully substantiated clinical assumptions. As a result of their findings, we suggest an adult ADHD screening to determine whether a recommendation to an ADHD specialist is warranted. The screening measure we recommend is the Adult ADHD Self-Report Scale—V1.1 (ASRS-V1.1) Symptom Checklist, available free online (www.hcp.med.harvard.edu/ncs/ftpdir/adhd/18Q_ASRS_English.pdf).

Additional Measures as Needed

Recent studies confirm a high prevalence of mood disorders, anxiety disorders, and substance-related disorders among patients seeking help for hypersexual behavior (Reid et al., 2013). We assume readers are familiar with mental and substance-related disorder measures and rely on training and clinical experience to identify relevant surveys for your practice. Online assessment measures that correspond to the *Diagnostic and Statistical Manual of Mental Disorders,* Fifth Edition (*DSM-5*; American Psychiatric Association, 2013) diagnoses can be found on the American Psychiatric Association website: www.psychiatry.org/practice/dsm/dsm5/online-assessment-measures. Practitioners might also consider the *Sexual Narcissism Scale* by Widman and McNulty (2010).

INFORMATION GATHERING: CLINICAL INTERVIEW

Psychotherapists typically obtain pertinent clinical information about client past experiences and current symptoms through a psychosocial assessment. The areas covered in the OCSB psychosocial assessment are family of origin, significant relationships, adverse experiences, mental health, relationship with drugs and alcohol, and medical history. Gathering additional information outside the general psychosocial information clarifies important details associated with the client's OCSB vulnerability factors. The goal of adding these additional areas of inquiry is to focus on the historical events that influence the client's self and attachment regulation and sexual/erotic-identity development. We recommend a few additional processes to gather the remaining OCSB assessment information.

Sexual and Erotic Development

Sexual and erotic conflict is the only clinical area during the OCSB assessment that relies solely on the clinical interview and depends on the therapist's ability to implement the sexual health conversation skills discussed in Chapter 2. Therapists will need to suspend judgment; avoid premature evaluation; and use accurate, clear sexologically informed language. There are various guides and techniques used to gather information about a client's sexuality. We recommend that all therapists develop a method for obtaining preliminary sexual health information for clients (see Barratt & Rand, 2009) as well as a process for conducting a thorough interview about client sexual and erotic development. An OCSB assessment offers just such a situation.

There are a variety of therapist resources that can be used to prepare and structure the interview. *What Every Mental Health Professional Should Know About Sex* (Buehler, 2014) and *Revisiting the Sexual Genogram* (Belous, Timm, Grace, & Whitehead, 2012) both identify and organize important content (e.g., sexual development, medical issues, relationship history, sociocultural influence, culture, community) and suggest a comprehensive range of human sexuality topics (e.g., gender, parental attitudes about sex, sexual education, masturbation, relationship with sexual imagery/media, sexual orientation, orgasm, early relationship crushes, sexual debut, body image, sexually transmitted infection, pregnancy, HIV, sexual functioning, sexual pain, nonconsensual sex, closely guarded sexual secrets, not keeping sexual relationship agreements, meaning of sex, peak sexual pleasures, and unconventional sexual interests). W. M. Edwards, Delmonico, and Griffin (2011) offer detailed instruction for creating an online sexual behavior timeline that is generalizable for an offline sexual history timeline. Risen's chapter "Listening to Sexual Stories" in *The Handbook of Clinical Sexuality for Mental Health Professionals* (Levine, Risen, & Althof, 2010) is a good resource to guide therapist language, flexibility, and sexual health conversation skills. She proposes a framework that interweaves sexual identity, sexual function, and the relational meaning of sex and provides specific open-ended questions that evoke a deep and contemplative consideration of these three areas of sexuality. Regardless of the interview structure you choose, we recommend modeling your interview on a source that encourages creating a reflective space in which clients review, disclose, and process important moments in their sexual and erotic development.

Fixed and Unconventional Turn-Ons

Gathering information about sexual and erotic development provides the backstory for understanding a man's difficulty integrating his sexual and erotic orientation into his self-concept and romantic relationships.

Childhood shapes orientation; each child simultaneously internalizes the sociocultural values of his or her family and the society in which he or she was raised. These external influences hold enormous sway and can either enhance or adversely influence sexual- and erotic-identity formation as well as contribute to the development of fixed or unconventional turn-ons. Money utilizes opponent-process models of behavior to understand the transformation of tragic childhood events into the triumph of orgasmic ecstasy. Morin (1995) correlated the impact of adverse child events, leading with the internalization of self-hating core beliefs and a sex-negative narrative that "lust is bad and love is good." Both researchers proposed that fixed arousal formation was an unconscious coping strategy that preserved one's sexual and erotic self, but "at the cost of separating it from love" (Money, 1999, p. 245).

People learn about their erotic orientations through a similar uncovering process that provides insight into sexual orientation. As the various sexual systems activate during childhood, individuals gradually develop a persistent direction for their sexual attractions. Over time, they may see a gendered pattern in their love and lust objects. The same can be said for one's eroticism. With exposure to an infinite amount of stimuli, people refine erotic self-concept through their awareness of the specific, reliable, and predictable stimuli that lead to their arousal responses. We draw comparisons to the sexual orientation identity development models with men in OCSB assessment who are concerned about their fixed turn-ons because these self-awareness processes are similar and lead to a sexual-minority status. Sexual and erotic minorities were likely raised with a presumed identity that conforms to traditional sexual behaviors and interests. Over time, they realize that they do not desire or identify with these presumed orientations. The excitement of sexual and erotic awakening is often paired with the existential dilemma that they are different than who they thought they were or believe they should be. Whether they judge that difference as positive or negative will significantly influence their identity development process.

The presence of any fixed or unconventional turn-on surfaces as clients share the details of their sexual thoughts, urges, and behaviors during the OCSB assessment. The unconventional or the rigidly fixed patterns of sexual arousal are more apparent when men describe their masturbation or partnered sex. Therapists need to remain curious about the themes that arise in the sexual images men watch and what specifically draws the most excited and arousing response. Men in OCSB assessment often articulate and discuss their peak erotic experiences either as a source of conflict or deep longing for acceptance. They may have sexual themes or objects that reliably bring them to orgasm. Ultimately, the OCSB assessment process is interested in determining the degree to which men's sexual desire, pleasure, and orgasms are fixed to a narrow range of stimuli that are predictable, reliable, and persistent.

Clients with fixed arousal patterns are likely aware of the difference in pleasure that they feel with and without the presence of their object of erotic attraction and excitement. When clients disclose a fixed turn-on, it is important for therapists to empathically explore the level of congruence between men's erotic orientation, erotic identity, and sexual expression. Said another way, to what degree has the client integrated his erotic orientation into his self-concept and intimate relationships? Exploring a client's erotic-identity development parallels the process used to discuss the client's sexual-identity development. For example, women's leather boots are a fixed erotic object commonly present among heterosexually identified men. When men disclose this erotic preference, we slow the process down to ascertain more details of their historical and current relationship with this source of erotic pleasure. When did you first notice that women's leather boots aroused you? How did you discover that? (For clients with fixed turn-ons, they frequently report a childhood awareness of their arousal, sometimes before they had an understanding that what they were feeling was sexual. And, with the introduction of the Internet, people are exposed to greater diversity of stimuli, which hastens the discovery of their turn-on.) What was it like for you to realize that you were intensely aroused by women's leather boots? When did you first share your turn-on with someone else? What was his or her reaction? When did you first have sex that involved leather boots, either with yourself or with one or more partners? The sexual and erotic milestone in the lives of people with fixed arousal patterns is an important timeline to understand the persistence and dependability of this specific turn-on for heightened sexual pleasure. Additionally, openly discussing his relationship with this erotic stimulus can raise awareness about how a man has internalized and navigated sociocultural biases that compete with a full integration of this erotic interest into his self-concept and sexual relationships.

The separation of lust and love is a common theme within sexual-arousal research (Bancroft, 2009; Money, 1999; Morin, 1995). Generally speaking, the long-term health of an intimate relationship is associated with people's ability to feel some degree of love and lust for their partner(s). There is, of course, a much greater variability within the degree of love/lust overlap among intimate couples once the conversation moves beyond this general statement. People with less love and lust overlap can form satisfying intimate relationships as can partners with a high degree of love and lust overlap. Most often, our clients present with a desire to feel lust with the person they love. If we suspect the client has a fixed arousal pattern, we explore the degree of separation between his love and lust. How much, if any, overlap does the client experience? How successful were attempts to integrate their turn-on in the past? How far do clients have to emotionally move away from their partner during sex to achieve or maintain their erections or to reach orgasm? (These dynamics are the moments when clients fantasize about or physically introduce their erotic object during partnered sex because they cannot reliably feel aroused without engaging it.)

Disseminating accurate human sexuality knowledge provides clinicians with opportunities to better understand the potential obstacles that impede each man's positive sexual and erotic-identity development. They may have misinformation or knowledge gaps about sexual and erotic orientation that the therapist can clarify. Clinicians can explore the client's underlying motivation to label themselves as sexually normal. What does the man value about being "like everyone else"? How does that belief influence their self-concept, sexual decision making, or relationship patterns? How would they treat themselves differently without that judgment? Clients may also carry false and negative beliefs about their sexual and erotic orientations. They may think that adverse childhood events warped their arousal pattern and may think of their sexual pleasure as a persistent reminder of being damaged. Some men want OCSB treatment to reunite them with the sexuality they perceive as lost and want it to be reclaimed. Restoring one's imagined and expected sexual self-identity is the unspoken treatment plan for getting rid of their disgraceful turn-on. The sexual health model for OCSB treatment offers men a different lens through which to view their eroticism. What if men began to appreciate their ability to preserve their sexuality in the face of adverse experiences? We invite men in OCSB treatment to appreciate and honor their erotic pleasures as evidence of the centrality of sexuality and their personal, resilient human spirit.

Sexual Problem Timeline

A sexual problem timeline establishes a linear trajectory of men's out of control sexual experiences from onset to the present day. The timeline gathers detailed historical information about the client's sexual problems. The clinical discussion that follows construction of the timeline presents an opportunity for men to identify the emotions connected with their sexual behavior, as well as to highlight strengths and useful coping skills during periods of sexual control. Typically, the timeline is the last component of the OCSB clinical interview.

To begin the timeline, clients are instructed to discuss the onset of sexual thoughts, urges, or behaviors that they identify as problematic. We advise them that we are interested in hearing about how their symptoms evolved over time, the frequency and intensity of their symptoms, the height(s) of their OCSB, and periods when they were not feeling out of control. We discuss the development of their motivation for change and listen for moments when their sexual behavior crossed a sexual health principle. For instance, OCSB treatment-seeking men who withheld information about extrarelational sex from their current or past partners are asked to describe their history of crossing the honesty sexual health principle. "When was the first time you were dishonest about not keeping your monogamy sexual agreement with an intimate partner?"

Clients may begin the sexual timeline with sexual memories that initially seem completely unrelated to their current OCSB symptoms. These sexual stories can reveal aspects of values conflicts and their self-judgment about early sexual and erotic development rather than a felt sense of being out of control. A client describes his adolescent masturbation fantasies of his teacher's breasts. He identifies his inability to stop staring and being aroused as shameful and disrespectful. The timeline discussion may be the first time he becomes aware of the relationship between his highly restrictive standards about lusting after someone and the origins of his current conflicts with his online sexual behavior.

As the sexual problem timeline is completed after the general biopsychosocial interview, therapists can make connections between out of control sexual experiences and overlapping life events. This linkage is an excellent opportunity to connect diverse and varied factors that contribute to sexual behavior problems. Questions like: Did the most serious OCSB symptoms occur after or before the client stopped drinking? How does the OCSB pattern of behavior overlap with the client's coming out as a gay-identified man? The sexual problem timeline is a thread that weaves the clients' disparate vulnerability factors, clinical areas, and life events into a narrative that completes their Unique Clinical Pictures.

Sexual Agreements

Saving a relationship or distress about not honoring an intimate partner sexual relationship agreement is a common motivation for OCSB treatment. These men are puzzled by the contradiction of committing to do one thing, yet doing another. Often these men find that they resolve unplanned or ongoing tantalizing situations by convincing themselves not to honor their relational sexual agreement. Their history of dishonoring sexual agreements carries inherent self-discrepancies that, when made conscious, can be a source of personal motivation. We examine what motivated them to make the partnered sexual agreement, to continue outwardly agreeing with the commitment despite not honoring it, and hiding their duplicity.

Looking at one's contradictory behavior can be a provocative moment in therapy. Contradictory behavior is especially humbling and difficult to face when it is framed as a decision or solution to resolve competing motivations. Clients frequently project onto the therapist their own fears about the moral implications, negative self-judgments, and perhaps antisocial traits that their contradictions reveal. We advise them that they are not condemned for the sexual symptoms they want to address in treatment and then help them identify the emotions that underlie their judgments. What is important in the assessment is providing a space for men to decide whether their current duplicity strategy and the concomitant consequences are something they want to change. It is good news when men decide they do not want to continue the avoidant and deceptive behavior that leads to hurtful and painful emotional consequences. This moment of self-discrepancy is an opportunity to access motivation for different choices. What is next usually involves two options: renegotiating the initial sexual agreement or finding new strategies to maintain the agreement. Obviously, easier said than done.

Maintaining the perspective of an intimate partner relationship as collectively created avoids colluding with narrative that places the OCSB client as the identified patient solely responsible for the current state of the relationship (Wiener & MacColl, 2012). This is a tricky balance because the client is the only person attending the assessment. As we nonjudgmentally and curiously gather information from our clients, we are available to encourage partners to consider help for themselves as well as to help the couple plan for relationship therapy. Besides the benefit of the support the partner would receive in managing the emotional consequences of the client's extrarelational sexual behaviors, the partner may benefit from a space to better understand her or his contribution to the relationship dynamics.

To be fair, relationship agreements often vary in clarity. Some are as clear as a highway median. Others are nothing more than an overgrown dirt path. In Jay's marriage, his wife was continually upset by his solo-sexual behavior, but they never explicitly discussed anything close to a clear boundary regarding masturbation. Despite not verbalizing a masturbation agreement, they did have an unspoken understanding. Each assumed the other masturbated but avoided discussing their differing opinions about what the other did for arousal and stimulation. This meant they never discussed Jay's use of sexual imagery in solo sex.

Jay had a vague understanding that Veronique disapproved of sexual imagery. They avoided conversations that would have made the situation much clearer and waited until she discovered his online sexual behavior. How did Jay contribute to the cocreation of this silent agreement with his wife? How aware was he about her wish that he did not watch online sexual videos? What prevented him from discussing his sexual practices or asserting his erotic interests? Did his passivity allow him to exploit the vagueness of the agreement? Without an explicit agreement, it is difficult to help clients determine whether they want to change and perhaps subscribe to an explicit solo-sex agreement that integrates the partner's shared values about solo sex. Throughout the assessment, the therapist and client collaborate to better understand the competing motivations in the descriptions about feared consequences of his sexual behavior. "I didn't want my relationship to break up." "I didn't want to lose access to my children." "I didn't want to be the first person in my family to get a divorce." "I wasn't ready to face that I was bisexual." Addressing client sexual relationship agreements enhances men's sexual and relationship communication skills as well as clarifies their sexual values. This is immeasurably important as men begin to transfer their sexual health plan and vision for sexual health in their current or future intimate partner relationship sexual agreements.

Sexual Narcissism

When assessing the contradiction between agreements and actions, we listen for narcissistic themes that may glean important insights. As we discussed in Chapters 4 and 5, *personality* is not the construct or terminology we regularly use to diagnostically label a client's sexual symptoms. We prefer the dual-process model of human behavior to provide the context in which to understand OCSB (Loewenstein & O'Donoghue, 2007). The dual-process model of human behavior and personality theory are not incompatible. On the contrary, we view personality traits as a set pattern of deliberative/affective interaction that produces the same interpersonal consequences. These enduring patterns may manifest sexual behaviors that are the source of distress and feel out of control. But in these situations, we find clients reporting that their personality traits feel out of control, not their sexual thoughts, urges, or behavior. In other words, they report not feeling in control of their narcissism.

We recommend that OCSB assessment look at a subset of clients with narcissistic traits as either pervasive (i.e., symptomatic of narcissistic personality disorder) or primarily activated in sexual situations (i.e., symptomatic of sexual narcissism). Widman and McNulty (2010) identified four traits that compromise sexual narcissism: sexual exploitation, sexual entitlement, lacking sexual empathy, and grandiosity in sexual skills. OCSB assessment focuses primarily on the first three as most salient to dysregulated sexual behavior. How often does the client remedy sexual dilemmas with unilateral, secretive, deceptive, or unspoken solutions? Clients often avoid or fear direct, honest, and vulnerable discussions about their solutions to sexual relationship or erotic conflicts. During the assessment, the goal is to familiarize clients with their reliance on unilateral and secretive decision making to manage their conflicts with their sexual agreements. Maintaining empathy, using precontemplative or contemplative interventions, and maintaining a stance of curiosity may lessen the activation of defensiveness or damaging rapport. Below are some questions to consider:

Sexual Exploitation: What strategies does the client use to have sex with others? What is his reasoning to justify lying, manipulation, or exploiting his position of power? If the client's sexual behaviors involve paying for sex, does he consider the feelings of the sex worker? How often does he think about the possibility that he may be exploiting another person for his sexual or relational needs? Does the money serve a function to avoid relational contact (i.e., I don't pay her for sex, I pay her to go away)?

Sexual Entitlement: Does he become frustrated or indignant when he is "denied sex"? How available does he believe his partner should be to *his* sexual advances?

Sexual Empathy: To what degree does he describe feeling emotionally connected during sex? Does he experience disappointment when there is little emotional connection with an intimate sexual partner? How invested is the client in his partner's sexual pleasure? Does the client hold a greater value for communal (e.g., shared intimacy) or individualistic (e.g., physical pleasure) rewards?

INFORMATION GATHERING: PROFESSIONAL CONSULTS

The final information-gathering segment of the OCSB assessment is exchanging collateral information with a client's medical and mental health providers. With the client's permission, we recommend consulting with all the professionals involved in the client's behavioral health care. The OCSB protocol was developed as an outpatient, mental health program. All other services for the diverse needs of our clients are provided through a local community of mental health and medical professionals.

Referring and Concurrent Providers

Drug and alcohol counselors, couple therapists, primary care physicians, psychiatrists, or individual psychotherapists commonly refer their clients for an OCSB assessment. We recommend that clinicians reach out to learn about the provider's reasons for the referral, his or her treatment history, and clinical impressions of the client. We educate the other providers on the OCSB screening, assessment, and combined treatment program. It is important to educate referring professionals that the OCSB screening appointment is not a group therapy preplacement appointment. Providers tend to appreciate knowing the purpose of the comprehensive assessment and the OCSB group treatment preparation process. For clients who plan to continue seeing the referring provider for individual therapy, it is important to clarify roles and treatment expectations. In that scenario, the main objective of the assessment is to determine whether specialized treatment for OCSB is warranted, and to provide treatment recommendations for the clients that can be folded into their work with their therapist.

After the assessment is complete, we consult with referring providers to discuss the outcome of the assessment. As we have previously addressed, all men in the OCSB group are required to continue their individual therapy. Clients have the option to create a treatment team. Clients can either continue with their referring therapist or choose to receive individual therapy from the group leader who conducted their assessment. For clients who are seen by an outside therapist, the group leader and individual therapist will collaborate from time to time regarding the client's treatment progress.

REFERENCES

Anda, R. F., Felitti, V. J., Bremner, J. D., Walker, J. D., Whitfield, C. H., Perry, B. D., ... & Giles, W. H. (2006). The enduring effects of abuse and related adverse experiences in childhood. *European Archives of Psychiatry and Clinical Neuroscience*, 256(3), 174–186.

Bancroft, J. (2009). *Human Sexuality and Its Problems* (3rd ed.). Edinburgh, UK: Churchill, Livingstone & Elsevier.

Bancroft, J., Graham, C., Janssen E., & Sanders, S. (2009). The dual control model: Current status and future directions. *Journal of Sex Research*, 46(2–3), 121–142.

Bancroft, J., & Vukadinovic, Z. (2004). Sexual addiction, sexual compulsivity, sexual impulsivity, or what? Toward a theoretical model. *Journal of Sex Research*, 41(3), 225–234.

Barratt, B. B., & Rand, M. A. (2009). "Sexual health assessment" for mental and medical practitioners: Teaching notes. *American Journal of Sexuality Education, 4*, 16–27.

Belous, C. K., Timm, T. M., Grace, C., & Whitehead, M. R. (2012). Revisiting the sexual genogram. *American Journal of Family Therapy, 40*, 281–296.

Berry, M. D., & Berry, P. D. (2013). Mentalization-based therapy for sexual addiction: Foundations for a clinical model. *Sexual and Relationship Therapy, 29*(2) 245–260.

Brenner, J. (2014). *The secret to better care: It really is all in your head.* Retrieved from www.philly.com/philly/blogs/fieldclinic/The-Secret-to-Better-Care-It-Really-Is-All-in-Your-Head.html

Buehler, S. (2014). *What every mental health professional should know about sex.* New York, NY: Springer Publishing, Company.

Chadwick Center for Children and Families. (2009). *Assessment-based treatment for traumatized children: A trauma assessment pathway (TAP).* San Diego, CA. Retrieved from www.taptraining.net/documents/Master%20TAP-12-09.pdf

Edwards, J. K., & Bess, J. M. (1998). Developing effectiveness in the therapeutic use of self. *Clinical Social Work Journal, 26*(1), 89–105.

Edwards, W. M., Delmonico, D., & Griffin, E. (2011). *Cybersex unplugged: Finding sexual health in an electronic world.* CreateSpace Independent Publishing Platform.

Felitti, V. J., Anda, R. F., Nordenberg, D., Williamson, D. F., Spitz, A. M., Edwards, V., Koss, M. P., & Marks, J. S. (1998). Relationship of childhood abuse and household dysfunction to many of the leading causes of death in adults: The Adverse Childhood Experiences (ACE) study. *American Journal of Preventive Medicine, 4*, 245–258.

Fonagy, P. (2008). The mentalization-focused approach to social development. In F. N. Busch (Ed.), *Mentalization: Theoretical considerations, research findings, and clinical implications* (pp. 3–56). New York: Analytic Press.

Fraley, R. C. (2010). *A brief overview of adult attachment theory and research.* Retrieved from www.internal.psychology.illinois.edu/~rcfraley/attachment.htm.

Fraley, R. C., Heffernan, M., Vicary, A., & Brumbaugh, C. (2011). The Experiences in Close Relationships—Relationship Structures questionnaire: A method for assessing attachment orientations across relationships. *Psychological Assessment, 23*, 615–625.

Fraley, R. C., Niedenthal, P. M., Marks, M. J., Brumbaugh, C. C., & Vicary, A. (2006). Adult attachment and the perception of emotional expressions: Probing the hyperactivating strategies underlying anxious attachment. *Journal of Personality, 74*, 1163–1190.

Fraley, R. C., & Shaver, P. R. (2000). Adult romantic attachment: Theoretical developments, emerging controversies, and unanswered questions. *Review of General Psychology, 4*(2), 132.

Graham, C. A., Sanders, S. A., & Milhausen, R. R. (2006). The Sexual Excitation and Sexual Inhibition Inventory for Women: Psychometric properties. *Archive of Sexual Behavior, 35*, 397–410.

Haidt, J. (2006). *The happiness hypothesis: Finding modern truth in ancient wisdom.* New York, NY: Basic Books.

Hook, J. N., Hook, J. P., Davis, D. E., Worthington Jr., E. L., & Penberthy, J. K. (2010). Measuring sexual addiction and compulsivity: A critical review of instruments. *Journal of Sex & Marital Therapy, 36*(3), 227–260.

Janssen, E., & Bancroft, J. (2007). The Dual-Control model: The role of sexual inhibition & excitation in sexual arousal and behavior. In E. Janssen (Ed.), *The psychophysiology of sex* (pp. 197–221). Bloomington, IN: Indiana University Press.

Janssen, E., Vorst, H., Finn, P., & Bancroft, J. (2002). The Sexual Inhibition (SIS) and Sexual Excitation (SES) Scales: I. Measuring sexual inhibition and excitation proneness in men. *Journal of Sex Research, 39*, 114–126.

Kessler, R. C., Adler, L., Ames, M., Demler, O., Faraone, S., Hiripi, E., Howes, …, & Walters, E. E. (2005). The World Health Organization Adult ADHD Self-Report Scale (ASRS). *Psychological Medicine, 35*(2), 245–256.

Loewenstein, G., & O'Donoghue, T. (2007). *The heat of the moment: Modeling interactions between affect and deliberation.* Unpublished manuscript. Retrieved from: https://odonoghue.economics.cornell.edu/heat.pdf

Miller, W. R., & Rollnick, S. (2013). *Motivational interviewing; Helping people change* (3rd ed.). New York: Guilford Press.

Money, J. (1999). *The lovemap guidebook: A definitive statement.* New York, NY: Continuum.

Morin, J. (1995). *The erotic mind: Unlocking the inner sources of sexual passion and fulfillment.* New York: HarperCollins.

Prochaska, J. O., Norcross, J., & DiClemente, C. (2006). *Changing for good: A revolutionary six-stage program for overcoming bad habits and moving your life positively forward.* New York, NY: HarperCollins.

Raymond, N. C., Lloyd, M. D., Miner, M. H., & Kim, S. W. (2007). Preliminary report on the development and validation of the Sexual Symptom Assessment Scale. *Sexual Addiction & Compulsivity, 14*, 119–129.

Reid, R. C., Davtian, M., Lenartowicz, A., Torrevillas, R. M., & Fong, T. W. (2013). Perspectives on the assessment and treatment of adult ADHD in hypersexual men. *Neuropsychiatry, 3*(3), 295–308.

Reid, R. C., Garos, S., & Fong, T. (2012). Psychometric development of the Hypersexual Behavior Consequences Scale. *Journal of Behavioral Addictions, 1*(3), 115–122.

Repetti, R. L., Robles, T. F., & Reynolds, B. (2011). Allostatic processes in the family. *Development and Psychopathology, 23*(03), 921–938.

Risen, C. (2010). Listening to sexual stories. In S. Levine, C. Risen, & S. E. Althof (Eds.), *Handbook of clinical sexuality for mental health professionals* (pp. 3–20). New York, NY: Routledge.

Stevens, J. E. (2012, October 3). The Adverse Childhood Experiences study—The largest, most important public health study you never heard of began in an obesity clinic. *ACES Too High News.* Retrieved from www.acestoohigh.com/2012/10/03/the-adverse-childhood-experiences-study-the-largest-most-important-public-health-study-you-never-heard-of-began-in-an-obesity-clinic/

Widman, L., & McNulty, J. K. (2010). Sexual Narcissism Scale. In T. D. Fisher, C. M. Davis, W. L. Yarber, & S. L. Davis (Eds.), *Handbook of sexuality-related measures* (pp. 496–497). New York, NY: Routledge.

Wiener, D. J., & MacColl, M. (2012). Co-creating reality: Acquiring mutual validation skills in couple therapy using theatre improvisation. *International Journal of Humanities and Social Science, 2*(23), 54–63.

CHAPTER SEVEN

ASSESSMENT—TREATMENT ELEMENTS

Therapy is energized when it focuses on the relationship between therapist and patient.

—Irv Yalom

In this chapter, we highlight the out of control sexual behavior (OCSB) assessment treatment elements for enhancing client motivation for change listed in Figure 6.1. Our overall intention in delving deeply into the assessment process is to organize the therapist's mind when listening to his or her clients and prioritizing clinical interventions. We conclude the chapter with a discussion on synthesizing the assessment information to construct the client's OCSB Unique Clinical Picture, which is the basis for treatment recommendations.

TREATMENT ELEMENTS: CHANGE PROCESSES

The transtheoretical model of health behavior change (TTM) defines human behavior change processes as overt and covert activities to help people modify thinking, feeling, or behavior (Prochaska, Norcross, & DiClemente, 2006; Prochaska & Velicer, 1997). TTM identified and organized principles and processes from every school of psychotherapy into a system that recommends the application based on the individual's stage of readiness for change. "Each process is a broad category encompassing multiple techniques, methods, and interventions traditionally associated with disparate theoretical orientations" (Prochaska, Norcross, & DiClemente, 2013, p. 13). In this model for behavior change, clinicians can flexibly use familiar therapeutic interventions tailored to the clients' individual needs to support their progress toward health. We highlight four of the 12 change processes that are pertinent to the OCSB assessment: consciousness-raising, emotional arousal, self-reevaluation, and social liberation. In general, most OCSB clients present with a mixture of precontemplative and contemplative readiness for change. The change processes we highlight are consistent with interventions that motivate precontemplators and contemplators to move to the next stage of change. The application of preparation- and action-stage change processes is discussed in the next chapter.

As with any generalization, there are exceptions. We conduct assessments with clients whose readiness is consistent with the preparation and action stages. These clients still benefit from the assessment process, but the duration of the assessment may be shorter as the clients typically present with greater insight and motivation for sexual health behavior change. We recommend readers familiarize themselves with TTM and motivational interviewing (MI) techniques. Besides offering flexibility and adaptability needed to successfully treat the variety of factors that influence their sexual behavior problems, the MI philosophy of "looking and seeing together" (Miller & Rollnick, 2002, p. 25) perfectly captures the disposition of an OCSB assessment.

Change Process: Consciousness-Raising

The OCSB assessment is an intense, consciousness-raising experience. Clients are carefully guided through a self-reflective process to understand the diverse factors that contribute to their sexual behavior problems. Raising client awareness about these factors helps clients evaluate their options for improving their sexual health. Rather than an assumed pathological process that will be uncovered, the OCSB assessment provides a reflective environment for the client to develop insights into his sexual problems. Michael is fond of telling clients that the clinical recommendations and conceptualizations summarized at the close of the assessment should not include any surprises. The purpose of the OCSB assessment is to ensure the clinical connections are made.

Therapist and client jointly explore contradictions among the client's actions, motivations, and values and the historical events that may have current relevance to his sexual health. The exploration may elicit uncomfortable or intense emotions. Since the dawn of psychoanalysis, therapists have observed the defenses clients deploy to avoid seeing and accepting painful truths about themselves. We understand these defenses as intrapersonal and interpersonal coping strategies that reduce anxiety stemming from unacceptable, threatening, or negative events. Less adaptive defenses are ways of mediating the emotions associated with threatening events and self-discrepant conflicts while keeping them out of the client's conscious awareness. The less adaptive defenses do not modify or ameliorate the emotional pain associated with the events (Juni, 1998/1999), but they are needed for people to avoid feelings they are unable to confront so they can continue with their lives. During the assessment, however, these defenses can be used to distract and avoid the uncomfortable task of self-analysis (Prochaska et al., 2006).

Assessment interventions that uncover irrational beliefs that focus client attention on relationship agreement violations may elicit uncomfortable emotions. Clients' in-session reactions present an opportunity to raise their awareness about the coping strategies they use during moments of distress. Because defenses function to avoid the emotional consequences of unacceptable or threatening events, exploring these moments can increase their awareness about what feels threatening to them. Are they defending against feeling guilt about their actions? Are they feeling shame because they judge themselves as deviant or perverted? Are they distancing themselves from the reality of their abusive childhood to avoid processing the residual hurt from those experiences? The OCSB assessment offers an opportunity to encounter client defenses so both client and therapist can learn about the emotional costs and consequences of change. In other words, therapists may be asking men to endure previously avoided uncomfortable emotions when evaluating the factors connected to their out of control sexual experiences.

Client defense may also be related to the therapist's stage-discrepant intervention. In the latest edition of *Motivational Interviewing*, Miller and Rollnick (2013) shifted away from labeling this defensive posture as "resistance." They wanted to avoid pathologizing a natural part of the change process. They saw how the term *resistance* fused two different concepts. One concept was the "sustain talk" clients exhibit when they are ambivalent about change. The other was the "discord" between the therapist and client. Sustain talk is "any client speech that favors *status quo* rather than movement toward a change goal" (p. 413). Discord is a relational event in which the client's behavior reflects dissonance in the working relationship with the therapist. Discord may be evident in therapy relationships that devolve into "arguing, interrupting, discounting or ignoring" (p. 408). Therapists can effectively respond to sustain talk and discord when they consider each as separate opportunities to change a client's patterned defenses and scripts, which repeatedly play out in their lives. When therapists can speak different lines from the role clients expect clinicians to play, the client's behavior and relationship script can change (Miller & Rollnick, 2013).

In this spirit, the OCSB assessment raises men's consciousness about factors contributing to their OCSB as well as the intra- and interpersonal defenses used to maintain their status quo. By integrating conscious-raising MI practices within the OCSB assessment, therapist and client become aware of the factors contributing to their OCSB and their relational patterns, which may interfere with the change process. Later in this chapter, we review some key defenses OCSB treatment-seeking men commonly exhibit during OCSB assessments and clinical responses to maintain the therapeutic alliance.

Change Process: Emotional Arousal

Emotions that are aroused during an OCSB assessment are a powerful force to motivate sexual health change. Throughout each assessment appointment, therapists shift their focus between gathering clinical information and attending to men's elicited emotions. Attending to their emotions during the OCSB assessment serves multiple purposes, of which we highlight two: helping motivate clients for sexual health change and assisting clients with affect tolerance.

Motivating Change

Many clients repeatedly engage in problematic sexual behavior because they defend against the very emotions that might motivate them to change. By walking clients through a paced and detailed OCSB assessment, we help men open themselves to their avoided affectations. For instance, they may begin to feel empathy for their intimate partner's pain after he disclosed breaking their relationship agreements. Men may begin to sense their fear of the physical or occupational consequences of continuing their OCSB patterns. Emotional activation paired with men who are deliberating their reasons for change energizes clients to move toward their sexual health goals.

Affect Tolerance

The OCSB assessment is an important opportunity to evaluate clients' window of affect tolerance within the relational container of psychotherapy. Some of the OCSB assessment tasks (e.g., Sexual Symptom Assessment Scale [SSAS]) examine how men manage the intensities and types of emotional activation that arise in therapy. The relational interaction between therapist and client is another process for gathering information on the client's affect tolerance. For example, when we observe a change in affect, we draw the client's attention to his experience in the moment. "Can you share what you just felt?" "When you started talking about your uncle, your face changed a bit, I am not familiar with that expression. What were you feeling?" OCSB treatment-seeking men frequently present with limited skills in identifying, labeling, and expressing emotions. They are more likely to respond with a statement about their thoughts or judgments. We acknowledge their attempt, but hold them to the question. "Bad is not a feeling. It is a judgment of your feeling. Can you find a feeling word such as *mad, glad, sad, fear,* or *shame*?" When men struggle with labeling their feelings, we ask the question again from a somatic perspective: "Where in your body did you feel something? Can you describe what it felt like?" This inquiry is motivated to help them increase their self-awareness capacity during moments of emotional arousal and provide the therapist with immediate experiences in which to gauge client readiness for this aspect of OCSB treatment. This treatment element provides early practice for men to prepare for individual and group therapy processes that will ask them to hold their focus on their emotions and to increase their tolerance of embodied feelings.

We frequently debrief the experience of identifying and labeling emotions as part of the OCSB assessment. "What was that like for you when I pressed you to find the feeling?" We explain the objective of holding their attention on uncomfortable emotions for less experienced psychotherapy clients who may be simultaneously learning about the therapeutic process while in the assessment. When men explicitly demonstrate higher levels of affect tolerance, the focus of this component of the OCSB assessment can review the experience in a more conscious manner. "You mentioned earlier that you were hesitant to revisit some of your life events because you were afraid of feeling overwhelmed. How overwhelmed did you feel?"

It is important to consider the timing of more direct exploration of clients' emotional arousal during the progressive sequence of OCSB assessment sessions. Men at the precontemplative stage of change may struggle more frequently with navigating emotional arousal connected with their sexual behavior. They can benefit from emotional regulation skills building before gathering additional information about their sexual histories. Emotional arousal is an effective change process for clients in the contemplative stage of change. When clients are less ambivalent about change and clearly moving toward taking action to change, then holding the client's focus on the negative emotional aspects of their problematic sexual behavior may demotivate them (Prochaska et al., 2006).

Change Process: Self-Reevaluation

An important change process for men considering changing their sexual behavior occurs when they examine the central values that conflict with their sexual behaviors (see Prochaska et al., 2006). An OCSB assessment integrates the client's self-appraisal of his sexual behavior in the larger context of his self-concept. The two aforementioned change processes, raising consciousness and eliciting emotional arousal, are used for self-re-evaluation. Men are provided a space to openly reflect on a life beyond feeling out of control in their sexual lives and to form beliefs about how much better life would be without sexual behavior problems.

Men frequently express confusion and frustration when they perceive contradictions between their values and their sexual thoughts, urges, or behaviors. In this moment of self-reflection lies the opportunity for therapists to guide men toward facing and exploring their contradictions. What is it about the sexual thoughts, urges, or behavior that a man does not like? Is his sexual value well defined or something that is more intuitive or reactive? Frequently, clients are uncertain about how they developed their sexual values or what standards they should use to evaluate them. Without a clear set of principles with which to evaluate their sexual thoughts, urges, or behavior, clients often rely on their emotional reactions to guide their decisions. "This sexual stimuli makes me feel disgusted, it must be bad." Or they may rely on the act-centered value system based on social conventions or the values of their intimate partner. This is where sexual health principles are helpful in evaluating clients' current sexual thoughts, urges, or behavior. The intention of the OCSB self-reevaluation is to help men develop principle-centered values that can function as a sexual ethic which guides decisions that, over time, more frequently align with their personal vision of sexual health.

Men frequently ask the therapist his or her opinion on what the client's sexual boundaries should be as they evaluate their sexual thoughts, urges, and behavior. "Do you think I should stop watching porn?" "Is it wrong to fantasize about my wife dominating me?" "Is it an addiction to want to have sex as much as I do?" Rather than reinforce an act-centered thought process, we advise them that the assessment process is designed to help them determine the forms of sexual expressions they find meaningful and important as part of their sexual health goals. The OCSB assessment is a guided process for men to determine the sexual behaviors or circumstances that they want to change.

A sexual self-reevaluation may lead to a dawning awareness of a man's deep disappointment with his sexual behavior. Within the confines of a confidential assessment, clients can seriously question the compatibility of feeling good about themselves and continuing their current sexual behaviors. Further, by reevaluating their sexual thoughts, urges, and behavior using the sexual health principles, they can develop the critical-thinking skills necessary to establish their sexual health plan and negotiate sexual value conflicts in the future.

Change Process: Social Liberation

Social liberation refers to the benefit of providing people with alternative choices to engage in nonproblematic behaviors, especially men who may be oppressed or deprived (Prochaska et al., 2006, 2013). Socially liberated spaces provide sexual health information and external support for sexual health behavior change. Examples vary from nonsmoking areas for people trying to quit smoking to peer support groups for people trying to improve their eating habits. We view the psychotherapeutic space as an example of social liberation for people trying to improve their sexual health. Therapists can provide external support and information for sexual health behavior change, while men gradually establish alternative spaces to support sexual health goals.

An OCSB assessment may be the first of its kind in which men have the privilege of honestly discussing their sexual health concerns with a sexologically informed professional who attentively listens to each man's concerns without judgment. Most sociocultural contexts for discussing OCSB may intersect with America's sexual illiteracy, misinformation, and sex-negative judgments. The OCSB assessment process protects the client's sexual autonomy and intrinsic motivation for sexual health behavior change from the undue influences of negative sociocultural sex messages. We contend that men entering OCSB treatment (along with their intimate partners and families) have paid a high price for the limited availability of sexual health conversations. Accessing a socially liberated space may offer the first safe harbor for men to have meaningful sexual health conversations that lead to lasting changes in their sexual health.

Change Process: Manifesting Sexual Health Change Talk

After reviewing the four change processes that commonly unfold during the OCSB assessment, we focus on several techniques to illustrate how processes might manifest in an assessment appointment. We highlight common client defenses and sexual language patterns that can obstruct the assessment process. We provide dialogue between Doug or Michael and one of the four case examples we introduced in earlier chapters to demonstrate our interventions.

Fleeing to Hopeless or Helpless

Hector, who is currently in an outpatient drug and alcohol treatment program, began his OCSB assessment concurrently. This is his second assessment appointment with Doug (group leader's name appears in bold type). He filled out the Adverse Childhood Experiences Study questionnaire (ACE) at home as requested. On his own, he asked his partner, Phil, to also fill out the ACE. Hector walked into Doug's office, threw the ACE form down on an end table and took his seat.

DOUG: What just happened?

HECTOR: What do you mean?

DOUG: Is the paper you put on the table your ACE survey?

HECTOR: (*sighing heavily*) Yes, I can't believe I scored so much higher than my husband.

DOUG: That was a pretty big breath. Can you tell me what the sigh was?

HECTOR: I got a 6 and he only had a 1. I am so fucked up. I don't know if I am cut out for all this recovery. I'm just fucked.

DOUG: What are you doing right now?

HECTOR: What do you mean?

DOUG: Well, you did a nice job of telling me what the sigh was about. I understand that part. I also understand you had a reaction to the different ACE scores between you and your husband. But what I'm curious about is if you know what you did when you talked about not being cut out for recovery.

HECTOR: I don't understand what you are talking about.

DOUG: That's OK, I just did not want to assume you didn't know about what I just observed. We find that men need to learn about two very important defenses early in the assessment process. We find that when men observe their use of these two defenses, they can increase their chances of changing their sexual health. Are you interested?

HECTOR: OK, but what about the ACE?

> **DOUG:** Yes, I know, we'll get to that in a minute. This is a bit of what the assessment is like. We will review the measures, but if something happens in the session between us, then we stop and discuss it. We can return to the measure later. We'll move back and forth throughout the assessment.
>
> **HECTOR:** OK, I'm listening.
>
> **DOUG:** Generally, I'm interested in drawing my clients' attention to how they act during the session, particularly how they react to uncomfortable feelings. I heard you say something pretty hopeless sounding just now. We find that men with OCSB, who are not aware of when they do this, who don't notice how they respond to difficult emotions, have a hard time achieving their treatment goals and maintaining their sexual health. So I was wondering if you could tell me a bit more about why you think you fled into hopelessness when you entered the room? Do you have any thoughts about that?

When a client in an OCSB assessment expresses forms of hopelessness or helplessness through his words or actions, it is an opportunity to educate the client about the function of this defense. What we have termed "fleeing to hopeless or helpless" exemplifies the intra- and interpersonal defense mechanisms that inhibit men moving past their status quo. It is also a common defense used among OCSB treatment-seeking men to dismiss their personal commitments or relationship agreements. They flee to hopelessness and helplessness as one of the final steps in their sequence of crossing their sexual boundaries.

We recommend that therapists refocus the client's attention on this defense and guide the dialogue on understanding the client's motive for relying on this emotion regulation tool. Viewing this moment through the lens of TTM processes of change, an aspect of the ACE discussion triggered an *emotional arousal* for which Hector's defense was a movement toward hopelessness or helplessness. Doug has an opportunity to *raise his consciousness* about this defensive coping and *reevaluate* his use of that response. Doug remained curious and open minded when inquiring about how Hector came to believe that his recovery was hopeless or that he was helpless to change. What was the function of his flight? Were Hector's helpless or hopeless feelings giving him permission to take action and cross his SHP boundaries? Hector's thoughts may be something like, "Since I'm hopeless, why bother maintaining my boundaries?" His reflexive flight to these interpersonal cognitive defenses may function to create distance with those close to him. Expressions of hopelessness or helplessness can also function as a form of communication that indirectly asked others for closeness or attention. How have loved ones responded to this expression in the past? Is he recreating these dynamics in the assessment as an unconscious education for Doug? These are only some of the directions in which the therapist can take the discussion.

At first it is important for clients to see and be able to understand that hopelessness and helplessness are activated feelings, not facts about their situations. When men start merging hopeless thinking with the activated feelings of hopelessness they tend to temporarily abandon motivation for change. The resulting void and concurrent tension that accompanies this sudden change in motivation is often expressed through a host of problematic sexual and nonsexual coping strategies.

We encourage men to conceptualize their fleeing to hopelessness and helplessness as a previously protective coping strategy that is now out of date. Their history of how they came to need this defense at one time in their lives is typically personal and idiosyncratic. Over the course of the assessment, the function of these defenses may become clear as the client's OCSB Unique Clinical Picture takes shape. We conceptualize the flight to a helpless/hopeless position as an important narrative for men to monitor. We explain to our clients that they obstruct their ability to change when they flee to a hopeless/helpless space because they will not change if they believe they cannot change. Psychotherapy is less effective when clients wrap themselves in this demotivating belief system. The OCSB assessment is designed to be flexible enough to both facilitate the change process as well as gather the essential OCSB clinical information.

Sex Talk

The use of direct and precise language in sexual health conversations has a variety of psychotherapeutic benefits. There are two specific benefits to discussing sexual activity in accurate and literal language: to enhance clarity for client self-reevaluation and to increase comfort and confidence when talking about sexual activity. When men avoid the details of their sexual urges, thoughts, and behaviors, intrapsychic and relational patterns remain hidden from view. Indirect sexual communication may reflect the client defenses against feeling negative emotions associated with his sexual decisions and behavior. Clients tend to avoid embarrassment, guilt, and rejection fears through indirect conversation about their

OCSB symptoms. Those who become more comfortable with frank sexual discussions will likely improve their abilities to establish a reasonable and an enjoyable sexual health plan and negotiate their sexual needs with others. Therefore, we use the assessment to develop men's skills of open and direct sex talk. In this section, we describe three therapist sex-talk skills to integrate within an OCSB assessment: using nonfigurative language, discussing sexual details, and using sexual health language.

Nonfigurative language

Assessment sex talk guides men away from their familiar figurative language, such as the use of metaphor, hyperbole, analogies, and euphemisms. Helping clients use accurate sexual language is consistent with the information-gathering and motivation-enhancing objectives of the OCSB assessment. By definition, when speaking in figurative language, clients use words and expressions that have different meanings than the literal interpretation, which leaves room for misinterpretation and false assumptions by the therapist. Some clients may express themselves with symbolism or cultural references unfamiliar to the provider. They may be unaware they are using words and expressions that are vague and unclear because that is how most people talk outside of a sex-therapy appointment. It is possible, however, that clients have been perfecting language that leaves ample room for misinterpretation and false assumptions by therapists, sexual partners, friends, and family. Either way, figurative language hinders a therapist's ability to clearly understand the factors contributing to the client's out of control sexual experiences.

Putting words to one's internal experience is a common struggle for many OCSB treatment-seeking clients, especially for those new to psychotherapy. When searching for the right words, clients may speak figuratively to communicate a thought or feeling for the first time or when their introspective skills are underdeveloped (Needham-Didsbury, 2012). We empathize with their difficulty but we do not stop inquiring when they figuratively describe unfamiliar or unexplored aspects of their sexuality or OCSB. We hear statements like: "My addiction took over," "I felt like my blood was boiling," and "It was like my computer was calling my name." These are vivid and colorful phrases but they do not clearly communicate what happened or what they experienced. What does it mean to the client when he says "my addiction"? Is he describing his sexual thoughts or urges? Does he believe that an internal system in his body took control of his deliberative system or is he struggling to see the choices he made leading up to sexual behavior? If boiling blood were an emotion, what would it be and where did he actually feel it? And, what did he mean that his computer was calling his name? Is that the client's way of describing a sexual temptation or his perception that he is powerless to control his deliberative mind when it is emotionally activated? If therapists want to understand the factors that contribute to their clients' OCSB symptoms, it is important to develop client engagement skills that address men's figurative sexual language.

We frequently interrupt the conversation when men use nonliteral sexual language and ask them for clarity. For instance, we may ask them to explain how they felt without using a metaphor or to describe their sexual behavior without euphemisms. Because the client is likely new to literal discussions about his sexual thoughts, feelings, and behavior, we remain patient as he searches for nonfigurative language without offering our interpretation. This moment is an opportunity to develop introspective skills, practice communicating thoughts and feelings directly, and concretize new insights developed in therapy (Needham-Didsbury, 2012).

Jay

Jay agreed to meet Michael for an OCSB assessment after the sexual discovery crisis with his wife, Veronique. The following dialogue occurred in the third assessment appointment while Michael was reviewing the SSAS measure with Jay. Jay read item #1 and described how his urges to engage in problematic sexual behavior were extreme because of his preoccupation with "porn."

JAY: I just watched porn all day.

MICHAEL: When you say "porn," what are you referring to? What exactly were you watching?

JAY: Well, this week, I watched video clips of men and women having sex. I streamed them on my phone from a couple of free sites.

MICHAEL: Any kind of sex in particular?

JAY: You know, the usual stuff.

MICHAEL: What's usual for you?

JAY: OK. I was watching men having anal sex with women.

MICHAEL: Have you ever been that specific about what sexual videos you watch?

JAY: Not really.

MICHAEL: What did it feel like to say?

JAY: A little embarrassing.

We are disinclined to use the word *porn* to avoid ambiguity and the cultural conflicts that surround explicit sexual media. The word *porn* can distract from details like how Jay was viewing the sexual images and the specifics about the images he wanted to view. If Michael left the original phrase unquestioned, he would have missed some details about Jay's behavior and erotic template, as well as the opportunity to desensitize Jay's embarrassment when he discussed the details of his preferred sexual imagery.

MICHAEL: You also mentioned that you were watching "all day"?

JAY: Yes, I'd watch it on my phone during my lunch break. I'd go to the bathroom a couple of times and watch … and on my drive home when I was stuck in traffic.

MICHAEL: Oh, so not "all day." There were periods of time when you weren't watching.

JAY: Well, yeah.

MICHAEL: What would be a more accurate description of how frequently you were watching sexual videos?

JAY: Off-and-on throughout the day.

MICHAEL: Off-and-on as in ….

JAY: Like, three to four times a day.

MICHAEL: Did you feel differently when you said that you watched sex videos "three to four times" versus "all day"?

JAY: Yes, it felt better.

MICHAEL: What emotion did you feel that you are describing as "better"?

JAY: It felt …

MICHAEL: (*interrupting*) Try using an "I" statement. I felt …

JAY: Oh, right. I felt … relaxed. Maybe a little relief.

> **MICHAEL:** Great, relaxed and relief are both feelings. What felt relieving?
>
> **JAY:** Well, it seemed less overwhelming.

There were several instances in which Jay was not speaking literally and thus less accurately. "All day" was hyperbolic and describing his feeling as "better" provided a judgment of his emotion (better) rather than the actual feeling (relief). By getting curious about what was meant by "all day," Michael developed a clearer picture of the sexual behaviors Jay considered problematic. Jay was also using his phone to view sexual media, not his computer. This may be important when developing his sexual health plan strategies to regulate and monitor his access to mobile sex videos. By exploring Jay's casual exaggeration of time spent watching videos, Michael subtly invited him to reevaluate distorted conclusions about his sexual behavior. This led to Jay identifying the inaccuracy of his statement and finding a nonfigurative description of his sexual activity. As with similar cognitive therapy techniques, the sex talk changed Jay's absolutist thinking with more accurate sexual behavior language, which generated a different and positive emotional consequence. When clients translate figurative language into literal meaning, it is easier to identity and reevaluate their negative and noncompassionate judgments about sexual activity.

> **MICHAEL:** Also, you said you were watching sexual videos all day. Were you just watching or were you also masturbating?
>
> **JAY:** Not always. Two of the times I went to the men's room, I masturbated. One time I watched at my desk for a couple of minutes and then went back to work. I also was masturbating when I was driving.

When Jay said "watching porn," it was unclear to Michael what he was actually trying to communicate. For Jay, the word "watching" was a euphemism that had a dual purpose to communicate both viewing imagery and masturbation. Euphemisms can be used to defend against negative judgments about sexual activity and the corresponding emotional consequences of these judgments. Euphemisms can also function as a way to withhold important clinical dialogue that can elicit change talk. When Michael asked Jay how he felt after being more transparent and honest, they were able to link an embodied feeling of relief as a consequence of moving from an avoidant discussion to a more detailed description of behavior. The clinical pursuit of literal sexual language raised Jay's consciousness regarding his avoidant defenses and elicited an emotionally calming consequence from a more thorough and honest self-reflection of his online solo-sexual behavior.

Sexual details

Sex talk is all about details. For an OCSB assessment, sexual details are not just important to ascertain frequency of behavior or intensity of urges, but also to learn the details of sexual activity, erotic arousal, and presence of conflicted feelings about unconventional turn-ons. Conversational norms about sex typically discourage revealing explicit details, even with long-time sex partners. Most couples talk about what they want for dinner more frequently and in more detail than what they want sexually. The OCSB assessment aims to disrupt set patterns of sexual discourse that contribute to avoidance of sexual problems.

Similar to figurative language, vague sex talk allows for ambiguity and contributes to obfuscation and clinical misinterpretation. Being vague when talking about sex is another defense men may have developed to regulate uncomfortable feelings experienced while being vulnerable in an assessment session. "It" is a perfect example of vague language that is pervasive in client sexual disclosures. "I didn't like it." "It felt terrible." "We did it." "I looked at it." "It was fun." "It" is a versatile word that can mean many things without revealing anything. Therefore, when clients use "it," we do not assume to know what "it" is.

For instance, the OCSB assessment commonly contains moments of sexual education. Men might say, "I never thought of it that way before." A typical response might be, "What is the 'it' that you had not thought of before?" or "What do you mean by 'it'?" Listen for the client's tendency to use pronouns when talking about new sexual information or content. Pronouns like "it" prematurely move the conversation to an assumed mutual understanding of the sexual content without first clearly stating the topic. It is important to listen for these moments early on in the OCSB assessment. The assessment is an important time for client's to increase self-awareness of their avoidance of more specific sexual language.

An important characteristic of the sex-talk skill used with men in OCSB assessment can be seen when a therapist expresses genuine curiosity rather than offers a corrective interruption. It is important that the therapist does not expect the client to paraphrase or repeat his newest insight perfectly or with ease. The client may have an affective response to the sexual-detail intervention. The activated feeling may need to be registered as an important aspect of his immediate response to this clinical clarification of the "it." The client feels unfamiliarly seen, understood, or stimulated by the sex-talk invitation. He may experience a feeling that he is not familiar with or cannot easily describe. Slowing this moment down to allow the client to provide a space for him to find his own words crystalizes the learning. The OCSB assessment will likely contain numerous collaborative exchanges to clarify sexual details. This requires a clinical style of engagement and curiosity about sexuality that draws a person out rather than activates distance. OCSB assessment incorporates stage-wise readiness strategies that elicit intrinsic motivation from within the person rather than instilling knowledge from an authoritarian position (Miller & Rollnick, 2002). Working with vague language is a process used to draw out the clients' perceptions of the content or emotion of the moment rather than a comprehension test of parroting imparted therapist information.

Hector

Hector's fourth and most recent SSAS score was 21. His previous three totals were typically around 30. Doug asked Hector to look over the questions and see which items had not changed much in all four totals. He identified Items 9 (On average, how much anticipatory tension and/or excitement did you have shortly before engaging in problematic sexual behaviors?) and 10 (How much excitement and pleasure did you feel when you engaged in problematic sexual behaviors?). Doug asked Hector for his thoughts about why these two items remained high when his urges and thoughts had decreased. Doug observed a small, almost unnoticeable change in Hector's facial expression in response to the question. Hector looked a bit glazed in the eyes, sat still longer than usual, stared at the wall to the left of the therapist, took a shallow breath and said:

HECTOR: I'm not sure.

DOUG: I noticed you became quiet, had a facial expression that is new to me. Can you tell me where you went just now?

(Hector hesitates and takes a deeper breath.)

DOUG: What was that breath just now? That was the biggest breath you have taken all session.

HECTOR: *(takes another breath and looks down)* I like to bottom.

DOUG: You stopped looking at me when you said that.

HECTOR: I'm a little embarrassed.

DOUG: What is it about saying that you like to bottom that is embarrassing for you?

HECTOR: Well, it's not that bottoming is embarrassing. What I really love is when guys cum inside me. I'm sorry. Can I say "cum"?

DOUG: Sure, if that's what's comfortable for you. Can you tell me what is embarrassing for you to tell me about enjoying men ejaculating inside you?

HECTOR: (*slightly surprised by the question, as if the reason he is embarrassed should be obvious*) Well, I know that it's risky but sometimes, I just want to have sex. I go online and find whoever is looking. I don't talk about their status or mine. I just imagine we are barebacking, so I just go for it.

DOUG: What is so important about this experience that you set aside your concerns about HIV?

(*There's a pause in the dialogue. Doug noticed that Hector was now sitting up, shoulders more squared, his feet planted on the floor, and leaning slightly forward.*)

HECTOR: It's always been that way. I remember seeing bareback VHS videos and I would pause the tape right when they ejaculated. My god, I can't believe I am telling you this! I have never told anyone this before.

DOUG: You're doing fine.

HECTOR: Well, I know this sounds really weird and demented, but I would imagine they would cum inside me, even before I had actually done it. What is that about?

By exploring the details of his SSAS score, Doug and Hector eventually uncovered a significant competing motivation. Hector had a highly arousing erotic interest in fluid exchange that conflicted with his motivation to avoid an STI/HIV infection. Hector had little knowledge that fluid exchange is a fairly common and meaningful aspect of sexual bonding. He had kept this private and had been conflicted about how to understand his contradiction between protecting himself from sexually transmitted infections and the pleasure of fluid exchange in intercourse.

Hector was isolated and alone with his conflict. He had not discussed this with his partner, Phil. He wondered whether his inability to stop his condomless sex was permanently altered by his crystal meth use. In his mind, any further discussion of his sexual intercourse practices had to be dismissed if he wanted to get clean and sober. He was even more afraid of discussing how much desired this turn-on was for fear of disapproval, disgust, or condemnation from his drug-treatment group and now in his OCSB assessment.

Hector's fluid-exchange erotic pleasure created a significant conflict and was a source of shame for him in this era of HIV. The OCSB assessment would be the first time Hector spoke so directly about his erotic conflict. He described his long history of deep sexual desire for anal intercourse fluid exchange while also wanting to avoid unwanted sexual health consequences. It is often difficult for men in the OCSB assessment to explore balancing their sexual pleasure with reducing harmful consequences because protection of unwanted consequences is often privileged over sexual desire and pleasure.

This conversation is an important expansion of our earlier discussion about the SSAS. It was a moment of confidence and rapport building as Hector was provided a moment of genuine therapist curiosity about this private and most pleasurable aspect of his erotic life. As Hector continued to speak in detail and described his sexual activity, Doug could match his empathy and curiosity with Hector's contemplative readiness for change. What if Hector had said: "Do you get off on this? What? Do you go home and tell all your friends about the sick things your clients tell you?" "It's just wrong, I don't want to talk about it. I just want to stop doing it!" The same curiosity could have been a stage-discrepant inquiry that inflamed precontemplative defenses that protected Hector from a premature exposure of his emotions and fears.

Sexual health language
Stephanie Buehler (2014), in her book *What Every Mental Health Professional Needs to Know About Sex*, identified therapists' personal attitudes, inadequate sexual knowledge, and lack of sexuality integration within psychotherapy as barriers in developing psychotherapy sexual health language. Barriers for sexual health language within psychotherapy stem in part from the therapists' personal histories of sexual abuse, unaddressed or avoided sexual dysfunctions, or low self-awareness of their own impeded or altered sexual development. She also holds the psychotherapy profession accountable for their unfortunate knee-jerk distaste in initiating discussions regarding the intimate details of their clients' sexual lives. Buehler identifies that some therapists retain unfounded fears of client

sexual misconduct allegations if they discuss sexual countertransference with other colleagues in case consultation or clinical supervision. Buehler is concerned that the psychotherapy office tends to mirror the existing sex-negativity endemic in the culture because of the low priority given to sexuality training and academic standards for sexual knowledge within psychotherapy education and licensure standards (Buehler, 2014). Therapists remain unprepared to integrate sexual health language into psychotherapy without fundamental changes in their sexuality education, training, and ongoing supervision.

Client acquisition of sexual health language requires vigilance by the therapist. Client sexual innuendo or veiled comments can be mutually ego-syntonic for both client and therapist (after all we all live in the same sexual-culture milieu). In OCSB assessment and treatment there are excellent opportunities to shape men's acquisition of sexual health language. The goal is to encourage assessment discussions that focus on terms and descriptions which foster an objective, observation-based discussion. Sexual health language does not include colloquial or slang terms and phrases. "I will be surrounded by debauchery" becomes "the bachelor party will involve hiring sex workers and group lap dances after everyone is drunk."

For example, a man reports high levels of anticipatory excitement on item #9 on the SSAS. He says that when he thinks about going online to sex chat with women, even though this is a secret and violates his relationship agreement, he continues to feel extreme levels of excitement.

CLIENT: I am just so hot for her. I can't believe some of the things we talk about.

THERAPIST: Can you describe "hot" to me?

CLIENT: What do you mean?

THERAPIST: Well, it seems there is a connection between what you chat about with her and feeling hot. I want to better understand what you mean by "hot."

The client goes on to describe how sexually excited he felt chatting with her about the details of his sexual fantasies. He was surprised to see that a significant part of his arousal was feeling liberated from having to worry about her judgments about his fantasies. As the client and therapist discussed in more detail what was so pleasurable about online sex chat, it became clearer to the client that what he desired was an environment free of immediate judgment about his desires from a woman. It was in this environment that he felt his most intense sexual excitement.

It was important for the therapist to listen to small culturally automatic phrases that avoided descriptions of the important pleasurable components of his online sex chatting. When the therapist slowed down the conversation to examine each statement, she helped the client begin to develop his specific sexual health language.

> THERAPIST: So, let me see if I am understanding you. You think the amount of excitement you feel when you focus on what really sexually turns you on is your sexual addiction. Is that what you think is your sexual problem?

> CLIENT: Well, when you put it that way, I guess I have to think about it. I am not sure. I always thought I was kind of sick and demented to want to say all these sexual things that I like out loud with my partner when we are having sex.

> THERAPIST: So, let's think about this. Is your arousal related to talking about your sexual fantasies when you are having sex that you think is the problem or is it that you have kept this a secret from your partners?

> CLIENT: I guess that's why I am here. I am just not sure how I feel about being so explicit. And I know my wife thinks it is pretty weird; she was so disgusted by what she read on my computer.

> THERAPIST: What we are not sure of though, and what may take some time to figure out between both of you, is how much of her disgust and hurt was the betrayal she felt from your keeping secrets and dishonoring your relationship commitment versus an erotic conflict between the two of you that has been avoided and remains unaddressed.

Therapist's sexual health language skills within the OCSB assessment can clarify men's competing motivations. In this situation, it became clear that the client lived with his erotic conflict through avoidant attachment patterns and poor self-regulation as a result of making sexual relationship agreements that directly competed with his peak erotic pleasure.

Change processes are integrated within the OCSB assessment and throughout treatment. The change processes, such as consciousness-raising, emotional arousal, self-reevaluation, and social liberation, are the foundations for manifesting sexual health change talk. Therapists will benefit from using practiced skills to effectively and confidently address client defenses that impede manifesting change talk as they are developing a new vision of sexual health.

TREATMENT ELEMENTS: FRAME PROCESSES

The treatment frame is a method used to understand the essential boundaries and agreements between client and therapist so as to provide an adequate environment in which to conduct OCSB treatment. Treatment frame processes are the fundamental clinical approaches the therapist uses for providing OCSB assessment and treatment. The treatment frame processes are methods used for treatment preparation as well as to provide additional assessment information to determine whether OCSB treatment would be recommended. OCSB assessment and treatment employ a range of clinical interventions that comprise the *frame processes.* As a part of the assessment process, men agree to discuss current moments in the relationship with the therapist during assessment sessions. These include the here/now interventions that address the inevitable transference, symptom presentation, and client frame crossings that occur during OCSB assessment sessions. Frame processes within OCSB assessment and treatment include explicit client agreements used to discuss treatment frame crossings and to explore the client's competing motivations, which emerge throughout OCSB treatment.

Client actions and emotions elicited by the OCSB assessment process are valuable clinical moments. Therapists can often draw direct parallels between the relational experiences they have with the client during the assessment with factors that contribute to the client's OCSB symptoms. For example, if clients reported difficulties regulating their sexual impulses, how are they regulating sexual and nonsexual impulses during the session? For clients who have had significant difficulties with honesty about their sexual activities, how honest are they during their assessment appointments? A frame process we work under is the assumption that clients knowingly or unknowingly display important components of their regulation, attachment, and erotic conflict throughout the OCSB assessment. This frame process is another avenue for gathering assessment information. Frequently, the parallel elements that exist between their behaviors and interpersonal patterns exhibited during the assessment process are indicative of similar patterns that exist outside the clinical hour. There can frequently be blind spots in the client's conscious awareness of his clinical picture. These implicit patterns can be brought to more explicit awareness by working with here/now interventions (Anderson & Przybylinski, 2012).

OCSB frame process interventions orient and prepare men for the interpersonal rigors of OCSB individual and group treatment. They learn the importance of tending to the therapeutic relationship and the value of relational agreements. Therapists have an opportunity to assess client readiness to manage and grow from the demands of OCSB treatment. Group treatment may not be a good fit for men who become highly reactive to self-awareness demands of here/now interventions or demonstrate a low capacity to develop regulation skills for managing their emotional intensity during sessions. Other men may report becoming increasingly unmotivated to be accountable for their sexual behavior or move toward a greater readiness for change.

Three frame processes are integrated within the assessment process as part of the assessment as well as the treatment preparation. We first review here/now interventions, then provide a general overview of methods for working with client transference, and end by working with inevitable treatment frame crossings of men in OCSB assessment.

Here/Now Interventions

One way to understand how here/now interventions facilitate growth is to see how they can function in the clinical hour as a means of understanding a man's window of optimal activation (Siegel, 2011). Here/now interventions, a form of improvisational observation about what is happening in the moment within a therapy session, have great potential to assist men in developing emotional tolerance (increase their optimal range of activation) for uncomfortable affect states and improve their intra- and interpersonal coping strategies to better regulate these emotional states.

The ability to self-regulate is a central focus of assessment and treatment for OCSB. As defined by Baumeister and Vohs (2007), self-regulation refers to one's capacity to alter/override or prolong/amplify responses to stimuli. During the assessment process, therapists can observe how clients alter or override their emotional responses to the various assessment measures and clinical interview. As we have stated, the overall goal of OCSB treatment is to help client's shift their affective–deliberative interaction to generate sexual health behavior change. We view here/now interventions as working directly with the affective–deliberative interaction. Emotional arousal is a form of affective activation and talking about what is happening in these moments is accessing the client's deliberative system. Discussing here/now experiences in the assessment is an activity that may provide an opportunity to change automatic client affective–deliberative interactions. Shifting these habitual patterns through shared clinical encounters with the client may create new ways to self-regulate the activation/deliberative balance. Here/now interventions generally follow a basic sequence: When clients experience an affective activation, the therapist directs his attention to the activation, investigates client internal experience, asks him to describe it, and debriefs this experience. In the debrief, the therapist helps the client articulate his explicit and implicit coping, especially when the client appears to be attempting to avoid or suppress the triggered affect. The here/now intervention also investigates how men experience staying with an uncomfortable emotion longer than their usual pattern as they continue to be introspective. The debrief is also a psychoeducational opportunity. The therapist may comment on how the intervention was motivated to help the client process his uncomfortable affect as an illustration to educate the client on future OCSB psychotherapy. And second, the debrief is a moment used to contrast what the client anticipated he would feel and how he actually feels now.

Frank

Doug was listening to Frank read aloud each Hypersexual Behavior Consequences Scale item and his number rating. They had completed 12 of the items, several of which dealt with financial, workplace, and relationship consequences, when he read item #13 (I have been humiliated or disgraced because of my sexual activities) Frank stopped and looked away from Doug.

DOUG: What is happening?

FRANK: My boss is such an asshole!

DOUG: What just brought your boss to mind?

FRANK: It asked if I felt disgraced by my sexual behavior. And I thought about the conversation I had with him after the IT [information technology] guys discovered what I was doing online.

DOUG: What feelings came up when you remembered that conversation?

FRANK: That he's an asshole.

DOUG: That may be true, but you also didn't answer my question.

FRANK: What do you mean?

DOUG: I asked you about what you felt and you replied with a judgment about your boss. Thoughts and feelings are different. Right now, I'm more interested in how you are feeling. And, since I'm just getting to know you, I'm not sure how you are feeling right now.

FRANK: I'm pissed! Is that a feeling?!

DOUG: Yes, like rage or anger.

FRANK: Yes.

DOUG: OK, what does your body feel like when you're angry?

FRANK: I'm getting hot. My heart is racing.

DOUG: How's your breathing?

FRANK: My what?

DOUG: Your breathing? I can't tell how you are breathing? Deeply or shallowly?

FRANK: Kinda shallow.

DOUG: OK. Let's take three deep breaths together before we proceed.

(Doug explained diaphragmatic breathing and returned to an earlier moment in the conversation.)

DOUG: Sometimes when people feel angry, there's another emotion underneath. Was anger all that you felt?

FRANK: No. I'm scared.

DOUG: What are you scared of?

FRANK: Of losing my job. Of having to explain to people why I lost my job. Of people looking at me like a pervert.

DOUG: When clients are worried about being seen in a negative way, that may also be a sign that they are feeling ashamed. Are you also feeling ashamed?

FRANK: Yeah.

DOUG: So, when you felt ashamed and afraid, you got angry. Has that happened before?

FRANK: All the time.

As Frank remained in the moment and explored his current feelings, Doug helped Frank raise his awareness of how his defenses protect him from naming uncomfortable feelings and emotions. The here/now exploration identified feelings of fear and shame that were outwardly expressed as judgmental anger. His judgment provided a view into how Frank may follow a pattern of externalizing responsibility for his actions. Frank judged the work consequences of his online sexual behavior as caused by his boss, not by his breaking the work policies regarding online behavior. Ultimately, without being accountable for his sexual behaviors, it is unlikely that Frank will achieve his sexual health treatment goals.

Transference

The definition and use of transference have evolved over time and vary across disciplines. Although commonly viewed as the purview of psychoanalysis and psychodynamic psychotherapies, evidence suggests working with transference is useful in any theoretical approach (Corradi, 2006; Marmarosh, 2012). Levy and Scala (2012) describe transference as a "tendency in which representational aspects of important and formative relationships (such as with parents and siblings) can be both consciously experienced and/or unconsciously ascribed to other relationships" (p. 392). This fundamentally unconscious process also occurs in relationships between therapists and clients. Transference often represents a distortion or cognitive bias that contains real aspects of the here/now therapy relationship. There are individual transference differences among clients in terms of the degree, extent, rigidity, and awareness of transference.

The therapeutic alliance, composed of transference and the collaborative working relationship between therapist and client, requires the capacity to form reasonable attachments by both parties and for the therapist to be aware of personally historic events that influence the alliance (i.e., countertransference; Corradi, 2006). The potential for internalized sociocultural sex negativity or unresolved psychosexual injuries that lead to countertransference is much greater among therapists who have avoided looking closely at their sexual development, sexual attitudes, and sexual health. Therapist comfort in facilitating sexual health conversations and developing a principle-centered approach when treating OCSB is also an important aspect of managing transference. By tending to the issues that trigger countertransference, therapists improve their ability to create the therapeutic conditions that effectively work with transference, and to develop "sufficient trust to allow the [client] to use the [therapist] as a therapeutic object" (Corradi, 2006, p. 421). OCSB treatment integrates here/now events in the therapy relationship to allow the therapist to provide insight into the client's maladaptive and repetitive relationship patterns. It's important for both the therapist and client to value the therapeutic alliance and to view the OCSB assessment as a process used to evaluate the client's motivation to establish and heal through the therapy relationship.

In a review of the empirical literature, Levy and Scala (2012) found transference-focused treatments to be equally effective in facilitating change, as compared to other empirically supported therapies. They identified important aspects of exploring transference, including the ability for clients to make use of transference interpretations, the accuracy of interpretations, and the context in which the transference takes place. Gelso and Harbin (2007) emphasize both cognitive and emotional insights that are developed from transference interventions. They promote transference interventions as opportunities to improve the client's ability to tolerate painful emotions as well as to us these moments to reflect on self and others.

The core material for psychotherapy is found within behavioral patterns associated with childhood attachment adaptions or past traumas that may recur in the therapeutic alliance (Corradi, 2006). An example of this can be seen when the assessment elicits interpersonal moments in which the client changes his emotional proximity to the therapist. The therapist may observe nuanced actions or statements that create distance or closeness that can be understood as a means of regulating his or her internal experience. In the language of the TTM change processes, OCSB assessments provide early opportunity in a therapy relationship to raise client consciousness about the relational reenactment patterns present during session, process the underlying emotions that were aroused, and provide the space for the client to evaluate changes to these attachment patterns. We provide a safe space for the client to stretch into new ways of interacting in a relationship (i.e., starting with the therapist) and to heal past relational injuries. Ultimately, we hope clients can apply those same skills to improve other relationships outside of therapy.

Will

Will is reviewing his SSAS with Michael. In earlier assessment appointments, Michael had reviewed Will's general psychosocial information and the sexual problem timeline. Michael asked a question to clarify details of Will's sexual behaviors in relation to an SSAS item when Will become outwardly upset.

WILL: Why do you need to know all this stuff?

MICHAEL: Which stuff are you referring to?

WILL: Like what kind of sex I was having with these guys? Do you get off on this?

MICHAEL: Before I answer your question, can you first share what you are feeling?

WILL: I'm getting annoyed. I don't see the point.

MICHAEL: It sounds like you are worried that I have another motive besides helping you.

WILL: Well, yeah.

MICHAEL: I'm glad you asked. I ask about the details of your sexual behavior so I can get a better understanding of what you are doing. It's hard to help people change their sexual behavior if I don't know the specific sexual activities they want to change. Have you ever discussed your sexual activity in such detail before?

WILL: Not really.

MICHAEL: I know you said it was annoying earlier. Were their other feelings?

WILL: Well, yeah. It's embarrassing.

MICHAEL: And it sounded like you were afraid that I was taking advantage of you?

WILL: (*silent*)

MICHAEL: How did it feel for you to hear me acknowledge your concerns?

WILL: I'm not sure.

MICHAEL: That's okay. It sounds like this might be a new experience. How often have you been able to express your concerns about what is happening and have those concerns respected?

WILL: Not often.

MICHAEL: What usually happens?

WILL: Well, I don't typically talk about my concerns with others. But when I do, people usually argue with me. Try to convince me that I'm wrong.

Having completed Will's psychosocial evaluation, Michael is aware of Will's family-of-origin history. Will is the oldest child. When his mother was unavailable, either because she was at work or spending time with a romantic partner, he was frequently placed in the role of caregiver for his younger siblings. Will was sexually assaulted by his mother's boyfriend. His mother blamed Will for the incidents and the subsequent ending of the relationship. Years later this blame narrative was reinforced when Will came out as gay. After additional processing, Will connected his distrust and anger reaction toward Michael with his resentment toward his mother. As another authority figure, Will feared Michael would exploit him if he revealed vulnerable elements of his sexual behavior. As a result of past events (e.g., disclosing details of his sexual assault and sexual identity), Will associated sensitive disclosures with rejection. Will's strategy to regulate this interpersonal threat transference in his relationship with Michael was similar to one he developed in childhood. Will regulated his emotional activation by increasing his relational distance from Michael. Will's provocative and distancing accusation regarding Michael's intention provided an opportunity for Will to experience his defenses being met with acceptance, curiosity, and empathy.

Client Treatment Frame Crossings

A variety of agreements are made between a therapist and a client prior to onset of an OCSB assessment. Common treatment agreements include the frequency and length of sessions, payment expectations, cancellation policies, and homework expectations. Establishing the treatment contract sets the stage for here/now interventions about client accountability.

Broken relational agreements are a common behavioral pattern among men with OCSB. Clients who want to change their sexual behavior report a long history of promises broken with themselves or their intimate partners. We assume clients will bring this relationship pattern into the therapeutic space. It is important to anticipate men in OCSB assessment not meeting one or more of the treatment frame agreements. How clients cross the treatment frame is a source of valuable insight into their OCSB symptoms. Assessment frame crossings provide an in vivo experience for the therapist to learn about how the client's self and attachment regulation patterns impact his personal and relational agreements. Once the precipitating details surrounding the frame crossing are understood and the conversation between the therapist and client reestablishes the frame, the therapist and client can discuss the parallels between not keeping the assessment agreement and similar patterns found in behavior with their partners, family, workplace, and friendships. In other words, how they mismanage assessment agreements likely indicates possible patterns in how they may mismanage group and individual treatment frame relational agreements. We suggest here/now frame-crossing interventions prepare men for important future treatment frame interventions.

Hector

Hector arrived late for several assessment appointments. Doug chose to inquire about this pattern when Hector arrived 15 minutes late for his appointment.

> **DOUG:** Can you tell me about what happened before you arrived that contributed to your being late?
>
> **HECTOR:** Well, I didn't mean to be late. I'm so sorry. Please know that I think these sessions are very important.
>
> **DOUG:** Thank you for the apology. But I'm more interested in your decision making prior to your appointment.
>
> **HECTOR:** Oh, OK. I was sitting in my office when my boss called me into her office. It was about an hour before I needed to leave. She was preparing for a meeting later this week and needed some information. It took longer than I expected and before I realized it, I left later than I wanted.
>
> **DOUG:** Before you realized it? I am not sure what you mean by this. Are you saying you were not aware of the time?

HECTOR: Not exactly. I was actually very aware of the time because I knew I was late twice before. But I couldn't say anything.

DOUG: Tell me more about "couldn't."

HECTOR: I'm so worried about losing my job so I want to make sure she knows I'm available.

DOUG: So, if I'm hearing you correctly, it's not that you couldn't tell her. It sounds like you decided not to tell her about your competing commitment with your assessment appointment as a way to manage what your boss thinks of you?

HECTOR: Well, yes.

DOUG: What does it feel like to hear your actions described that way?

HECTOR: I'm worried that you think I don't care about your time.

DOUG: That's interesting. I hear the exact opposite. You sound really worried.

HECTOR: Yes. It's nonstop.

DOUG: What's nonstop?

HECTOR: My thoughts. I'm constantly worrying about something. Either losing my job. My partner leaving me. Testing positive.

DOUG: When you say "constantly," are you being literal?

HECTOR: Just about. And it's gotten worse since I stopped using.

Doug reasserted the OCSB assessment treatment frame by initiating a discussion about Hector's behavior that did not honor his agreement to be on time for appointments. This frame discussion opened up two important aspects of Hector's OCSB clinical picture, his constant worrying and attachment-related anxiety. He seemed to experience excessive worrying and to have difficulty regulating his racing thoughts. His poor anxiety management impacted his decisions to set boundaries to protect his time commitments when they competed with the content of his racing thoughts. In this case, the false choice with which Hector struggled was between arriving for his therapy session on time or losing his job. Because of the intensity of his anxiety, Hector was unable to see the irrationality of his fears and find another solution to this bind.

Hector's anxiety was evidenced in his attachment patterns. The assessment revealed how he was regularly worried about what others thought of him and, when he experienced someone as distant, he feared the relationship ending. Most relationship tensions and distress felt to him like emergencies that needed immediate resolution. Doug could see this in the assessment sessions when Hector verbalized his worries about what Doug was going to think of him. Doug gained insight into how difficult it was for Hector to remain relationally present and connected in his moments of intense anxiety. Hector defended against feeling the intensity of this interpersonal fear and talking about the thoughts in his mind by moving quickly to receive reassurance from Doug that everything between them was fine. It was as if Hector would borrow Doug's less anxious mind to coregulate his runaway fears and anxious thoughts. Hector was unfamiliar with someone remaining present and empathically interested in his experience despite Hector's not honoring the relational agreements.

Identifying Competing Motivations

Listening for competing motivations is a frame process used to assess a client's acumen for verbalizing his affective–deliberative imbalance. We recommend clinicians educate their clients about the importance of identifying and labeling competing motivations. With practice, men can learn to articulate their inner tensions and feelings of ambivalence. They may defend against being curious about their conflicted motivations and ambivalent feelings regarding changing their sexual behavior with comments such as "I don't know, I was just being stupid" or "I couldn't help myself." The OCSB assessment offers an opportunity for therapists to listen for men's ambivalence and remain curious and resolute in helping them move past subtle defenses against accountability. The goal is to use this frame process to develop a more nuanced understanding of the competing motivations that drive men both toward and away from sexual health.

As we discussed in Chapter 3, we conceptualize problems with OCSB as an outcome of multiple, coexisting affective and deliberative motivations—combinations of "we want" versus "don't want" and "we like" versus "don't like." Miller and Rollnick (2013) describe four variations of motivational conflicts. First, the approach–approach conflict is exhibited when a person is faced with a choice between two attractive options. Second, an avoidance–avoidance conflict involves choices between options that all have negative consequences. The third variation is the approach–avoidance conflict. In this scenario, one is "both attracted to and repelled by the same object" (Miller & Rollick, 2002, p. 14). The last conflict, the double approach–avoidance, is when both options have powerful positive and negative aspects. Clients seeking treatment for problematic or out of control sexual behavior frequently present with the latter two internal conflicts. These men are motivated by the pleasure of sex while being concurrently determined to avoid the painful consequences of their sexual behavior. The assessment is a time to look closely at each man's unique motivational conflicts in relation to sexual pleasure. Is it the pleasure of sex that is motivating him, or the gratification of distress relief that accompanies the sexual activity? Is he focused on the specific pleasure of the release of orgasm or is he motivated by the feelings of relationship security he feels when having partnered sex? Deconstructing colliding or counterintuitive motivations for sex becomes the task for each man seeking treatment for OCSB.

Competing motivations are found in all three clinical areas. Internal conflicts influence how men self-regulate and coregulate their emotions. Sexual/erotic conflict often involves motivations related to self and attachment regulation. For instance, a client reports that he really enjoys watching and masturbating to online videos of people having sex but dislikes the amount of time spent on this sexual activity. His dislike for the amount of time spent competes with his intense feelings of pleasure when viewing sexual imagery (clinical area: self-regulation). Another man is ambivalent about his frequency of casual sex but he continues this behavior because partnered sex helps him feel loved and less lonely. Not wanting to feel lonely competes with wanting to stop casual sex (clinical area: attachment regulation). Another man feels intense arousal when being dominated by his sexual partner. He withholds this from his mate to avoid the anticipated judgment and rejection from his partner knowing about this erotic desire. His motivation to avoid rejection competes with deeply felt desires for erotic satisfaction (clinical area: erotic conflict). The process used to investigate competing motivations involves regularly slowing down key assessment moments when men seem to be "of two minds" about a particular aspect of their sexual behavior.

OCSB treatment-seeking men often struggle because they erroneously believe they are capable of managing coexisting competing motivations without negative consequences. Therapists may need to repeatedly normalize this dilemma. Empathy perspectives that frame their actions as a flawed solution to a need rather than an indication of a pathological disorder may need to be clearly explored. During the assessment, therapists can inform men that it is quite human for people to be motivated by deeply felt sexual and erotic desires and by their drives to avoid uncomfortable affect such as loneliness or rejection. What started as a wrenchingly painful contradiction eventually becomes an understandable human attempt to resolve an internal conflict with the skills and capacities they had at the time.

Jay

Jay's disclosure of finding pleasure in viewing sexual videos of men having anal sex with female partners led to further clarity about his competing motivations, which influence his out of control sexual experiences.

MICHAEL: When you are watching sex videos, how frequently is the content specifically about men having anal sex with women?

JAY: It's not all the time.

MICHAEL: OK. But how often do you watch videos with this sexual activity?

JAY: I don't know. Is it that important?

MICHAEL: The details of what you find arousing are important. It lets me know what you are motivated to watch.

JAY: Alright. It's the majority of what I watch. Like almost daily.

MICHAEL: So watching anal sex is really appealing for you?

JAY: Yes.

MICHAEL: How often have you acknowledged this to another person?

JAY: Not very.

MICHAEL: And to your wife?

JAY: Sort of.

MCHAEL: Meaning?

JAY: Well, I have tried to, you know, test the waters when we were having sex. And she kinda freaked out.

MICHAEL: "Test the waters?"

JAY: You know, while having sex or going down on her, I would try to finger her to see if she was interested. She slapped my hand away.

MICHAEL: So, I'm assuming you hadn't talked with her about what you wanted to do before you tried?

JAY: No, no, no!

MICHAEL: What just happened. You got more animated.

JAY: Oh God, the thought of talking to my wife about having anal sex. She'll feel disgusted. I mean, can you blame her?

MICHAEL: Blame her?

JAY: I mean, it is kind of disgusting.

MICHAEL: Is that what you think?

JAY: Sorta.

MICHAEL: But it also sounds like it's something that's very arousing for you. What's that like for you? To be aroused by something that you also find disgusting at the same time?

In this dialogue, Michael was exploring Jay's competing motivations related to his erotic interests. Jay was highly turned-on by anal intercourse with women but, at the same time, believed it was disgusting. This presented an opportunity to empathize with his bind about asserting his erotic interests when harboring his own belief that these needs are unworthy of respect. Jay identified this competing motivation with Michael and was able to more clearly see how he has avoided direct discussions about this sexual interest to avoid his wife's disapproval. This competing motivation emerged through first addressing Jay's figurative language and then identifying the competing motivation. Through this assessment process Jay was able to discern the conflict between his erotic desires and disgust defenses. Identifying his competing motivations led Jay to see his anticipated thoughts of his wife's disdain regarding his desire for anal intercourse as his defensive projection, not his wife's actual feelings. Remaining unaware and avoidant of his competing motivations prevented Jay from integrating his erotic interests within his erotic identity and honestly exploring these with his romantic partner.

> **MICHAEL:** So, your solution to avoid the potential of your wife's disgust was to touch her anus during sex and hope for the best?
>
> **JAY:** (*laughing*) Well, yeah. But I only did that when we were dating. I haven't tried it since.
>
> **MICHAEL:** Now your solution to this conflict between your erotic pleasure and avoiding disgust is to enjoy anal sex by watching videos and masturbating?
>
> **JAY:** Yeah, there's no other option.
>
> **MICHAEL:** Wow. That sounds pretty grim for you.
>
> **JAY:** But it's true.

Jay's long-term avoidance not only led to poor sexual decisions, but he coped with this emotional fallout by using the hopelessness defense. In this state of hopelessness Jay resorted to crossing boundaries that exploited the vulnerability of his partner during sex. His solution was to take advantage of his wife's distracted and sexualized state by nonverbally initiating anal sex, hoping she might be more responsive and less judgmental because of her own state of arousal. He concluded that his surprise attempt at digital anal play resulted in his wife, Veronique's, generalized and rigid disapproval of anal sex. It's not that she may not have been ready for anal sex at that moment or was reacting negatively to his approach. She might be open to anal play with some discussion, forewarning, or collaborative preparation. His solution to his hopelessness was not to check with his wife to confirm she actually was not interested in anal sex. His avoidance of this disappointment was to channel this erotic interest into his solo-sex life without any involvement with his partner; as a result she could have no way of understanding his motivation for online sexual imagery and solo sex. In other words, it was easier to masturbate to videos of anal sex than to move toward his vulnerability and fears.

COMPLETING THE ASSESSMENT

The therapist determines whether OCSB treatment is recommended before transitioning along the OCSB Clinical Pathway (see Figure 5.1) by using the assessment to create a unique clinical profile. The OCSB Unique Clinical Picture (Figure 7.1) is the first treatment area of the OCSB Clinical Pathway. This transition is visually represented on the OCSB Clinical Pathway by the gray rectangular background, which represents OCSB treatment.

There are three possible outcomes to an OCSB assessment. Two assessment conclusions are indicated by "Yes" on the Pathway figure; the other option is "No." One outcome of an OCSB assessment is that the client enters OCSB treatment with concurrent psychiatry, medical treatments, couple therapy, drug and alcohol recovery, or other adjunctive services. The alternative "Yes" on the pathway is to recommend OCSB-combined treatment when no other concurrent services are indicated or are currently provided (less frequent than the first option). The third option is not to recommend OCSB treatment and to refer the client to an alternative service that is more appropriate.

At the end of the assessment process (i.e., the clinical interview, completion of the measures, collaboration with other professionals), the therapist and client meet to summarize the assessment information and discuss the therapist recommendations. The OCSB Assessment Summary (Figure 7.2) is a resource for the therapist to use to organize the assessment information and clinical impressions within each of the Unique Clinical Picture categories.

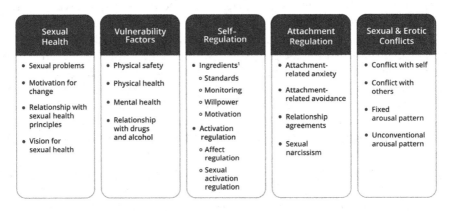

Figure 7.1 *OCSB Unique Clinical Picture.*

[1]Baumeister and Vohs (2007).

OCSB ASSESSMENT SUMMARY

Client Name: _____

Sexual Health

1. What are the sexual behaviors the client wants to change?
2. Client's motivation for change
3. Sexual symptoms involve nonconsensual sex? Concerns regarding the other sexual health principles?
4. Vision of sexual health

Vulnerability Factors

Does the client present with symptoms, concerns, or diagnoses in the following areas?

1. Physical safety
2. Physical health
3. Mental health
4. Relationship with drugs and alcohol

Clinical Areas

Self-regulation

Question 1: How are OCSB symptoms related to self-regulation ingredients?

1. Overly rigid or under developed sexual *standards*?
2. *Self-monitoring*
    a. Self-observation impairments?
    b. Capacity to view distal concerns beyond immediate gratification
    c. Degree of habitual sexual thoughts and behaviors
3. Managing *willpower* resources
    a. Willpower limitations and strengths
    b. Sexual behavior linked with depleted willpower reserves?
4. *Motivation*
    a. Current state of readiness for changing sexual behavior

Question 2: How are sexual urges, thoughts, or behavior solutions to regulating uncomfortable activation?

Question 3: Are the OCSB symptoms an outcome of hyper/hypoactivated states?

Question 4: How does the client regulate sexual activation?

Figure 7.2 *OCSB Assessment Summary.*

1. What is the client's sexual excitation level?
2. What are levels of inhibition (i.e., threats of performance failure, threats of consequences)?
3. Is there an imbalance between the client's sexual excitation and inhibition capacities?

Attachment Regulation

Question 1. How do the OCSB symptoms reflect the client's attachment style?

1. OCSB related to relationship-anxiety management?
2. OCSB related to relationship-avoidance strategies?
3. Outcome of attachment style measure (e.g., mother, father, significant other, and friends)

Question 2. How does the client maintain relationship agreements?

1. Sexual relationship agreements
   a. Agreements not kept in relationship
   b. Agreements kept in relationships
2. Sexual relationship agreements to negotiate

Question 3. Does the client have traits of sexual narcissism? (low partner empathy, sexual exploitation, and sexual entitlement)

Sexual and Erotic Conflicts

Question 1. Are the OCSB symptoms related to sexual or erotic conflicts that the client has with himself?

1. Obstructed sexual- and erotic-identity development
2. Degree of love/lust split in erotic orientation

Question 2. Are the OCSB symptoms related to sexual or erotic conflicts that the client has with others?

1. Degree of sexual and erotic integration in intimate relationships
2. Attachment threats with partner, family, religion, and community related to sexual and erotic orientation

Question 3. Does the client experience a fixed or unconventional arousal pattern?

Figure 7.2 *(continued)*

Determining Treatment Recommendations

The decision to recommend or not recommend OCSB treatment represents the summation of the man's sexual health vision, readiness for change, vulnerability factors, and the subjective clinical opinion of the therapist in the three OCSB clinical areas. At this point in the assessment, the therapist uses the OCSB Assessment Summary to organize the assessment information and to formulate his or her recommendation. This summary sheet is a tool for organizing the clinical interview, measures, and professional consultation components of the OCSB assessment. We propose a contemplative process for the therapist to use to organize the assessment process, a process not too dissimilar from what we believe is essential for the client to follow in considering treatment.

Postassessment Review

Acuity-related questions are central to formulating OCSB assessment recommendations. The guiding ethic for the therapist in contemplating levels of acuity is to protect the client from unnecessary levels of treatment. We have discussed our observation that current treatment practices for sexual behavior problems risk promulgating a premature evaluation and movement to specialized sexual behavior treatment. At this stage of the assessment, it is vital to return to this ethic as a guide for moving forward. A few common questions have emerged over the years that have proved to be helpful prohibitions that protect the client from prematurely entering an extensive course of sexual behavior therapy.

Is he still feeling out of control?

The OCSB assessment measures and treatment elements help the therapist to make a clinically informed recommendation. The felt sense of being out of control may have subsided as the client focused on the assessment tasks and weekly session dialogues. The SSAS scores provide a barometer for symptom acuity. How much a client continues to feel out of control can be seen in his self-regulation patterns, both in the client–therapist relationship and the week-to-week reports of sexual urges, thoughts, and behaviors. How often has he commented on his concern about his ability to regulate his behavior? How many of his sexual behavior symptoms have persisted throughout the assessment?

Is he likely to benefit from OCSB therapy?

The treatment elements of the assessment are valuable resources for addressing this question. How did he respond to the change process elements of the assessment? Did he demonstrate a capacity for being curious about his defenses? What was his capacity for listening to feedback in here/now moments with the therapist? Did he seem interested and intrigued by the potential benefit of having more of these interactions? Was he interested in how his emotions in the assessment meetings provided information about how he feels and functions in other relationships? How did he respond to frame crossings that emerged over the course of the assessment? Was he interested in expanding his understanding of himself? How well did he maintain the concurrent services in conjunction with the OCSB assessment? Are the OCSB vulnerability factors stable enough to proceed with the additional clinical work of combined individual and group treatment?

How motivated is he to change?

OCSB treatment offers a self-discrepant model for behavior change. The treatment depends on the man's commitment and sustained motivation for change. The multiple-session assessment offers a window into the client's strengths for sustaining motivation over time. How were his personal values and interests in improving sexual health reflected in his language and behavior? Did the assessment process strengthen his commitment to change? How tolerant was he of ambivalent feelings and uncertainty? What collaborative conversation skills did he demonstrate during the OCSB assessment measures?

Is he amenable to the OCSB Model?

How cooperative and responsive was the client to the various aspects of the assessment? How open was he to considering self-regulation, attachment style, and sexual/erotic conflicts in his conceptualization for changing his sexual behavior? How interested was he in the sexual health principles used to direct his behavior and attachments? Does he demonstrate malleability for integrating his current 12-step fellowships (Alcoholics Anonymous [AA], Narcotics Anonymous [NA], various sexual recovery 12-step groups) within the nonaddiction disease paradigm of OCSB treatment?

These questions exemplify the range of perspectives that a therapist can incorporate when reviewing the assessment summary; they also help the therapist review his or her clinical impressions resulting from the assessment relationship. There is no avoiding the subjective elements of determining whether to recommend OCSB treatment. The art of therapy is inextricably linked with clinical assessment and symptom data. Transparency about the subjectivity of the clinician's informed opinion is important to include in the feedback. OCSB is a human behavior problem that, for some men, can resolve without specialized outpatient combined individual and group therapy. The question for us in determining whether to recommend clients to enter combined OCSB outpatient therapy comes down to determining whether this man will benefit from this approach at this time.

OCSB Assessment-Summary Appointment

This appointment summarizes the assessment process within the organizational structure of the OCSB Unique Clinical Picture. We organize the assessment impressions, data, and observations using the OCSB Assessment Summary (see Figure 7.2). The Assessment Summary organizes all five elements of the Unique Clinical Picture discussed in both the OCSB screening appointment and throughout the OCSB assessment.

When OCSB Treatment Is Not Recommended

Several key factors may lead to not recommending OCSB treatment. Each situation is discussed in a collaborative conversation with the client. Lack of sufficient motivation to change, although uncommon, can be one of the conclusions of an assessment. Inability to maintain a commitment to the assessment appointment schedule or significant change in motivation during the assessment may lead to this recommendation. A client may agree to an assessment as part of a child custody evaluation. It may be clear that the client is not motivated for treatment, but is simply motivated to provide family court with a record of attending specialized sexual behavior assessment to give the court documentation that treatment for OCSB is not recommended. A client may agree to an assessment to "save his marriage" and a few weeks later the couple decides to separate or divorce. This will likely lead to an open discussion to discern what self-discrepancy remains to foster a motivation for sexual health behavior change. Clients may have a change in health insurance, employment, or a family emergency. Over the years, men have been diagnosed with a major medical condition or faced an unexpected pregnancy that shifted their life priorities.

Men who engage in nonconsensual sexual behavior are not recommended for OCSB treatment. Men may disclose nonconsensual behavior patterns after the assessment has commenced. Other times, the screening appointment is followed up by a series of appointments to facilitate the transition to a nonconsensual specialist for further assessment. One of our initial case examples involved Anthony, who had a long-established pattern of nonconsensual public masturbation. Specially trained professionals in the clinical evaluation of nonconsensual sex are the qualified professionals to determine the best course of treatment for him. It was emphasized to him that he should seek help without waiting to be arrested. He learned that there are professionals with whom he could receive treatment to stop his illegal and nonconsensual sexual behavior.

Other clients will not be recommended for OCSB treatment because they fail to meet the clinical threshold for combined individual and group OCSB treatment. If a client presents with SSAS scores below 15, an Adverse Childhood Experiences (ACE) score of 1, indicates few consequences on the Hypersexual Behavior Consequences Scale (HBCS), reports diverse attachment styles within all four relationship dimensions, and has a fairly balanced excitation and inhibition sexual response system, but yet is expressing concern about his sexual behavior, more often than not there is significant distress about a sexual behavior value conflict that can be addressed in individual therapy.

A heterosexually identified man with strong, deep attachments to his religion is engaged in having sex with men with some frequency. He believes his same-sex sexual behavior is an "addiction." Some clients have presented for an OCSB assessment with instruction from their religious leader that diagnosis of a sexual addition will prevent them from being ejected from their religious institution. Clients may be highly motivated for treatment, not because their symptoms require this level of care, but because the treatment reduces their risk of being rejected by their religious community because of their nonexclusively heterosexual orientation. It would be misguided and potentially harmful to recommend OCSB treatment as a solution to this painful attachment dilemma.

OCSB treatment is not an "erotic-ectomy." If the only OCSB symptom is a significant erotic conflict without other elevated symptoms, then OCSB treatment is not indicated. For example, a man has worn women's clothing for sexual pleasure and arousal while masturbating since his early teens. He is married with two young children and has recently disclosed this behavior to his wife. They both perceive his behavior as out of control. The unconventional turn-on is a direct threat to the marriage and the couple's narrow standards for appropriate sexual expression. He sought treatment for the "compulsion" to wear women's clothing, to stop the behavior, and to focus on "normal" sex with his wife. Disappointing clients who are invested in a specific course of treatment or diagnosis as a solution to an attachment fear or to sever an unwanted sexual turn-on will lead to an alternative course for treatment other than OCSB outpatient group and individual therapy.

When OCSB Treatment Is Recommended

Recommending OCSB treatment is the step that follows the therapist outlining the Unique Clinical Picture and collaborating with the client in building his sexual health plan. Common factors that support this recommendation are as follows: an ACE score above 3, SSAS weekly scores between 20 and 35, numerous consequences for sexual behavior, high risk for additional negative consequences, one or more co-occurring clinical disorders (anxiety disorder treatment, depression, early substance abuse recovery, etc.), underdeveloped capacities in self and attachment regulation, and unresolved sexual/erotic-identity conflicts. The unique combination of these clinical areas frames the client's out of control sexual experiences and provides the basis for OCSB treatment recommendations.

OCSB treatment-seeking men often feel hopeful after participating in an OCSB assessment. They learn about the factors contributing to their sexual problems, clarify their vision of sexual health, and enhance their motivation for sexual health behavior change. Clients will most likely benefit from the OCSB combined treatment program when they are ready to change their sexual behaviors, agree to maintain their individual and adjunctive treatment, and commit to the OCSB treatment agreements.

After clients complete their sexual health plans, we offer a conjoint session with the (nonsingle) clients and their romantic partners. The objective of this session is to orient the partner to the assessment process and treatment recommendations. The agenda of the meeting is for the therapist to review the assessment procedures and for the client to share any information about the sexual health plan and lessons learned from the assessment that he chooses. Any clinical information that is discussed about the client must be predetermined so the therapist knows what information is unauthorized for release. Intimate partners may have completely different views than the client of the sexual symptoms, the appropriate course of treatment, and level of confidence and trust in the therapists each has chosen to see for professional help. For some partners, OCSB treatment's lack of a disease model is a significant source of distress. The conjoint session can be an opportunity for the partner to learn more about the OCSB Model, which should ease the tension, and to learn more about the reasons for the treatment recommendations. We often recommend that the partner consider individual therapy if he or she does not currently have a mental health professional with whom to consult about having a partner in treatment for OCSB. We encourage couples with persistent sexual value conflicts or who are struggling to repair their relationships after sexual infidelity to consult a couples therapist.

REFERENCES

Anderson, S. M., & Przybylinski, E. (2012). Experiments on transference in interpersonal relations: Implications for treatment. *Psychotherapy, 49*(3), 370–383.

Baumeister, R. F., & Vohs, K. D. (2007). Self-regulation, ego depletion, and motivation. *Social and Personality Psychology Compass, 1*(1), 115–128.

Buehler, S. (2014). *What every mental health professional should know about sex.* New York, NY: Springer Publishing Company.

Corradi, R. B. (2006). A conceptual model of transference and its psychotherapeutic application. *Journal of the American Academy of Psychoanalysis and Dynamic Psychiatry, 34*(3), 415–439.

Gelso, C., & Harbin, J. (2007). Insight, action, and the therapeutic relationship. In L. Castonguay & C. Hill (Eds.), *Insight in psychotherapy* (pp. 293–311). Washington, DC: American Psychological Association.

Juni, S. (1998/1999). The defense mechanism inventory: Theoretical and psychometric implications. *Current Psychology, 4,* 313–332.

Levy, K. N., & Scala, J. W. (2012). Transference, transference interpretations, and transference-focused psychotherapies. *Psychotherapy, 49*(3), 391–403.

Marmarosh, C. L. (2012). Empirically supported perspectives on transference. *Psychotherapy, 49*(3), 364–369.

Miller, W. R., & Rollnick, S. (2002). *Motivational interviewing: Preparing people for change* (2nd ed.). New York, NY: Guilford Press.

Miller, W. R., & Rollnick, S. (2013). *Motivational interviewing: Helping people change* (3rd ed.). New York, NY: Guilford Press.

Needham-Didsbury, I. (2012). The use of figurative language in psychotherapy. *UCL Working Papers in Linguistics, 24,* 75–93.

Prochaska, J. O., Norcross, J. C., & DiClemente, C. C. (2006). *Changing for good.* New York, NY: William Morrow.

Prochaska, J. O., Norcross, J. C., & DiClemente, C. C. (2013). Applying the stages of change. *Psychotherapy in Australia, 19*(2), 10–15.

Prochaska, J. O., & Velicer, W. F. (1997). The transtheoretical model of health behavior change. *American Journal of Health Promotion, 12*(1), 38–48.

Siegel, D. J. (2011). *Mindsight: The new science of personal transformation.* New York, NY: Bantam Books.

Yalom, I. (2003). *The gift of therapy—An open letter to a new generation of therapists and their patients* (1st ed., p. 64). New York, NY: Harper Perennial.

CHAPTER EIGHT

THE SEXUAL HEALTH PLAN

FROM ASSESSMENT TO TREATMENT

Men formulate a sexual health plan (SHP) when the client and therapist agree with the recommendation to enter combined individual and group out of control sexual behavior (OCSB) treatment. Writing an SHP is the last step before transitioning into an OCSB group. Having engaged in a rigorous self-examination process beginning with the initial screening appointment and the subsequent OCSB assessment sessions, this step is to be acknowledged and commended. Because the client was not asked to change his sexual behavior to participate in the assessment process, this step in the pathway also marks a change in the treatment frame. Establishing an SHP clarifies the client's commitment to sexual health behavior change and introduces accountability into the therapeutic relationship.

The Sexual Health Plan

Writing and committing to an SHP is consistent with an action-stage intervention. The SHP is an outcome of a collaborative planning process between therapist and client that develops a man's initial sexual boundaries and sexual health goals for beginning OCSB group treatment. It incorporates the insights and observations from OCSB assessment to guide the client when operationalizing his sexual health vision. The SHP is a written document composed of three side-by-side columns. The first SHP column, Boundaries, is populated by the specific sexual and non-sexual behaviors the client is ready to change in order to maintain his vision of sexual health. The next column is Ambivalence (or High-Risk

Behaviors). The assessment will likely reveal some behaviors that men are not ready to change. The Ambivalence column normalizes different stages of readiness for the various clinical areas and the vulnerability factors identified in the assessment. This section identifies potentially problematic behaviors that the client is not ready to change, but is willing to monitor. Over time, these items are typically reconsidered and may evolve into SHP boundaries or are removed from the SHP because the client does not consider them problematic. The last column is Health. This column includes client sexual and nonsexual behaviors that the client is ready to implement and that support sexual health behavior change.

The initial SHP is developed at the conclusion of the assessment and is typically revised throughout OCSB treatment. The SHP is designed to shift the deliberative–affective interaction to help men regain sexual control. The document offers written accountability for men that helps them to gradually and more consistently align their sexual behavior with the sexual health principles and personal vision of sexual health. Clients write this concrete plan to clearly outline the behaviors they are committing to stop and the activities they are committing to pursue. It integrates the relevant clinical issues identified through the OCSB assessment as well as the therapist's suggestions for skills and tools that foster behavioral change. Before we discuss the process writing the SHP, we first discuss the change processes on which the SHP relies and how the SHP works as a tool to change sexual health.

THE SEXUAL HEALTH PLAN: CHANGE PROCESSES

The assessment process facilitates movement from contemplating change to preparing to take action for change. Creating the SHP is an action that prepares men to begin their change process and move toward entering the action stage of change. Prochaska, Norcross, and DiClemente (2006) identify five change processes well matched for people at the preparation and action stages of readiness for change: (a) commitment, (b) countering, (c) environmental control, (d) reward, and (e) helping relationships. *Commitment* is the process of taking responsibility for your actions and choosing to change. *Countering* is the term for substituting old behaviors with healthy behaviors. *Environmental control* involves external changes to avoid triggering stimuli. *Rewards* are positive reinforcements. *Helping relationships* involve enlisting people to support a client's desired changes. These change strategies inform the clinical dialogue for constructing the SHP. We present case examples of this dialogue later in the chapter.

Accountability and Commitment

We return to the OCSB treatment frame to describe how we use the SHP. The SHP establishes two additional treatment frame agreements and conditions for entering OCSB individual and group psychotherapy. First, the client agrees to maintain his SHP boundaries. Second, the client agrees to disclose crossing any of his SHP boundaries at his next individual and group therapy appointment. The SHP treatment frame sets the conditions for clients to improve self-regulation skills and change attachment patterns.

Accountability

Clients agree to reveal an SHP boundary crossing in their next OCSB treatment session for practical reasons. An SHP boundary crossing is a significant event for the therapist, client, and group to deconstruct collaboratively so that men can understand their behavior, reflect on their decisions, and identify potential new strategies to honor their commitment to the SHP. At first, some clients are confused by the contradiction of discussing broken agreements. They are concerned that we are undermining their commitment to upholding their boundaries in the first place by openly acknowledging the possibility of crossing a boundary. Is this agreement giving men permission to cross their sexual health boundaries? Their concern reveals a misunderstanding about how OCSB therapy works, which starkly contrasts the dynamics in other relationships in which they broke agreements. As a result, men often project fears of being punished for their "disobedience." They may also not realize that lapses and relapses are sometimes a part of clients' sexual health change. OCSB treatment acknowledges that possibility and establishes a relational commitment that expects men to get curious about their symptoms and engage their therapeutic support for assistance. Sexual health conversations in response to client SHP boundary crossings are a collaborative discussion rather than a punitive response. Furthermore, OCSB treatment does not automatically require clients to fully disclose their actions to their intimate partners immediately after discussing the boundary crossing with the group or individual therapist. Men learn to follow their SHP boundaries and to disclose when they do not keep their boundaries.

These treatment frame agreements offer opportunities to help men improve self-regulation capacities and emotional activation coping skills. The SHP accountability commitment supports men in developing their self-monitoring and sexual-inhibition skills. Self-monitoring skills can improve when men know they agreed to be accountable to the therapist and group. It introduces a consequence (i.e., reporting to treatment) that can gradually alter their consciousness (i.e., self-monitoring) in the moments preceding boundary crossings. As clients become more aware of their sexual urges or thoughts and link them with their anticipated feelings when disclosing an SHP boundary crossing to the group (e.g., disappointment, fear, shame, sadness, embarrassment, guilt), they improve their deliberative systems balance with the sexual activation. From the perspective of the dual control model of sexual response, men are predicting the negative consequences of sex to inhibit levels of sexual excitation that were difficult to regulate previously. In OCSB treatment, thinking about the feelings associated with a sexual boundary disclosure in therapy prior to engaging in problematic sexual behavior is a sign of progress. It is a self-monitoring success. Men slowly and gradually develop these transcendent thoughts and feelings prior to crossing a sexual boundary. OCSB SHP accountability sows the seeds for improving self-monitoring capacity and altering the affective–deliberative sexual decision-making process.

Commitment

The SHP agreement uses therapeutic relationships to evoke client attachment-style patterns that they are attempting to understand and change. As you might imagine, OCSB clients frequently struggle to honor this SHP boundary crossing disclosure agreement. Clients often report their conflicted thoughts driving to the therapy appointment and sitting in the waiting room. They describe vacillating between honoring the treatment frame agreement and withholding the information. A decision not to honor this agreement (consciously or unconsciously) injects the client's anxious or avoidant attachment traits into the individual or group treatment space. This situation, referred to by Langs (1992) as a "secure frame moment," is an opportunity for the therapist to respond with curiosity and explore the motivations that competed with the client's disclosure commitment. What priority was the client considering when he decided to withhold the boundary crossing? What was he attempting to accomplish? To avoid feelings of shame or guilt? To avoid projected judgment or disappointment of the group or therapist? We have interpreted a systems perspective to not disclose an SHP boundary crossing. The sexual secret injects into a system, in this case the group, a familiar homeostatic recreation of familiar emotional tensions that may be paradoxically more comfortable for some men than transparent honesty. Men's solutions to their competing motivations in OCSB therapy often parallel the interpersonal patterns found in their current and historic primary attachments. Each time a client reports an SHP boundary crossing and honors his accountability commitment, he is cultivating self- and attachment regulation skills. When men do not cross an SHP boundary, they are building on the developing self and improving attachment regulation.

SHP accountability creates opportunities for men to practice aligning their behavior with sexual health principles of nonexploitation and honesty. Group members and therapists assume clients are maintaining their boundaries when men do not report boundary crossing. Dishonoring the accountability agreement is contrary to the honesty and nonexploitation sexual health principles. Allowing his support system to maintain the impression that he is keeping his relational commitments exploits the group's trust while accessing the supportive and caring group environment. In essence, the member recreates the withholding patterns in the group that he displays in his significant relationships. The therapist and group provide the opportunity for the client to vicariously empathize with his intimate partners, family, and others who have experienced the same emotional and relational consequences from his exploitative withholding when the group openly processes his choice to dishonor his accountability commitment.

For people familiar with 12-step sexual recovery programs, the Three Circle plan is similar to the SHP; both are tools used to identify and organize behavior health change (Sex Addicts Anonymous [SAA], n.d.). There are significant differences in goals and implementation of an SHP and a 12-step fellowship circle plan. The goal of the OCSB SHP plan is to define and maintain a personal vision for sexual health, not to abstain from specific sexual behaviors to achieve a form of sexual sobriety. As we discussed in Chapter 2, definitions of sexual health have expanded beyond the absence of disease or unwanted pregnancies. Much like mental health or physical health, sexual health is a condition to maintain and continually shape. Crossing an SHP boundary or failing to align with one or more of the six sexual health principles is not equivalent to a relapse in a disease process and loss of sexual sobriety. During OCSB treatment, we track the duration of maintaining SHP boundaries to chart progress and inform treatment decisions, but we do not frame it as a sexual sobriety date. We contextualize the client's actions in the larger process of maintaining sexual health and do not consider that the client is starting over or request that he reset his sobriety date when SHP boundary crossings are discussed and explored. Rather than consist of three concentric circles, the SHP is a chart containing three columns. The items in the inner circle list sexual abstinence behaviors that are considered addictive, harmful, or unacceptable and that led the person to "hit bottom" (SAA, n.d.). The SHP does not illustrate a self-representation in which there is a core of one's self that contains an addictive, harmful, or unacceptable sexuality. We avoid this style for outlining sexual health to avoid implying an inherent deviance or degeneracy.

Writing a Sexual Health Plan

Column One: Boundaries

A question from the consultation guides clients when they start their SHP: What is your vision of sexual health? They are likely more prepared to articulate an answer to this question after they have completed the OCSB assessment. The therapist will have reviewed the clients' Unique Clinical Pictures, including the three OCSB clinical areas, the vulnerability factors, and the competing motivations that influence their sense of feeling out of control in their sexual behavior. The assessment summary organizes a range of new insights that men can use to draft and refine their initial sexual boundaries. Clients face the reality that their SHP boundaries inherently lead to them forgo previously pleasurable sexual activities. The Boundary column is a tangible acknowledgment that certain sexual behaviors are problematic for him and that he is ready to change them. Setting and committing to sexual health boundaries may activate feelings of shame, disappointment, grief, or fear. This is a moment in treatment to handle with care and compassion because it is vital for clients to believe that they have the ability to follow through and are agreeing to be responsible for the changes to which they are committing (Prochaska et al. 2006). Miller and Rollick (2002) warned of three hazards when clients are committing to behavior change: (a) underestimating ambivalence, (b) overprescription, and (c) insufficient direction. The OCSB SHP preparation and commitment process attempts to circumvent these vulnerabilities to successful behavior change decisions by focusing on the men's readiness for action, flexibility, and attention to language.

Readiness for action

SHP is not meant to compromise client sexual autonomy by establishing boundaries that the client feels ambivalent about changing or to establish restrictive boundaries that are unreasonable to meet. During the process of establishing sexual boundaries, it is important for the therapist to provide sufficient guidance for the clients to avoid the inherent traps present when forming new sexual boundaries. It is common for clients to conform the act-centered values system asserted by sociocultural forces rather than the less common principle-centered framework promoted by the sexual health field. Therefore, prior to firmly committing to any one SHP boundary, the client and therapist evaluate whether the proposed boundary is reasonable and review the client's readiness and responsibility for establishing the boundary.

The pace of the OCSB assessment is designed to reduce premature movement toward action as a protection from underestimating men's ambivalence about changing their sexual behavior once the initial shock, pain, and shame caused by the precipitating crisis subsides. Normalizing ambivalence is essential when evaluating client readiness to establish new sexual health boundaries. Client and therapist utilize the OCSB assessment summary to collaborate and determine sexual boundaries they both agree he is ready to follow. Part of the purpose for this discussion is to avoid boundaries the client agrees to set because he is seeking approval from the therapist.

Together, the therapist and client explore ideas and language for sexual boundaries. Each boundary is reviewed by the therapist for clarity and congruence while keeping in mind the client's action stage of readiness. As each boundary is presented or proposed, the therapist can explore the client's reason for this boundary. Defensive responses like, "Isn't that what I'm supposed to do?" or "My wife doesn't want me to," require deeper exploration. The therapist can remind him that the SHP is the client's plan to achieve sexual health and is not designed to please another person's external ideal. It is not his partner's plan, his therapist's plan, his clergy's plan, and so on. SHP boundaries that the client feels torn about establishing and that are primarily motivated to please his partner require further discussion to elucidate and resolve the competing motivations. There could be a significant empathy gap or a continued avoidance of establishing relationship agreements that are motivated to restore the intimate partner's need for safety. The SHP boundaries are established when client and therapist agree that the client is ready for that change.

Flexibility
The first SHP is just a starting point of OCSB outpatient therapy. An SHP can always be revised. Once it is completed and OCSB treatment begins, clients agree not to revise their SHP without first collaborating with their therapist and group.

An SHP must be flexible enough to prevent rigid or unrealistic sexual standards that work at cross-purposes to improve men's self-regulation. As a living document and tool used to support men changing their sexual health behavior, normal scrutiny of the SHP will evaluate whether the boundaries are sufficient for achieving behavior change. Clients who have a high frequency of crossing one or more SHP boundary can benefit from reevaluating their plan. New sexual or behavioral boundaries may be considered, as well as specific sexual behaviors moved from Ambivalence to Boundaries.

Collaborative sexual health conversation skills are vital for every person in treatment for OCSB. As such, clients are to communicate any sexual health boundary changes to all members of their treatment team (e.g., individual, group, couples, medication management). Revising the SHP provides men with uncommon opportunities to develop sexual health communication skills with their intimate partners and the OCSB group. Involving others in changing sexual health boundaries disrupts long-standing patterns of unilateral decisions to change sexual agreements with their romantic partners without telling them. Men with dismissive attachment styles can learn new skills when discussing a change in their sexual boundaries before engaging in the prohibitive behavior. Other men may benefit from interrupting the internal negotiation that frequently occurs during heated sexual moments. They can rely on a decision that was made during a calm moment and, if they want to engage in that sexual behavior again in the future, they have agreed to first talk about it with the group or their therapist. The agreement puts a step between the sexual urge and sexual action.

Notes about language
The terms and behavioral descriptions used in each SHP column should be written in clear, accurate, and detailed sexual health language. The OCSB assessment process can increse men's awareness of their use of terms that are sex negative, vague, or of sex talk that overly relies on sex euphemisms, metaphors, and pejoratives. For example, a client lists: *No longer see prostitutes*. Sexual health translation: *I will not pay for sex*. To "see a prostitute" is too vague. It relies on the infinitive "to see" to denote "to have sex with." The main objective of this boundary is to clearly convey the boundary as an agreement to discontinue paying for sex. Avoiding the locations frequented by sex workers may be a legitimate strategy to prevent high degrees of sexual activation when literally seeing a sex worker. If that is the case, another boundary can be included that states: *I will avoid areas frequented by sex workers* (e.g., specific freeway exits or surface streets).

The original statement (*No longer see prostitutes*) is a phrase that relies on a derogatory term (*prostitutes*). The word *prostitute* describes someone who is paid for sex and it contains a moral judgment about using one's sexual skills for an unworthy or corrupt sexual purpose (synonymous with: cheapen, sell-out, degrade, or debase). The moral judgment regarding who is being paid for sex is irrelevant to the SHP boundary and may indicate a subconscious moral judgment about the client himself. Men in OCSB treatment can use the SHP wording to displace feelings of disgust and disdain about their sexual behavior onto others. Therapists have an opportunity to raise the client's awareness about his moral self-judgments by reframing and processing the use of derogatory language. As a general rule for developing an SHP, the more accurate the sexual health language, the less likely the language promotes sex-negative messages or attitudes.

Examples of boundaries our clients have agreed to (in no particular order)
No paying for sex; no being paid for sex; no searching on Craigslist for anonymous sex partners; no viewing sexual imagery when masturbating, or only view sexual imagery when masturbating _____ (fill in the blank) times per week; no viewing of sexual imagery on my work laptop, not viewing sexual imagery at work; no viewing of sexual imagery that depicts sex/drug-linked interactions; no masturbating at work; no sex outside my relationship, or no sex outside of my relationship that has not been agreed to by my partner; no condomless sex; no sex without a contraception plan; no sex with a new partner until I have addressed my relationship with HIV; only have sex with people I'm attracted to; stop pursing a casual or one-time sexual partner if I do not find the person attractive; no stealing of women's underwear; no reading of my partner's e-mails; no drinking or drink only _____ (fill in the blank) times per week; no driving past (insert location where client engaged in problematic sexual behaviors); only carry $20 cash.

Column Two: Ambivalence

Clients are often not ready to change every factor that the assessment suggests contributes to their OCSB. After all, clients are describing their feeling out of control as the sense of "being of two minds" about their sexual behaviors and that ambivalence does not disappear because they started treatment (Miller & Rollnick, 2002). In one recent study, 70% of the sample of treatment-seeking clients were highly ambivalent about sexual behavior change (Reid, 2007). The SHP Ambivalence column normalizes and welcomes client ambivalence and the problematic sexual and nonsexual behaviors that men are hesitant to change.

The Ambivalence column often lists situations, attitudes, emotions, behaviors, and interpersonal relationship patterns that increase the risk for crossing one or more SHP boundaries. Items in the Ambivalence column have the potential to disrupt men's affective and deliberative systems, which in turn, influence their regulation of behaviors, situations, and feelings. Although clients are not agreeing to change any of these items, they are agreeing to monitor and evaluate these items as long as they are included on the plan. Reviewing thoughts, feelings, and behaviors from the Ambivalent column in group and individual therapy can increase men's understanding of how these factors contribute to their SHP boundary crossings or to maintaining their boundaries over time. The Ambivalence column provides both individual and group therapy a space for an ongoing sexual health conversation to collect evidence about specific behaviors that may impede changes in sexual health.

The Ambivalence column allows time for sexual health boundaries to unfold without forcing men to make immediate or premature changes. It offers a reminder that change is a continual work in progress. For example, a man may have a goal to learn his HIV status and if he does not have the virus, to remain HIV negative. His SHP boundary may be "no condomless anal intercourse with anonymous partners." The Ambivalence column behavior was to take PrEP (preexposure prophylaxis—when taken regularly, this medication prevents the HIV virus from establishing a permanent infection; Centers for Disease Control and Prevention [CDC], 2014). He was not sure whether he wanted to take a daily medication and was concerned about contracting other sexually transmitted infections (STIs) not prevented by PrEP. He felt ambivalence because he also enjoyed anal sex without condoms. At the time of establishing his plan, he was able to acknowledge his ambivalence and agreed to include taking PrEP to process that sexual health intervention. Men can increase a sense of responsibility and self-efficacy when they have sexual health conversations that honestly process their ambivalence about some of their sexual health goals. Over time, these vulnerable conversations, conducted in a safe, informed, and respectful space, may lead men to resolve their ambivalence and move a specific sexual behavior into the Boundary or Health column.

Column Three: Health

The Health column translates OCSB assessment information into behaviors, psychotherapy interventions, regulation skills, and interpersonal attachment dynamics that support sexual, mental, and overall health. General questions may help the transition into discussing supportive actions: "What activities support the changes you would like to make in your sexual health?" and "We know the sexual behaviors you want to stop, what are the sexual behaviors you want to continue to enjoy and explore?" The discussion that centers around the Health column identifies the strengths and social supports that can form client's initial reinforcements for sexual behavior change. The transtheoretical model of health behavior change (TTM) change-process strategies (countering, environment control, rewards, and helping relationships) provide guidance for defining Health column actions that are relevant for the preparation and action stage of readiness of change

Health column change processes
The TTM identifies overt and covert activities relevant for each stage of readiness for change (Velicer, Prochaska, Fava, Norman, & Redding, 1998). OCSB treatment integrates a collaborative mind-set between client and therapist that is used to apply these well-established psychotherapy change processes. Five cognitive/experiential change processes that have been found to be more relevant in the early stages of contemplating change are consciousness-raising, dramatic relief, environmental reevaluation, social liberation, and self-reevaluation (Velicer et al., 1998). These processes are the primary treatment elements integrated within the OCSB assessment process. Transitioning from the assessment to establishing the SHP moves one into the action stage of change, which benefits from other behavioral methods associated with a commitment to change. The Health column uses these stage-concordant behavioral methods associated with taking action to create and maintain change over time. We introduce each of the five change processes to elucidate how they are included in the Health column. In the final section of the book, we describe group and individual treatment approaches using these processes to address vulnerability factors, self- and attachment regulation patterns, sexual/erotic-identity development, and aligning sexual behavior with the sexual health principles.

We review the relevant change processes of TTM of health behavior change to organize the item options for the Health column (Prochaska et al., 2006):

Countering behaviors are healthy substitutes for problem behaviors. Many of the following countering techniques may be familiar to therapists who work with clients attempting to change any problematic behavior like eating, drinking, smoking, or managing anger.

1. Active diversion—These are behaviors that preclude sexual behaviors men want to stop. An active diversion could be anything, preferably a fun, healthy behavior unrelated to the sexual behavior the client is trying to avoid.
2. Exercise—"There is no more beneficial substitute for problem behaviors than exercise" (Prochaska et al., 2006, p. 177). The mental and physical benefits of exercise are so important that to not include even minimal exercise is like benching your best player. Intentional physical activity strengthens the deliberative and affective systems' biological foundations, which can improve OCSB

self-control and affect regulation. Furthermore, both immediate and long-term exercise are positively correlated with improving willpower (McGonigal, 2011).

3. Relaxation—This is another technique that works to improve the capacities of the deliberative and affective systems. Prochaska et al. (1994) include meditation as a form of deep relaxation providing mental and physical benefits. Haidt (2006) describes meditation as one of the three most effective ways to change one's affective patterns; the other two are psychotherapy and psychopharmacology.

4. Counterthinking—This technique targets the unhelpful thoughts generated by the deliberative system by evaluating and replacing these irrational or distorted thoughts. This category can be filled with any cognitive counseling technique used to address a man's irrational belief system. An important skill for OCSB treatment-seeking men is to replace their judgmental and distorted thoughts about sex with beliefs that are more accurate, effective, and kind. Anecdotally, OCSB clients report greater ease with improving their self- and attachment regulation patterns and erotic conflicts when they learn counterthinking techniques for their sex-negative judgments and narratives.

5. Assertiveness—This refers to a relational behavior that involves an active stance of communicating one's thoughts, feelings, and desires. Assertiveness is often necessary to implement and maintain one's sexual health principles. For instance, a mutually pleasurable sexual encounter relies on communicating what is sexually pleasurable and highly desired along with listening to one's partner assert what he or she finds pleasurable. Assertiveness may also involve following other health behaviors, like declining a drink when the client has a history of poor sexual decision making when drunk or taking a "time out" to prevent a heated discussion from escalating into a verbally abusive argument.

These countering behaviors are important SHP tools employed throughout OCSB treatment as well as being essential for ongoing maintenance of one's sexual health.

Establishing *environmental controls* is another strategy used to maintain sexual health boundaries. Men who have not developed an internal self-regulatory capacity can rely on environmental controls to maintain their sexual behaviors, especially early in the implementation of their SHP. This behavior change strategy is intended to remove potentially triggering stimuli when men do not have adequate internal deliberative processes that balance the sudden onset of emotions within a given situation. Internet filters that restrict access to sexual imagery or social media sites, avoiding situations or locations where the client has regularly engaged in problematic sexual behaviors, leaving his work laptop at the office, and so forth are strategies used to control environmental triggers. It may be important to help men who are early in treatment process to define clear external controls so they can build their confidence and experience periods of time without feeling sexually out of control. The client's motivation may improve when he feels relief from the stress of maintaining his SHP boundaries because he successfully implemented environmental controls. Most men in OCSB treatment are unfamiliar with the concepts of allostatic load and ego depletion. Prior to treatment, they had limited success with willpower approaches to changing their sexual behavior. Environmental controls can provide a newfound sense of safety that allow men to learn about their willpower capacities and how to best utilize this finite resource.

As an environmental control strategy, avoidance has a bad reputation and some men protest against it. "I don't need an Internet filter, that's cheating!" or "I shouldn't have to avoid the bookstore, I should be able to walk past it without going in." These statements are derived from their false beliefs about their willpower capacities. These beliefs can be interwoven with their sense of masculinity, autonomy, and shame avoidance. They may erroneously believe that avoiding these triggers is not "manning up" and truly dealing with their problems. Men who merge a sense of toughness and brave adversity by testing their willpower without respecting its limitations may use a range of defenses to protest against this change practice. They may be disappointed, embarrassed, and ashamed that they cannot simply "white knuckle" their way through their SHP boundaries.

Information about self-control can be useful for men contemplating using environmental control to decrease their exposure to environmental triggers. Research suggests that sexual activation is correlated with more difficulty resisting temptation (Ariely & Loewenstein, 2006; Blanton & Gerrard, 1997). Although it may seem quite reasonable to implement strategies that decrease exposure to tempting stimuli to maintain sexual boundaries, men often comment that these controls are not failsafe. With enough persistence or technological skill, anyone can circumvent an Internet filter. This is true and also not the point. External controls are not used to sexually sanitize every aspect of their daily lives. They are intended to decrease the frequency of spending unnecessary energy on easily avoided situations to reserve ego strengthen for the sexual situations that are less avoidable. They are implemented to conserve the resources that will be called on in other circumstances and that require internal regulation. These environmental controls can also establish small buffers that create time between urge and action. This newly established, yet brief, window provides the space for the deliberative system to influence their behavior and stop the momentum toward crossing a boundary.

Rewards are Health column items that reinforce behavior change. They bring pleasurable consequences to new and difficult behaviors. They would be unnecessary if resisting temptation was its own reward (Prochaska et al., 2006). The SHP can include rewards for avoiding pleasurable behaviors to decrease feelings of apathy that can occur when clients make changes toward fulfilling their sexual health goals. Rewards can either be overt positive acknowledgments of progress or preplanned responses earned when they achieve a specified length of boundary maintenance (Prochaska et al., 2006). The reward center of the brain motivates people toward a particular action that has the promise of a reward. People who are unable to anticipate the pleasure of an action, such as those who experience anhedonia related to Parkinson's disease or other neurological conditions, lose motivation and develop depression (Heller et al., 2009). With that in mind, we shape each man's rewards to motivate him toward sexual health.

Change does not happen instantly despite the client's urgency. As a result, clients frequently have the implementation of rewards backward. "Why should I celebrate for doing the right thing?" "It's terrible that I need to reward myself when I don't cheat on my wife." Clients tend to be more familiar with negative reinforcements for boundary crossings (i.e., negative self-judgments, romantic relationship problems) rather than with positive reinforcements used to maintain sexual health. As such, these clients are prepared to belittle or berate themselves for their willpower failures or dismissive attachment styles as a strategy to motivate themselves toward sexual health. It may feel counterintuitive to them, but motivating clients with positive reinforcement is usually a more effective approach than relying on negative reinforcement.

Change does not happen in isolation. Whether people enlist friends, family, or therapists, *helping relationships* are a vital component of the change process. The Health column often includes social elements that are either directly or indirectly related to supporting men's sexual health boundaries. Using helping relationships as a sexual health change strategy is not without its challenges. Revealing that one has a sexual problem is difficult for many people, as it carries with it a degree of shame, regret, and disappointment. Men may defend against these negative feelings by avoiding exposure and hiding their sexual behavior problems. When men ask for help it often engenders a vulnerability with which they have limited experience. This results in some men having less life experience in tolerating the emotions that accompany their vulnerable disclosures.

Avoidance and lack of experience with vulnerability does not teach men about the benefits of connection. When men are not ready to disclose the details of their sexual health beyond the treatment circle, consider an emphasis on team exercise, meditation classes, and other countering activities that can indirectly expand their social network. During the course of treatment, clients will have the opportunity to process the negative emotions they are avoiding, which may increase their willingness to make direct requests for help.

THE SEXUAL HEALTH PLAN: CASE EXAMPLES

In this section, we provide sample OCSB Assessment Summaries and client SHPs that reflect starting points for treatment. We also include details of treatment that reflect the Unique Clinical Picture of each client. We present case summaries of four men we introduced to you on the day they disclosed their concerns with out of control sexual behavior. The treatment summaries for Jay, Hector, Frank, and Will provide a sample documentation process that organizes key aspects of each man's sexual health, vulnerability factors, and OCSB clinical areas that emerged during the assessment.

OCSB ASSESSMENT SUMMARY

Client Name: Jay

Sexual Health

A 35 y/o, White, heterosexual-identified, married man with 2 children under 7, presenting for OCSB treatment involving masturbation to online sexual imagery and online sexual behavior with other women (online text and video chats), which violates his marital agreement.

Client Motivation: The client's stated motivation for treatment was to maintain his relationship agreements and to remain married to his wife. Secondary motivation was to be more honest about his erotic interests with his wife in order to integrate them into his marriage.

(continued)

OCSB ASSESSMENT SUMMARY (*continued*)

Sexual Health Principles: Behaviors incongruent with non-exploitative and honesty principles by not honoring his relationship agreements. Also not mutually pleasurable because he does not disclose his erotic interests with his wife.

Sexual Consent: Denied nonconsensual sexual behavior.

Vulnerability Factors

1. *Physical Safety*: Reported several incidents in which his wife pushed and hit him since learning about his sexual behavior. No reported injuries. Some occasional incidents of violence between the couple prior to the precipitating incident. Recent incidents occurred after wife suspected the client was engaging in sex chats with other women again. No police involvement or injuries. Client believes that his children have never witnessed any violence between the couple. No Suspected Child Abuse Reported filed at this time; continue to monitor.
2. *Physical Health*: Client denied medical problems; HIV negative, no other current STIs.
3. *Mental Health*: Moderate symptoms of anxiety and depression; client denied history of adverse events.
4. *Relationship With Drugs and Alcohol*: Alcohol abuse; adult child of an alcoholic

Clinical Areas

1. *Self-Regulation*
   A. Four ingredients:
      a. Standards—client held clear standard against dishonesty and online sexual behavior that violated his marital agreement.
      b. Monitoring—impacted by alcohol. Alcohol was identified as a contributing factor to the relationship violence in marriage. Client was less able to identify signs of escalation when drinking.
      c. Willpower

(*continued*)

OCSB ASSESSMENT SUMMARY (*continued*)

- Client frequently experienced ego depletion. Described persistent behavior restricting at home as a strategy to manage wife's unpredictable reactivity. "It's like walking on eggshells."
- Client reported a permission-giving pattern that preceded sexual boundary crossing after marital conflicts.

   d. Motivation

- Client reported competing motivations between erotic interests and managing wife's reactivity.
- Client not motivated to limit his weekly drinking at the conclusion of the assessment

  B. Regulating activation:

   a. Client is frequently managing his hyperactive states triggered by marital tension and violence.

  C. Regulating sexual activation:

   a. Levels of sexual excitation and inhibition do not seem out of balance, supported by Sexual Inhibition/Sexual Excitation Scales (SES/SIS) survey results.

   b. Worries his wife's rejection may inhibit his desire to assert his erotic interest.

2. *Attachment Behaviors*

  A. Attachment style:

   a. Father—secure

   b. Mother—fearful

   c. Close friendship—fearful

   d. Romantic relationship—dismissive

   e. Global—dismissive

   f. Client struggled to manage wife's episodic reactivity that occasionally escalates to violence.

   g. Client experienced a familiar emotional tension: managing the unpredictability of his mother's untreated alcoholism felt similar to managing his wife's unpredictable reactivity.

  B. Relationship agreements:

   a. Client was interested in having a monogamous relationship. His only expression of his erotic turn-on has been through masturbation and online chatting.

(*continued*)

OCSB ASSESSMENT SUMMARY (*continued*)

> b. The client's solution to his relationship bind has been to not assert himself sexually with his wife, explore his erotic interests through masturbating to sexual videos, and hide his fantasy chatting from wife; both are strategies to avoid conflict.
> C. Sexual narcissism:
> a. Client reported feeling empathy fatigue toward his wife's reactive emotional process.
> 3. *Sexual and Erotic Orientation Conflict*
> A. Conflict with self:
> a. Client reported shame regarding his intense turn-on with anal sex. Client held act-centered value that vaginal intercourse is normative and proper.
> B. Conflict with others:
> a. Client reported limited experience having anal sex with women. Client indicated he has felt too nervous in the past to initiate anal sex. He believed his wife finds the behavior disgusting, expressed feeling too afraid to mention it previously and, since she discovered his turn-on, feared that she will end the marriage.
> b. Client also reported difficulties feeling turned on by wife, possibly related to lack of emotional tension in the relationship.

Jay's Sexual Health Plan

Boundaries	Ambivalence	Health
• I will only sex chat with my wife. • I will only have sexual relations with my wife. • I will not engage in physical or verbal violence with my wife. • I will not use sexual imagery when masturbating.	• I will evaluate my sexual imagery boundary in 6 months. • I will monitor my relationship with alcohol for the next 3 months.	• I will install a computer filter. • I will develop and implement a safety plan when relationship violence is feared. • Individual, group, and couple therapy • Bibliotherapy • Masturbation without sexual imagery • Play time with children

Notes About Jay's SHP

Vulnerability Factors—Items to address included *relationship violence* and alcohol abuse. Client committed to no physical and verbal violence, the implementation of a safety plan, learning strategies to de-escalate arguments, and couple therapy to learn new ways of communicating. Jay was not ready to discontinue or limit his alcohol consumption when he was establishing his first SHP. *Alcohol abuse* was a contributing factor to their violent interactions and preceded numerous online sex-chatting episodes. Jay was ready to monitor his use and reevaluate the consequences of his drinking in 3 months. Reading materials were suggested around safe, intimate communication and the experiences of an adult child of alcoholics.

When creating Jay's SHP, using accurate language was important. An initial boundary of not having sex outside his marriage was not specific enough. Does online flirting count as sex outside of his marriage or is sex confined to oral sex and vaginal intercourse? Because Jay's behavior never manifested in offline sexual intercourse, specifying "Only sex chatting with my wife" avoided the debate around what constitutes sex and accurately targeted the presenting problem.

Sexual Health—Jay wanted to disrupt his chatting routine and was motivated to stop masturbating to online images. The assessment identified an unrealistic expectation for internal regulation. Jay was unable to maintain his online chat boundary when he was sexually aroused by viewing online sexual images. He acknowledged it was unrealistic for him to internally self-regulate his boundary to not open his instant messenger and initiate a sexual conversation. By avoiding online sexual images, Jay wanted to use external controls to successfully manage these boundaries. Jay wanted to construct situations that provided him with more time to regulate his behavior in response to sexual urges and excitement.

Jay made clear that his children were highly rewarding (hence a potentially useful countering behavior). He made a direct connection between time spent chatting online and less time spent with his children. Jay began to see how his sexual behavior competed with his motivation to be an engaging father. Spending time with his children was a positive reinforcement and a significant motivation for Jay to maintain his SHP boundaries. Jay was honest about his current ambivalence about spending time with his wife. At the start of OCSB treatment, the couple had a few moments without hostility or contempt. Jay agreed to work in couples therapy to establish a mutual safety agreement and improve the emotional tone and quality of his relationship.

OCSB ASSESSMENT SUMMARY

Client Name: Hector

Sexual Health

A 42 y/o, Mexican American, gay-identified married man presenting for OCSB treatment involving sex–drug-linked behaviors and sexual behaviors with other men that are not within his current relationship agreement.

Client Motivation: Client was motivated to maintain his sobriety from alcohol and drugs and was motivated to remain married.

Sexual Health Principles: Behaviors incongruent with non-exploitation, the need to be protected from HIV, and honesty in marriage by not honoring his relationship agreements with his husband.

Sexual Consent: Denied nonconsensual sex.

Vulnerability Factors

1. *Physical Safety:* Denied safety concerns.
2. *Physical Health:* HIV status is unknown; recent condomless receptive anal intercourse.
3. *Mental Health:* Symptoms of anxiety; rule out generalized anxiety disorder or posttraumatic stress disorder (PTSD), delayed onset; reported childhood nonconsensual sex history involving incest/rape with an older brother. Other adverse childhood experiences included witnessing domestic violence between parents and experiencing caregiver neglect.
4. *Relationship With Drugs and Alcohol:* Newly in recovery from alcohol and drugs. Client considered alcohol his main addiction and reported sporadic history of abusing marijuana, methamphetamine, and gamma-Hydroxybutyric acid (GHB).

Clinical Areas

1. *Self-Regulation*
   A. Four ingredients:
      a. Standards
         - Clear standards against: contracting HIV, infecting his partner with an STI, and dishonoring relationship agreements.

(continued)

OCSB ASSESSMENT SUMMARY (*continued*)

---

 b. Monitoring
 - Impaired when intoxicated
 - Underdeveloped self-awareness and accountability for self-monitoring.
 - Impaired at times by dissociation defenses potentially related to past sexual abuse involving sibling incest and witnessing violence between parents.
 c. Willpower
 - Highly reliant on external controls and other people's boundaries during sexual encounters.
 d. Motivation
 - Client seemed more motivated to not infect his partner than to avoid contracting HIV himself.
 B. Regulating activation:
 a. Learning to manage high- and low-activation levels without alcohol and drugs
 C. Regulating sexual activation:
 a. Learning to regulate sexual activation when sober
 b. Client may have underdeveloped sexual inhibitors regarding the behavioral consequences of dishonoring sexual agreements and condomless anal intercourse.
2. *Attachment Behaviors*
 A. Attachment style:
 a. Father—fearful
 b. Mother—dismissive
 c. Close friendship—secure
 d. Romantic relationship—fearful
 e. Global—fearful
 f. Underdeveloped skills in asserting protective boundaries
 g. Recreated the emotional tension of holding a secret that was familiar in a violent and incestuous family system.
 B. Relationship agreements:
 a. Client engaged in sex that was inconsistent with relationship agreements. Client's solution to manage fear of losing his relationship was by withholding information from partner.
 b. Sexual behavior (e.g., sexual attention and touch from others) possibly in service of his dependency needs and self-soothing attachment distress.

(*continued*)

OCSB ASSESSMENT SUMMARY (*continued*)

C. Sexual narcissism:
   a. Client reported sexual activity consistent with exploitation of romantic partner's trust and permits assumption of fidelity to relationship sexual agreement.
   b. Client is unfamiliar with empathy capacity during sexual activation given the pervasiveness of sex/drug-linked patterns of behavior.
   c. Client does not express a strong sense of entitlement to sexual expression.

3. *Sexual or Erotic Orientation Conflict*: Reported fluid exchange as highly erotic, which motivates him to have sex without condoms. An extremely pleasurable activity, does not currently present as fixed and necessary for orgasm.
   A. Conflict with self:
      a. Conflict with self regarding the erotic pleasure of fluid exchange
   B. Conflict with others:
      a. Partner held similar value about having a fluid-bonded relationship, conditional on only exchanging fluid with each other.

Hector's Sexual Health Plan

Boundaries	Ambivalence	Health
• I will not use drugs or alcohol. • I will keep my sexual behavior agreement with my husband and only have sex with him. • I will not look at, download, or maintain membership with sex websites [specific names] or mobile apps. • I will not visit my family for the next 3 months.	• I will discuss with therapist and group my thoughts and feelings about my current relationship agreement. • I will complete a psychiatric medication evaluation. • I will meditate beginning with 5 minutes in the morning and 5 minutes after dinner. • I will talk with family on the phone and be honest about not visiting in person. • I will use a nonsmart phone for 6 months.	• I will test for HIV after 3 months from the last condomless sexual encounter. • I will attend individual therapy twice a month and weekly group therapy for the next 6 months. • I will attend three AA/NA meetings per week. • Bibliotherapy • I will learn and practice sexual assertiveness skills to increase honesty with husband about sexual desires and turn-ons. • Plan fun events together with husband • Sleep 8 hours minimum per night • Charge phone outside of bedroom at night

Notes About Hector's SHP

Vulnerability Factors—Multiple vulnerability factors required assessment given the various co-occurring issues common to a person new in drug and alcohol recovery. Abstinence is the recommended behavioral boundary for OCSB clients who identify being in recovery from *drugs and alcohol*. They agree to participate in a drug and alcohol recovery program while they are in OCSB treatment. This may range from inpatient or outpatient treatment to 12-step or SMART Recovery (Self Management and Recovery Training) meetings (http://www.smartrecovery.org/professionals/). Hector was referred for the assessment by his drug and alcohol counselor and agreed to follow an aftercare plan once he completed the program. To meet a sexual health goal for knowing his relationship with HIV (*physical health*), Hector planned to take an HIV test at the start of the assessment as well as 3 months after his last exposure. Diagnostic refinement to address a possible untreated psychiatric disorder (*mental health*) was also indicated because he was no longer using drugs or alcohol, which could have masked or exacerbated an undiagnosed mood disorder.

Clinical Areas—Hector and his partner agreed to close the sexual boundaries of their relationship. The goal was to allow themselves time to repair the relationship ruptures of the past several years. Hector was clear that he was not interested in a long-term monogamous agreement, but was willing to close the relationship for now and reevaluate the boundaries once they have rebuilt confidence that both partners will follow their sexual agreements.

Hector decided to discontinue family contact for a brief period. He found that he became too agitated whenever he spoke or visited with his family and wanted to decrease unnecessary stressors in his life. They were unsupportive of his decision to enter recovery, unwilling to look at their relationship with drugs and alcohol, and unwilling to acknowledge his childhood molestation experience. He chose to focus his energy on mending his marriage and maintaining his sexual health and drug and alcohol treatment goals. He was interested in reevaluating this boundary when he reached his 1-year sobriety anniversary.

The helping relationships of his recovery community were an important source of support for Hector. Brainstorming sexual and nonsexual rewards were a struggle for Hector. He feared not being able to find the same excitement in life that he experience when having sex high. Meditation was recommended, but Hector struggled with seated practices and was quickly discouraged. He was more interested in moving meditation practices, but was not ready to pursue them.

During the assessment, Hector struggled to break his habitual cruising on mobile social apps when he was bored. He would frequently delete and reload the applications and occasionally contact new or former sex partners. After making contact, Hector would get scared and delete the app before meeting anyone in person. Hector was ambivalent about temporarily switching to a nonsmart phone because he used it for work during the day. He was willing to distance himself from the phone after work by charging it in another room where he did not have easy access.

OCSB ASSESSMENT SUMMARY

Client Name: Frank

Sexual Health

A 56 y/o, multiracial, heterosexual-identified, single (divorced with one adult daughter) man, presenting for OCSB treatment involving online sexual behavior at work.

Client Motivation: Client is motivated to remain employed and would like to discontinue his online sexual behavior at work. Client was ambivalent about his pattern of paying for sex.

Sexual Health Principles: Behaviors incongruent with non-exploitation, protection against HIV, sexual principle of mutual pleasure and shared values by paying for sex with potentially trafficked sex workers.

Sexual Consent: Denied nonconsensual sex.

Vulnerability Factors

1. *Physical Safety:* Denied safety concerns.
2. *Physical Health:* Reported good health. HIV status unknown; reported not having an HIV/STI test after last time he had partnered sex, which was with a sex worker.
3. *Mental Health:* Generalized anxiety disorder, currently seeing a psychiatrist, prescribed antianxiety medication. Reported taking medication as prescribed. Reported history of attention deficit hyperactivity disorder (ADHD) treatment, denied current medications. Reported father was inconsistently treated

---

(continued)

OCSB ASSESSMENT SUMMARY (*continued*)

for bipolar disorder and was aware that he had multiple affairs before divorcing his mother when Frank was 10 y/o.

4. *Relationship With Drugs and Alcohol*: Denied drug use and reported drinking socially.

Clinical Areas

1. *Self-Regulation*
   A. Four ingredients:
      a. Standards
         i. Clear standards and agreed with his employer's policies prohibiting workplace sexual behavior.
         ii. Client standards about paying for sex were less developed.
      b. Monitoring
         i. Self-monitoring situationally impaired during heightened states of anxiety and sexual arousal.
      c. Willpower
         i. Pattern of permission giving when sexually aroused or feeling hopeless about being single
      d. Motivation:
         i. Client struggled to manage competing motivations between regulating his emotional distress in a manner that doesn't endanger his employment and finding a relationship but wanting to being sexual in the meantime.
   B. Regulating activation:
      a. Client globally struggled to regulate his anxiety. Client reportedly more sexual during hyperactive states.
      b. Online sexual behavior may be related to boredom regulation.
   C. Regulating sexual activation:
      a. Possible activation transference; when client feels sexually excited, he wants to have partnered sex. He feels frustrated because he is single and worried about never getting married again.
      b. High levels of sexual excitation with moderate levels of sexual inhibition

(*continued*)

OCSB ASSESSMENT SUMMARY (*continued*)

2. *Attachment Behaviors*
   A. Attachment style:
      a. Father—secure
      b. Mother—on border between fearful and dismissive
      c. Close friendship—on border between fearful and dismissive
      d. Romantic relationship—secure
      e. Global—fearful
      f. Client reported history of feeling motivated to soothe anxiety by being sexual with ex-wife.
   B. Relationship agreements:
      a. Behavior not crossing current relationship agreement because he is single.
      b. Client reported that he would masturbate to online sexual images or pay for sex at massage parlors when ex-wife was sexually unavailable.
   C. Sexual narcissism:
      a. Low empathy for sex workers present. Defended against the possibility of sexual exploitation.
      b. Entitlement displayed during the assessment process.
      c. Spending money for sex used as a partnered-sex shortcut, avoiding having to establish a relationship in order to have sex.
3. *Sexual or Erotic Orientation Conflict*: No unconventional or fixed arousal patterns.

Frank's Sexual Health Plan

Boundaries	Ambivalence	Health
• I will not view sexual imagery at work. • I will not visit sex websites at work. • I will not masturbate at work.	• Paying for sex • Masturbating with sexual imagery	• I will get tested for HIV and STIs. • I will install an Internet filter. • I will attend individual and group therapy. • I will masturbate to manage sexual temptations to pay for sex. • I will continue to see my psychiatrist and follow medication regimen as prescribed. • I will attend structured social events. • I will meditate for 10 minutes twice a day.

Notes About Frank's SHP

Vulnerability Factors—Frank agreed to an HIV/STI test as a part of his SHP (*physical health*). Frank was concerned that his psychiatric medications were not effective enough and he screened positive for ADHD during the assessment. Frank decided to fully disclose his concerns and behaviors with his psychiatrist and authorized communication between his psychiatrist and his individual and group therapist to coordinate treatment (*mental health*).

Clinical Areas—Frank was ready to discontinue his workplace online sexual behaviors. He installed an Internet filtering program on his work laptop to block general sex sites and the specific sites he visited. Frank was interested in learning techniques to disrupt the unconscious habits that contributed to mindless Internet surfing. He was motivated to meditate at work and identify the triggering emotions that contributed to his online sexual behavior.

Frank's main challenge was resolving his ambivalence around paying for sex. He struggled to identify other behaviors that would be as pleasurable as partnered sex. Frank reported a sense of sexual entitlement to partners that influenced his decisions to pay for sex. In particular, he became defensive when invited to consider exploitative aspects of his paid sexual activities. Frank was not ready to subtract paying for sex from his life, but he was ready to add social activities to address his loneliness.

He reported avoiding social settings to regulate his anxiety. During the assessment, we identified that he was less anxious in structured or semistructure social settings, particularly if he had a role or function at the event (e.g., volunteering at charity or political events, poker night with his friends or hosting small dinner parties).

OCSB ASSESSMENT SUMMARY

Client Name: Will

Sexual Health

A 29 y/o, African American, gay-identified single (heterosexual divorce) man, HIV positive, presenting for OCSB treatment regarding casual and anonymous sex with other men.

(*continued*)

OCSB ASSESSMENT SUMMARY (*continued*)

Client Motivation: Motivated to reduce frequency of sex that interferes with work; conflicted about disclosing his HIV status. Motivated to enter into long-term romantic relationship with another man.

Sexual Health Principles: Sexual behavior risks contracting STIs and reports general dissatisfaction with sexual pleasure.

Sexual Consent: Denied nonconsensual sex.

Vulnerability Factors

1. *Physical Safety:* Denied current violence. History included exposure to community violence throughout childhood.
2. *Physical Health:* HIV positive, newly diagnosed; receiving medical treatment, not taking medications regularly, viral load was undetectable. Reported regular STI testing. All results have been negative.
3. *Mental Health:* Symptoms of depression, rule out major depressive disorder (MDD); adverse childhood experiences include molestation by mother's boyfriend as a young adolescent, growing up gay in a homophobic family and church; and exposed to community violence.
4. *Relationship With Drugs and Alcohol:* Reported frequent social drinking to intoxication; stepfather was an active alcoholic.

Clinical Areas

1. *Self-Regulation*
   A. Four ingredients:
      a. Standards
         i. Internalized homo-negativity from family and community
      b. Self-monitoring
         i. Does not have a sense of his future since living with HIV or managing tension between sexual and ethnic identity.
         ii. Impacted by trauma-related defenses.

(*continued*)

OCSB ASSESSMENT SUMMARY (*continued*)

> c. Willpower
> > i. Potentially impacted by untreated depression (rule-out MDD).
> > ii. Permission giving is related to beliefs about a life with HIV.
> d. Motivation:
> > i. Experiences competing motivations between living as an openly gay man and his identity as an African American man. He questions how to remain attached to important figures in his life (i.e., mother, sister, childhood friends, and church).
> > ii. Is interested in developing a long-term, monogamous relationship.
> B. Regulating activation:
> > a. Used online and mobile cruising to elevate low mood, internalized shame and loneliness
> C. Regulating sexual activation:
> > a. High levels of sexual excitation with moderate levels of inhibition; quickly sexually excited when accessing sex apps
> 2. *Attachment Behaviors*
> > A. Attachment style:
> > > a. Father—dismissive
> > > b. Mother—preoccupied
> > > c. Close friendship—preoccupied
> > > d. Romantic relationship—fearful
> > > e. Overall—preoccupied
> > > f. Preoccupied with approval from mother, loyal to her as a single mother, conflicted about being a disappointment to her (i.e., HIV positive, being gay). Reported feeling guilty about his depression—doesn't think she will understand.
> > > g. Is attuned to rejection so he withholds information in all relationships.
> > B. Relationship agreements:
> > > a. Single. However, history of not honoring relationship sexual agreements. Was having sex with men outside of his marriage. No long-term relationship with men reported.
> > > b. Ex-wife tested positive for syphilis, which prompted confrontation about the client's extrarelational sex.

(continued)

OCSB ASSESSMENT SUMMARY (*continued*)

> C. Sexual narcissism:
>   a. Narcissistic traits do not seem to apply.
> 3. *Sexual or Erotic Orientation Conflict*
>   A. Conflict with self:
>   a. Internalized homo-negativity obstructing positive sexual-identity development.
>   b. Unclear about his erotic identity and interests.
>   c. Struggled with figuring out how to develop his erotic identity living with HIV.
>   B. Conflict with others:
>   a. Client reported feeling frustrated by persistent objectification by White men who are interested in being dominated and/or topped by a Black man, which does not always match his sexual interests.
>   b. Has fear of rejection from family and African American community.
>   c. Inconsistently out; is divorced, disclosed being gay and his mother had a high rejection response. He told his family of origin that he was HIV negative, which was true at the time. Since he has not had a boyfriend, his identity is dismissed.

Will's Sexual Health Plan

Boundaries	Ambivalence	Health
• I will not have sex without condoms. • I will not visit sexual social media during work hours. • No partnered sex during work hours. • Suicide is not an option to manage my depression or relationship problems.	• Disclosing my HIV status to family, friends, and sex partners • Evaluating my relationship with my church community • Evaluating the consequences of childhood non-consensual sex • Monitor drinking pattern	• I will follow my HIV medication regimen. • I will follow my psychiatric medication regimen. • I will make changes only after consulting with my psychiatrist. • I will attend individual and group therapy. • I will read about the experiences of openly gay African American men living with HIV. • I will monitor my pattern of withholding my needs in relationships. • Regular exercise

Notes About Will's SHP

Vulnerability Factors—Assessing Will's persistent depressive state for a potential untreated mood disorder and the ongoing factors associated with minority stress were issues that presented themselves early in treatment (*mental health*). Will's depressive symptoms seemed compounded by multiple stressors, including adjusting to his HIV diagnosis, experiences with racism in the society and the lesbian/gay/bisexual/transgender (LGBT) community, and experiences with homophobia within the African American community and his family. Will may have used sexual behavior to elevate his depressed mood and upregulate the lethargy associated with depression. He agreed to several mood-stabilizing behaviors as a part of his SHP, including a psychiatric referral, a no-harm contract, and regular exercise. Will also agreed to monitor the self-regulation effects of alcohol by including drinking in the Ambivalence column of his SHP (*relationship with drugs and alcohol*). Will was also concerned about other STIs and infecting others with HIV, so he agreed to discontinuing condomless sex (*physical health*).

    Clinical Areas—Managing rejection was a major theme in Will's assessment. His primary coping strategy was withholding aspects of himself to manage other people's reactions. It was a defense he learned growing up as a gay child in a homophobic family and community. He remained closeted through his adolescence and young adulthood. Although he was out to his family about being gay, he was in another closet about his HIV status. He was anxious about being rejected by his mother should he disclose his HIV status. This strategy was also similar to how he was sexual with other men. He would not disclose his erotic interests and mainly engaged in sex the way his partners wanted. His preoccupation about relationship rejection was a significant stressor, which he historically soothed with anonymous sex prior to his HIV diagnosis. Will's HIV treatment went well and was a bright spot during his OCSB assessment. His body tolerated the medications, and his viral load was undetectable when he started writing his SHP. This improved his outlook on his future and his willingness to date improved. He began to explore sex with other HIV-positive men he was dating, with full disclosure of his health status. This gave Will opportunities to explore his erotic template.

REFERENCES

Ariely, D., & Loewenstein, G. (2006). The heat of the moment: The effect of sexual arousal on sexual decision making. *Journal of Behavioral Decision Making, 19*(2), 87–98.

Blanton, H., & Gerrard, M. (1997). Effect of sexual motivation on men's risk perception for sexually transmitted disease: There must by 50 ways to justify a lover. *Health Psychology, 16*(4), 374–379.

Centers for Disease Control and Prevention. (2014). *Preexposure prophlylaxis for the prevention of HIV infection in the United States: A clinical practice guideline.* Retrieved from http://www.cdc.gov/hiv/pdf/PrEPguidelines2014.pdf.

Haidt, J. (2006). *The happiness hypothesis: Finding modern truth in ancient wisdom.* New York, NY: Basic Books.

Heller, A. S., Johnstone, T., Shackman, A. J., Light, S. N., Peterson, M. J., Kolden, G. G., ... Davidson, R. J. (2009). Reduced capacity to sustain positive emotion in major depression reflects diminished maintenance of fronto-striatal brain activation. *Proceedings of the National Academy of Sciences of the United States of America, 106*(52), 22445–22450.

Langs, R. J. (1992). *A clinical workbook for psychotherapists.* London, UK: Karnac.

McGonigal, K. (2011). *The willpower instinct: How self-control works, why it matters, and what you can do to get more of it.* New York, NY: Penguin.

Miller, W. R., & Rollnick, S. (2002). *Motivational interviewing: Preparing people for change.* New York, NY: Guilford Press.

Prochaska, J. O., Norcross, J. C., & DiClemente, C. C. (2006). *Changing for good.* New York, NY: William Morrow.

Reid, R. C. (2007). Assessing readiness to change among client seeking help for hypersexual behavior. *Sexual Addiction & Compulsivity, 14,* 167–186.

Sex Addicts Anonymous. (n.d.). *Abstinence, sobriety and the three circles.* Retrieved from http://saa-recovery.org/OurProgram/AbstinenceSobrietyAndTheThree Circles.

Velicer, W. F., Prochaska, J. O., Fava, J. L., Norman, G. J., & Redding, C. A. (1998). Smoking cessation and stress management: Applications of the transtheoretical model of behavior change. *Homeostasis, 38,* 216–233.

Out of Control Sexual Behavior Treatment

CHAPTER NINE

OCSB GROUP THERAPY—PRINCIPLES

The combined group and individual outpatient out of control sexual behavior (OCSB) treatment is the focus of the remaining three chapters. Implementation of the OCSB Clinical Pathway integrates a range of best-practice clinical interventions to help men regain sexual control and achieve their personal visions of sexual health. In this chapter, we review the group and individual psychotherapy principles that serve as the foundation for the program. We continue to apply the transtheoretical model of health behavior change (TTM; Prochaska & Velicer, 1997) and to use motivational interviewing strategies as our preferred method for facilitating sexual health behavior change. Therapists are not expected to maintain absolute fidelity to the treatment techniques, exercises, or clinical goals that we outline. We share our approach so therapists can learn from our experience and enhance their skills.

COMBINED TREATMENT

Combined treatment, in which clients attend group and individual psychotherapy with the same therapist, is the primary modality for OCSB treatment. Every OCSB group member agrees to concurrent individual psychotherapy for as long as he participates in the group. Combined therapy is a potent modality because it uses two change mechanisms. One mechanism is the complementary function between each modality and the other potentiates the therapy of both individual and group work (Porter, 1993). OCSB *individual therapy* provides clinical management, treatment planning, and in-depth focus on intrapsychic concerns associated with dysregulated sexual behavior. OCSB *group therapy* provides in-the-moment relationship events in which members explore defenses and interpersonal patterns, and expand relational capacities for intimacy and closeness. Each modality provides different opportunities to engage the complex interaction of diverse factors that influence a client's sexual health. The process group becomes a mechanism for communicating, fostering, and deepening an investment in sexual health that grows far beyond the walls of weekly group therapy. Individual therapy provides a strong clinical backstop that allows clients to process and work through interpersonal or psychological issues that could lead to dropping out of group. Of the more than 200 men treated in OCSB combined treatment, less than 10% have failed to complete the initial 6-month commitment. An even smaller percentage of men dropped out of group treatment for failing to complete treatment goals or because of an irreconcilable conflict with the group. The weekly OCSB group therapy session is typically the primary treatment modality, and individual therapy frequency varies depending on symptom acuity. In particular, early stabilization of sexual impulses, urges, behavior, and affect regulation is more effectively accomplished with weekly individual and group treatment.

Confidentiality

Before we discuss clinical application, it is important to briefly clarify confidentiality issues when clients participate in group therapy and when multiple therapists are involved in their care. For group participants, we cannot guarantee that clients' information will remain confidential in group therapy as we can with individual psychotherapy. Group members are not licensed therapists bound by law to keep information confidential. This is a risk that exists with OCSB group therapy that is not faced in OCSB individual therapy. During the appointment that precedes entrance into the group, we advise clients that group therapy, by its legal standing and very nature, presents an additional risk. Although our track record with clients upholding the spirit and intention of confidentiality has been high, it remains a risk for every person entering OCSB group. The group agreement document that members sign states, "Group members are expected to protect the names and identities of fellow group members. Please be advised, confidentiality in group therapy cannot be guaranteed because the members are not held to the same legal and ethical expectation as the group leaders. However, prior to entering the group, each group member is informed of the importance of confidentiality and has agreed to the confidentiality expectation."

In the combined approach, the therapist who conducts the assessment transitions into the client's individual and group therapist. The information discussed during the assessment and concurrent individual sessions must remain confidential unless the client provides written authorization to share that information. We ask clients to sign a written authorization for the OCSB individual therapist to be able to discuss protected health information (PHI) with the group coleader. This release of information is necessary for treatment coordination and planning within the combined OCSB Model. However, the authorization does not extend to the group-as-a-whole. The client retains the privilege of confidentiality, which means only the client can reveal the content of his individual therapy sessions to the group. As with any PHI, the client is free to discuss as much or as little of the individual therapy content as he pleases, but the therapist cannot provide additional information to the OCSB group. The group coleader cannot use disclosures from a client's individual session to start an OCSB group topic, report a boundary crossing by a group member disclosed in his individual appointment, or correct misinformation or contradictions in a client disclosure that he either intentionally or unintentionally provided to the group. The therapist waits for the next individual therapy session to discuss the client's content discrepancies between group and individual therapy and collaborates with the client to discuss specific content with the group. The OCSB therapist must respect a client's decisions to reveal information even when the client is not honoring the accountability agreement. Ultimately, it is the client's choice to share the content from individual therapy with the OCSB group.

A Shame-Reduction Process

Combined therapy has been described as a transformative shame-reduction process (Cadwell, 2009). Individual OCSB psychotherapy is a vital space for men to "come out" to themselves about highly conflicted or secretive erotic turn-ons. The therapist and client codevelop a personal language in which the client can organize and honestly express sexual desires. We start this identity process during the individual therapy relationship, after which we encourage men to bring their disclosures to group. The long-term objective is to integrate his sexual and erotic orientations within his self-concept and current or future relationships. For most men, the first step toward a positive sexual or erotic identity is revealing highly shameful sexual details in the safety of individual therapy.

After clients disclose conflicted or shameful aspects of their sexual/ erotic history in individual therapy, we prepare them to bring these sexual narratives to group. For instance, during his assessment, Jamie disclosed his lifelong erotic interest in smelling men's unwashed underwear, which had escalated to stealing clothes from gym bags and hampers. His friend recently found him rummaging in the clothes hamper when Jamie was visiting. Demoralized and ashamed, he entered OCSB treatment to understand his behavior and his sexual excitement. Through his combined therapy, he identified distorted beliefs about his erotic orientation and slowly processed his fears of the judgment and shame he anticipates when he discloses his erotic turn-on to the group. Individual therapy provided the first glimpse into Jamie's defenses and disgust toward his turn-on. His motivation to tell the group increased after months in individual therapy reevaluating his irrational beliefs about his orientation and processed his rejection fears. Once he disclosed his unconventional turn-on to the group, they responded with curiosity and supported his honesty. The group experience provided a useful map for future shame-reduction work directed toward integration of his turn-on within partnered relationships.

Combined therapy is not for everyone seeking OCSB treatment, nor do all clients agree to that level of care. Combined individual and group treatment is only recommended for men who are ready to change their sexual behaviors. Group cohesion is enhanced when clients acknowledge that they need help managing their sexual behavior and are personally motivated to improve their sexual health. Their precontemplative defenses would likely dominate the group's attention and impede the group process. Group treatment can be added if the client moves toward contemplation and preparation stages for changing his sexual health. In the meantime, individual therapy can focus on developing his self-discrepancy and raising his self-awareness about his sexual behavior problems.

Conjoint Treatment

Some men in OCSB group see an individual psychotherapist who is not one of the coleaders to meet the requirement for individual therapy. This concurrent individual and group therapy configuration is *combined* rather than *conjoint* treatment. Although we prefer combined treatment, we have seen positive treatment outcomes with conjoint treatment as well. An important condition for effective conjoint therapy is a respectful professional collaboration between the individual and group therapists (Yalom, 1995). Conjoint treatment also promotes developing a diverse local network of mental health professionals capable of effectively addressing out of control sexual experiences. In this section, we examine several clinical issues that help establish and maintain conjoint treatment.

Clients choose to divide their individual and group psychotherapy between two clinicians for various reasons. They may have a well-established working relationship with another therapist, which is likely the therapist who initially referred them for an OCSB assessment. If these men feel confident that their therapist can complement their OCSB group work, they often choose to continue seeing the referring therapist for individual therapy. Other times, it may be less expensive to see a different clinician for individual therapy. When clients begin the OCSB assessment and they have a separate individual therapist, we strongly recommend that both therapists coordinate the treatment relationship before clients join the group. Will clients continue in individual therapy with their current individual therapist? Or will clients combine their therapy with an OCSB group therapist who conducted the assessment? We encourage clients to choose the arrangement that best supports their sexual health goals.

Within a conjoint OCSB therapy arrangement, it is important to monitor client use of splitting defenses. Conrad was seeing his psychiatrist for both individual therapy and psychiatric management. Michael, who conducted the OCSB assessment, obtained authorization from Conrad to discuss his case with his psychiatrist. Michael and the psychiatrist coordinated Conrad's conjoint treatment through regular phone discussions. The authorization, similar to a combined treatment agreement, did not extend to group therapy. Information exchanged between Michael and the psychiatrist was kept confidential from the group members and they relied on Conrad to bring this content to the group. Coordination discussions emphasized the OCSB group treatment frame and Conrad's sexual health plan (SHP) boundaries. They discussed any SHP boundary crossings and relevant clinical and medication issues. Conrad agreed to discuss his SHP in both individual and group treatment, which provided sexual health conversation practice for relationships beyond the OCSB group.

Early in his OCSB group therapy, Conrad disclosed an SHP boundary crossing, but did not honor his treatment agreement and withheld this information from his individual therapist. He explained to the group, "I feel so embarrassed to go into the details with her, I would rather leave it to group." Conrad disclosed to group that he was attracted to his psychiatrist and said he feared a more detailed sexual health conversation because "she will be disgusted." The group challenged Conrad's compartmentalization as a defense against his fear of being the object of disgust while reinforcing his honesty with the group about his fear of his psychiatrist's antipathy. One group member observed, "If you can't be honest with your psychiatrist, why see her?" Another group member eloquently described his relief after he talked about the sexual images he looked at to reach orgasm while masturbating. "It wasn't until I disclosed the details of the images that I was able to use therapy to understand why these turn-ons excited and repulsed me at the same time. It was after this discussion with my therapist that I eventually came to group and was really honest about the kind of images that turn me on." With further inquiry, Conrad began to see that he was attempting to manage a familiar relationship pattern. He was attempting to manage his psychiatrist's emotions by withholding information he assumed would trigger a negative reaction. The group invited him to look at this pattern and the consequence of not fully engaging his individual therapist with his sexual health problems.

Individual OCSB therapy provides focused diagnostic and treatment planning for each man's unique clinical profiles. OCSB group members often have a diverse range of psychiatric diagnoses, from posttraumatic stress disorder, mood disorders, anxiety disorders, alcohol and substance addiction, to personality disorders. Not every therapist has the adequate training and experience to treat the diagnostic combinations of OCSB clients. Conversely, not every therapist who specializes in individual psychotherapy for a common OCSB co-occurring disorder is up to date in OCSB treatment. When this skill and specialization gap exists between the individual and group therapist, conjoint OCSB individual and group treatment may be the best approach to take to meet the client's needs. The individual and group therapist form an important relationship in the client's life. Resembling an arranged marriage with the client as matchmaker, the therapists must keep in mind that together they are meeting a larger systemic goal of improving their shared client's treatment outcomes. The individual provider targets the co-occurring issue, the group therapist focuses on the client's OCSB, and together they help the client achieve his vision of sexual health while living with a mental health disorder.

Objectives for OCSB Groups

OCSB groups have three primary objectives:

1. To help clients maintain their SHPs
2. To improve client self- and attachment regulation
3. To facilitate a positive sexual/erotic-identity development

Once established, the group objectives are integrated into the group guidelines, for which the leaders are accountable. Just as a clear and specific SHP, combined with treatment goals, is crucial to improving sexual health, well-articulated group objectives are vital to the success and value of OCSB group treatment. When the group leader or coleaders have a clear understanding of the purpose of their group, they possess a map to guide group formation and facilitation. Clear group objectives provide the necessary guidance for determining selection criteria, group size, start and end times, fees, and guidelines. Many structural elements for OCSB group therapy derive from the methodologies that best meet these objectives. The OCSB groups we discuss in this book are long-term, semistructured process groups with no more than eight members. Group membership is separated between heterosexual- and gay/bisexual-identified cisgender (people whose gender identity is congruent with their sex assigned at birth) men over the age of 18. A member's length of group participation is open ended, with a minimum commitment of 6 months. Group meetings are 90 minutes long and new-member admission is staggered. Clients also agree to attend individual psychotherapy at least once per month while they are enrolled in the OCSB group. Fees are within the average to below-average range. Because the program is a combined treatment program, clients commit to both a monthly charge of group therapy and typically twice-monthly individual therapy. Many clients also have to pay for psychiatric appointments and couple therapy, along with a spouse attending his or her own individual therapy. The ability to access affordable group therapy allows men to use a variety of recommended mental health services in conjunction with the group. This is a philosophy that we have never regretted. It allows for clients who are diverse in terms of socioeconomic status, race, ethnicity, age, and marital status, which generates a dynamic group process.

Cotherapy Relationship

We recommend that two leaders facilitate OCSB groups due to the complex and diverse clinical profiles of OCSB treatment-seeking men. There are practical and clinical advantages to coleadership. In practical terms, a group does not lose momentum if one leader is sick, traveling, or otherwise unavailable. Clinically, members have two leaders on whom to place their projections or recreate familiar relationship patterns. Coleader teamwork forms an accountability system that maintains the leadership commitments with the group. Group members experience the security of the leaders' investment in honoring their agreements, especially if leaders are transparent about conferring with each other between group meetings and discussing their strategies for facilitating group. Members in a co-led group gain from complementary approaches to OCSB treatment that a well-paired cotherapy dyad can provide.

The group coleader relationship is an additional clinical component of OCSB groups with important developmental trajectories, tasks, and challenges. To aid therapists who are forming a co-led group, we review the first three stages of Dugo and Beck's (1997) nine-stage model of coleader relationship development. The first stage creates a contract, develops the formal norms of their relationship, and discusses their views on strategies of individual and group change. In the second stage, the leaders develop an identity as a team. This usually involves a degree of conflict, as the leaders identify differences in leadership style, personality, and theoretical orientation. The important tasks in this stage are to identify the issues on which they differ and to develop a working relationship that respects the differences and similarities between the leaders. The third stage is team building, in which the pair learn about and from each other in practice, not just in theory. Coleaders ideally move into the third stage prior to convening a psychotherapy group or receive supervision until they reach that stage if coleading an existing group (Dugo & Beck, 1997; Wheelan, 1997). The underlying assumption is that a group cannot achieve a higher level of development beyond that of its coleaders. When the leaders focus on developing as a team, the co-therapists model and exemplify emotional congruence, high self-esteem, and clear and direct communication within the group process (Roller & Nelson, 1991).

Michael and Doug co-led two different OCSB groups for over 8 years. These groups were a vital forum in which we developed the OCSB Model and Clinical Pathway. The 8 years of coleading groups was a weekly affirmation of the investment we made in our cotherapy relationship. Combined individual and group therapy is complicated, takes focused energy and practice, and benefits from the diverse range of clinical skills that two clinicians can bring. Retrospectively, we have developed a few suggestions we have found helpful in maintaining our cotherapy relationship.

We structured time to connect and check in to discuss the overall group development. We met briefly prior to each group session to shift into our roles as group coleaders. Debriefing after group provided us valuable time to immediately process each group session and plan strategies for subsequent group and individual sessions. During our pre- and postgroup meetings, it was important to prioritize member frame crossings that may be brought to the group's attention (e.g., attendance, keeping group agreements, payment). We often used these meetings to prepare clear explanations for the group and to discuss our process as coleaders by exploring the dynamics and meaning, for instance, of a member's repeated lateness. Especially when considering the safety needs of a new group, "a united front, clarity of purpose, a consistent, and a shared plan of action on part of the co-therapists are essential" (Wheelan, 1997, p. 308).

The boundaries of outpatient private practice therapy influence the cotherapy relationship in a different way than community agency or inpatient group therapy settings. In a private practice situation, each cotherapist is leading a group with clients from both of the leaders' practices, as well as group members who see other individual therapists. The coleaders must have written authorization from every group member in order to discuss his individual therapy with the group coleader. How each cotherapist manages the mutual client relationships and separate individual therapy relationship boundaries is essential to group safety. Many times, after a group session, one leader may review with the other how "I had to not say anything about Willard's recent herpes eruption because he just talked about this in individual therapy and was ambivalent about whether he would share it with group. I had to wait for him to bring it to group." In this way, the coleaders respect the client's readiness to reveal vulnerable content from individual therapy to group but remain united in the information they share.

Disagreements between coleaders are likely to emerge. Open dialogue about a disagreement between leaders can be helpful for long-term group, but may be unhelpful in the early weeks of group formation (Yalom, 1995). For example, open dialogue about disagreements may sound like: "I remember this differently. I do not think Maxwell reported on his boundaries last week." "Doug, before we move on, I would like to first hear from the group about their response to Maxwell's word *whatever*." Or "Michael, let me interrupt you. Victor, how are you feeling about Michael's questions regarding your decisions this week?" Groups that witness leader mistakes, leadership differences and imperfections, and the leaders' own discomfort can humanize the therapists beyond their facilitation role and coleader function.

Last, group therapy is full of surprises. No matter how long a group leader has been facilitating groups or how much clinical training or expertise he or she has in OCSB clinical treatment, groups present new situations that require private deliberation or open discussion in front of the group. "This is a new situation for us. We need to confer after group and we will revisit this topic at next week's group." "I noticed there is no call or voicemail from Gary, will you check your voicemail as well in case he may have called you?" "Can you remember a situation like this coming up before? I don't remember." We often looked across the group treatment room when we recognized that the group was in new territory while also observing that there was no need to have an immediate response. Much like we tell our clients "there is no such thing as a sex emergency," it is equally important for coleaders to know that few group circumstances require an immediate response, even when group members demand clarity about a specific group guideline or process.

OCSB GROUP TREATMENT FRAME

The group treatment frame consists of the boundaries and commitments that members agree to honor and process while they attend group, and serves as the essential relationship covenant within the OCSB group. Establishing and maintaining the group treatment frame develops group safety and trust within a wide range of theoretical orientations or group types (Beck, 2008). These agreements are fluid expectations of group relationships and are open for discussion, revision, clarification, and individual processing. They are often a source of group contention, heightened emotions, and the genesis of new relationship patterns. Exploring and deepening men's commitment to group relational agreements is the currency for improving their individual relational capacity. Every phase of group development involves establishing and maintaining agreements among the therapist(s), the members, and the whole group. Without group agreements, psychotherapy cannot happen.

Modus operandi in all groups: frame challenges and boundary maintenance. Making clinical use of and successfully resolving frame violations is the therapeutic work of both the leader and the group. Violations likely have multiple meanings, are often repeated, and require delicate negotiations (Pearlman & Courtois, 2005). They provide important here/now allegorical narratives to provide sources of insight into the OCSB clinical areas of self-regulation, attachment patterns, and sexual/ erotic-identity development obstacles. The treatment frame discussions bring to light a client's attempt to resolve competing motivations, which often generate therapeutic possibilities for psychological and interpersonal maturation. Failing to adequately negotiate and maintain emerging group treatment frame issues will likely contribute to poor treatment outcomes and client dissatisfaction.

Consistently honoring agreements is at the heart of sustaining sexual health. Group treatment is a weekly opportunity for men to practice core skills of honoring agreements and maintaining their SHPs. Clients who enter OCSB groups have historically failed to honor a wide range of intra- and interpersonal agreements. It follows that OCSB group members will likely respond to these explicit treatment agreements in a similar fashion at some point. Leaders monitor group relationship agreements, encourage group members to hold each other accountable for their group agreements, and discuss their successes and challenges in maintaining these agreements. Processing frame crossings present clinical opportunities to develop new strategies to maintain relationship agreements and one's sexual health. The leaders can explore comparisons with their sexual behavior and increase members' self-awareness, confidence, and ability to discuss maintaining the sexual agreements with each group treatment frame discussion.

Written Group Agreements

All groups need written, straightforward agreements to establish stability and safety. Clear agreements support the layered relationship dimensions that exist among members, coleaders, and the group-as-a-whole. The group guidelines list expectations for each group member and are developed by the group leaders. It is not a document that is cocreated with group members, although it can be modified over time based on group events or suggestions for improving the clarity and usefulness of the document. "Appropriate boundaries are a means of meeting the client's need for safety, not simply in order to be able to explore painful aspects of their lives, but also to ensure ethical practice that protects the client from abuse by the therapist" (Symons & Wheeler, 2005, p. 19). Protecting the client from injuries by the therapist is a strong theme that runs throughout this book. Just as we spend a considerable amount of time during the assessment preparing clients for OCSB treatment, we prepare therapists to establish an ethical foundation for safe and effective sexual health-based treatment.

OCSB group guidelines provide the leader and members with an essential relationship dimension for the group to explore and learn about themselves (Black, 2008). Commonly, OCSB treatment-seeking men have violated central commitments in their romantic relationships as well as with themselves, and may have denied their commitment violations through a myriad of defenses. OCSB groups incrementally rebuild men's confidence and ability to maintain agreements, which starts with their accountability to attend all group sessions, to participate, and to honor confidentiality agreements. Practice maintaining these commitments increases the clients' likelihood of maintaining SHP boundaries and moving toward their personal vision for sexual health. Thus, the group commitments are the mechanism for OCSB behavior change. In this section, we highlight several agreements vital to managing OCSB group therapy.

First, it is important to understand that a frame lapse is not an emergency unless the safety of a client or the group is a factor. Second, the group treatment frame is best seen as what Lucas (2004) calls a "gentle envelope" (p. 3) or a flexible container. Group leaders strive to maintain a balance between upholding adherence to the frame and curiosity when the group structure is tested. When the leader or members are overly rigid about the rules or guidelines, a compliance fixation may develop among the members that collapses the space for group exploration about client motives for crossing the treatment frame. Third, hold the perspective that a frame crossing is an opportunity to advance the purpose of the OCSB group. Keep in mind, a frame crossing in an OCSB group is an expected symptom rather than an exception; it is rarely a reason to terminate someone's group membership. The OCSB group leader values the group contract as an ethical group practice and as a central source for clinical understanding and relational insight for the entire group. (The complete listing of the group guidelines is available in the Appendix.)

The SHP Commitments

The primary driver of group process involves the client's SHP. In the written group guidelines, OCSB group members agree to follow their SHP boundaries *and* to disclose any boundary crossings at the next group and individual session. We anticipate group members will either momentarily cross an SHP boundary or return to old patterns at some point while enrolled in an OCSB group. It is unlikely that clients will immediately and consistently accomplish lasting change without returning to familiar coping defenses as part of establishing their new sexual health behavior. When clients meet the group agreement by reporting SHP boundary crossings to the group, the leader's interventions are guided by the group's primary objectives. The first objective is to help clients maintain their SHPs; therapists can facilitate a discussion that deconstructs the event. That discussion usually provides information regarding the unsuccessful strategies the client used to manage the competing motivations he experienced prior to crossing his boundaries, followed by recommendations for improvement. The second objective is to use group process to improve the factors identified in the client's Unique Clinical Picture that contribute to his OCSB. In the discussion that examines the precipitating experience, therapists can listen for themes that reveal what clinical issue needs attention (e.g., sexual health principles, vulnerability factors, client self- and attachment regulation, or sexual/erotic-identity development).

For instance, a client discloses that he underestimated his ability to maintain his boundaries when he was near a familiar sex venue. The therapist observes that the client is discussing his difficulties with self-regulating his activation when in close proximity to a sexual stimulus and invites the group to focus on that aspect of the client's disclosure.

The group empathizes with the reluctant acceptance of his need for additional external regulation (e.g., taking an alternative route) and challenges his self-judgment regarding his lack of willpower in moments of high activation (e.g., I'm weak). Group members offer some pragmatic solutions such as amending his SHP to include "driving past exit ramp" in the Ambivalence column and adding "monitoring negative judgmental thoughts when taking the alternative route" in the Health column. Honest group conversations about SHP boundary crossings provide the entire group an opportunity to uncover more details about group members' conflicted motivations, which frequently lead to improvements in sustaining treatment goals and SHP commitments. Further, welcoming and encouraging the SHP boundary-crossing conversation may reduce client isolation and increase the recognition that other people also struggle to change their sexual behaviors. Members inspire one another through their progress and increase their confidence by sharing concerns and support. This is a benefit that group therapy provides more directly than individual services can (Wagner & Ingersoll, 2013).

A sexual health focus provides the group with ample opportunities to explore the inherent and inevitable tensions created between newly formed health behaviors and well-rehearsed historical sexual patterns. The self-discrepancy focus is a subtle difference from a clinical disorder treatment model. Other treatment models may facilitate a group process that labels this self-regulation failure a symptom of a pathological process and whose interventions serve to ameliorate a diseased state. OCSB group interventions are grounded in the client's motivation for change as the impetus for the discussion. It was his choice to seek treatment because he felt sexually out of control. We are helping him change his sexual behavior because he was motivated to improve his sexual health. This means we can frame his choice to discuss his boundary crossing as the outcome of his decision to take responsibility for his sexual health rather than evidence of a diseased state that requires therapeutic intervention. By not relying on a disease model, we avoid inadvertently colluding with the commonly held shame-based narratives that exist around deviant sexuality and offer an esteem-building framework for sexual health responsibility.

Accountability

The second part of this agreement is to report any sexual boundary crossings that have occurred between sessions. The minimum expectation for honoring this group agreement is to verbally self-report crossing an SHP boundary. Any discussion beyond the initial disclosure is optional. Some treatment groups use sign-in systems (I kept/did not keep my boundaries this week), others have a structured "check-in" at the opening of group. The OCSB group structure does not include any of these reporting systems intended to ensure SHP compliance. Each group member is responsible for initiating this discussion, which means that every weekly meeting contains the possibility of a member reporting or hiding an SHP boundary crossing. OCSB groups are intentionally structured to provide a weekly experiment in self-regulation (e.g., managing boundaries between sessions) and attachment regulation (e.g., opportunities to regulate emotional proximity). This continuous choice is intended to incrementally build men's ability to take responsibility for their personal vision of sexual health.

As we mentioned earlier, only the clients who are committed to changing their sexual behavior are enrolled into OCSB group treatment. To participate in this group, they all made the decision to follow the agreements outlined in the guidelines. As a result, the decision to not follow their disclosure agreement is framed as a contradiction between their commitment to change and their decision to cross this group agreement. Their self-discrepancy serves as the entrance point to evaluate their choices and manage their defenses. Clients who report that they did not hold to this agreement in a previous session often respond as if they are in trouble, fear they will be exited from the group, or deflect their responsibility for upholding the agreement. Before processing the underlying meaning of their defense, we reassure them that we do not terminate group participation for not honoring the agreement. Instead, we invite him to be curious about what happened and to approach disclosure agreement avoidance as an opportunity for him to use the entire group to discuss and better understand his choices.

When a group member withholds his sexual behavior, the leader focuses the group on how the member resolved his competing motivations. We know one of his motivations was his desire to attend group to improve his sexual health. Deconstructing his choice to withhold information from the group will likely reveal the motivations that competed with honoring his agreements. What consequences was he trying to avoid? Did he withhold information to regulate his uncomfortable feelings (e.g., shame, guilt, fear) or to manage the reactions of others (e.g., disappointment, rejection, anger)? Did withholding information serve a similar function to his pattern of not honoring commitments in other relationships? By exploring the client's contradictory behavior, the leaders have an opportunity to develop the client's self-discrepancy about his choices. The process can raise his awareness of his strategies to resolve his binds and develop into new and direct solutions to his competing motivations.

Group Time

Reduced to its primary structures, a group meeting is a regular time in which people agree to meet. The group starts and ends at the same time each week and lasts for a limited duration. The time commitments within OCSB treatment groups provide opportunities for relational and clinical insight regarding how the members honor their timeliness commitments and how they manage the finite amount of time in which to talk. As we like to say to members during the group preparation meeting, "If the group is boring we don't end early and we don't stay longer if the group is particularly interesting."

A pattern of tardiness presents a contradiction that warrants group investigation. Each member has agreed to arrive on time to group, not following through with this commitment is another opportunity to explore how the client resolves competing motivations. Clients likely have other uses for their time or have made other commitments that complicate their ability to attend group. Occasional tardiness may not provide fruitful insight other than underestimating traffic. But patterned tardiness may indicate larger themes connected to their OCSB, even if the reason is traffic. What is preventing them from adapting to the actual amount of time it takes to arrive at the office? How are they asserting their boundaries in order to arrive on time? What are the consequences they are trying to avoid by not asserting their boundaries? Here/now group interactions can clarify the nature of the competing motivations, which could stem from ineffective self-regulation or avoiding relational consequences.

Each week, the finite amount of group time creates a controlled tension between group members requesting time to talk about their needs and sharing the group time with others. How they respond to this act of intimacy likely reflects their attachment styles. Did they withdraw and allow the time in the session to expire? Did they feel disappointed by missing the opportunity to speak? Did they explicitly blame the group leaders for not structuring the group so every member has the same amount of time to speak? Any one of these reactions provides clinicians with valuable insights into the group member's internal experience with emotional proximity.

Another common treatment frame issue is a member requesting to leave before the group session ends. The OCSB group guidelines do not establish a time at which it is too late to attend the group session. However, members are expected to remain in the group for the full 90 minutes. Meaning, we ask that members not leave group early if they are upset, bored, or ashamed. Viewed another way, members do not leave the group as a solution to regulate uncomfortable emotions. By leaving early, they avoid the moments to learn self- and coregulation skills. Whatever emotions, thoughts, urges, or perceptions are experienced in the group, members experience them together in the therapy session. To be clear, group members have the legal right to leave group at any time. But we ask members to make every effort to remain for the entire session as a regulation tool. Clients learn to rely on the leader(s), members, as well as the group-as-a-whole for guidance when experiencing uncomfortable affect states that arise in session. Over time, group members continue to process strong feelings; they learn how maintaining contact with others can be a source of empathy and improves self-efficacy in building more secure attachments.

Occasionally, group members request to leave a future group in advance. "I have a grandchild's 5th-grade promotion." "I need to leave early to get to a concert." "I have my parents coming into town, and I need to pick them up at the airport." Here, members are requesting to attend part of the group and then leave. Despite the clear guideline, members still ask. Often the member presents the request as if leaving early is a benign event, not really that significant. "I'll just leave 20 minutes early." However, leaving group early is not inconsequential. It inserts a tension into the group as we wait for the member's time to leave. The group takes responsibility for managing the disruption of the member's departure by monitoring time and avoiding intense conversation that might be interrupted. But, just like other challenges to the treatment frame, this request offers an opportunity to get curious about group member strategies for resolving competing motivations.

For instance, a planned early exit may reflect the member's dismissive attachment style. The request contains significant defenses. He is both minimizing the consequences of his departure and demonstrating entitlement by changing his agreement with the group. The client may think the open negotiation with the group represents clinical progress to be rewarded with permission to leave group early. However, the request represents a solution to a problem that has not been fully revealed to the group. This can be an opportunity for understanding interpersonal patterns when coping with competing needs: The member wants to be in the group and he wants to attend another event. The client's solution is an attempt to do both and avoid the feelings associated with loss. By leaving early, he attempts to reduce his negative affect (e.g., disappointment from missing the other event) while remaining unaware of the relational consequences he is expecting the group to absorb. After all, the other members remain in the room after he leaves. By failing to endure the feelings connected with loss, the member reveals a common empathy gap. What might seem like a trivial request offers an excellent opportunity to raise awareness about the relationship consequences of his defenses against uncomfortable affects.

Screening Criteria

The screening criteria, first reviewed during the consultation, are monitored throughout group membership. The criteria remain significant clinical distinctions and factors for organizing treatment and determining levels of care. For instance, clients occasionally enter an OCSB assessment with a problematic relationship with alcohol. A portion of the assessment is dedicated to investigating the symptom acuity and the connection between their drinking and out of control sexual experiences. Increasing self-awareness about their drinking patterns may lead clients to limit their use or discontinue alcohol consumption as a strategy for improving sexual health. Clients with a problematic relationship with alcohol may enter the OCSB group with a predetermined agreement to be evaluated by a substance abuse treatment professional if unable to adequately maintain their alcohol use/abstinence boundary. The client, leaders, and group members observe the maintenance of his SHP alcohol boundaries over the course of treatment. Some men have discontinued OCSB group and entered into a residential substance abuse program when their relationship with alcohol became increasingly problematic.

Of course, symptoms that were either missed or not present during the assessment process may emerge in the group. A client might report a physical altercation with his intimate partner for the first time. He may be diagnosed with a medical condition unrelated to his OCSB. Anecdotally, one of the most common problems we see is clients who engage in sexual behavior that risks HIV infection. They may have engaged in condomless sex with an anonymous partner or had sex with a sex worker. After these encounters, their relationship with HIV moved from negative to unknown and getting tested became a priority. Confidently knowing one's current relationship with HIV is a sexual health priority for men in OCSB treatment. The group therapist has the responsibility to draw attention to this change if the client is not considering the sexually transmitted infection (STI) consequences of his sexual behaviors.

GROUPS WITH SPECIFIC DEMOGRAPHICS

Gender

Men are the predominate consumers of problematic and OCSB treatment despite their lower rate of mental health treatment compared to women (Addis & Mahalik, 2003). Integrating gender awareness and the male socialization process are important preparatory steps for OCSB treatment. Traditional male socialization values toughness and independence; failure to meet these gender norms risks ridicule, ostracization, or violence (Good & Robertson, 2010). Masculine socialization often discourages men from self-disclosure and emotional expression, which contributes to social isolation, restricted interpersonal skills, and decreased self-awareness. Although the past 30 years provide limited research on male psychology, studies emphasize the need for applying knowledge of male psychology to better engage men in treatment and to adapt specific clinical practices when treating distinct male subgroups (Robertson & Williams, 2010; Wade & Good, 2010).

Larger societal and systemic forces affect the social construction of masculinities, and the maturing male, in psychologically significant ways (Kingerlee, 2012). This concept suggests that some men exhibit a male-specific personality profile that is identifiable across clinical disorders. This is not to suggest that *all* men exhibit these personality traits, but rather that men are subjected to "neurological, developmental and cultural factors that impact their functioning in characteristic ways, notable under distress" (p. 88). In the following summary, we review the four traits that form the male-specific profile: status-seeking, empathic potential, emotional potential, and shame-avoiding.

There is evidence to suggest that men tend to be more concerned with *seeking status* and rank when compared to women (Baron-Cohen, 2003; Sax, 2007). In a stable situation, this pattern is largely unproblematic. During a crisis, however, men may be vulnerable to serious psychological difficulties, such as suicide (Kolves, Ides, & DeLeo, 2010) or perpetrating violence (Gresswell & Hollin, 1994), when this status is perceived as threatened.

Some evidence suggests that men are less empathic, scoring lower than women on empathy measures (Baron-Cohen & Wheelwright, 2004). Men's *empathic potential*, or undeveloped empathic skills, may be seen across clinical disorders in two ways. Men traditionally believe they will be deprived of care from others. As a result, they are initially more reluctant to seek help and if they access support, they remain reluctant to discuss their problems (S. V. Cochran & Rabinowitz, 1996). Second, despite experiencing high distress, men tend to deprive themselves of empathy. Men who are status aware or socialized to value personal strength and toughness may perceive social and public failure as unacceptable. This makes men intolerant to their own emotional and psychological vulnerabilities. Their vulnerability, intolerance, and common lack of self-soothing capacities (Gilbert, 2007) can lead men to push themselves harder, rather than to treat themselves empathically by seeking care (Kingerlee, 2012).

Men tend to have underdeveloped emotional skills or, said in a positive way, they have the *emotional potential* to develop their emotional skills. Compared with women, men tend to be more emotionally controlled or inhibited. Research suggests that women are freer with expressing emotions through words, body language, and facial expression than men (Goleman, 1996; Gottman, Katz, & Hooven, 1996). Evidence also supports the notion that men are less skilled at identifying and reflecting their emotions than women (Levant, Hall, Williams, & Hasan, 2009). Men's tendency for emotional inhibition may be disadvantageous if they are less emotionally skilled to cope when serious problems arise.

The last characteristic in the male-specific profile is a link between psychological distress and *shame aversion*. It has been observed in clinical practice that men struggle to discuss their symptoms or negative feelings without experiencing a strong sense of shame (S. V. Cochran & Rabinowitz, 1996; Pollack, 2005). Shame aversion may be associated with avoiding perceptions of failure, which may be related to their tendency to avoid help seeking (Addis & Mahalik, 2003).

The male-specific profile and the factors that shape characteristic male behavior provide a context to understand the competing motivations and sexual symptoms that surface in an OCSB men's group. Men garner social status and rank through normative sexual expression and acquiring sexual prowess. Social rewards may incentivize high-frequency sexual behavior for those whose self-esteem and masculine self-concept are sensitive to status and rank. Men who are motivated to enhance their sexual knowledge and skills but are without sexual partners may watch explicit sexual material as vicarious learning and a substitute for partnered sexual experiences. Men's sexual urges and desires may not be as restricted during the male socialization process as other emotions, thereby becoming one of the few emotional states men feel more free to express. But for men who judge their emotional distress as a weakness and deprive themselves of emotional caring or empathy, negative feelings and self-judgment may be combated with sexual behaviors they deem more masculine and therefore worthy of esteem.

David Wexler (2009) promotes psychotherapy for men that increases empathy through raising men's awareness of cultural influences on their gender-role expectations. In his book, *Men in Therapy: New Approaches for Effective Treatment*, Wexler organizes four common male gender-role conflicts with these mentalization sentences:

1. I have difficulty expressing my tender feelings.
2. Affection with other men makes me tense.

3. I worry about failing and how it affects my doing well as a man.
4. My work or school often disrupts other parts of my life such as home, health, or leisure.

Wexler's gender conflicts are commonly found among the competing motivations men bring with them to an OCSB group. Although gender expectations may have different consequences between clients, the imprimatur of gender seeps into the lives of every OCSB treatment-seeking man. OCSB group therapy is one of the few informed, respectful, and safe spaces for men to explore their sexual health values, aspirations, and disappointments. At times, the themes discussed and dynamics observed in OCSB groups seem indistinguishable from those of a general men's process group. The group process can be a powerful vehicle for men to expand their emotional and empathic potential beyond the restrictions of masculine socialization. It is a social laboratory used to address their difficulties experiencing tender feelings and affection with other men. As leaders, we regularly help clients re-evaluate beliefs that equate emotional vulnerability with weakness or empathy seeking as shameful. OCSB group leaders who develop a gender-aware approach may notice their groups move beyond the uniting theme of sexual behavior problems to foster a deeper intimacy that has been absent in men throughout their lives.

Gender Aware Therapy offers several clinical guidelines for psychotherapy (Brooks & Good, 2005; Good, Gilbert, & Scher, 1990):

1. View gender as an essential aspect of psychotherapy.
2. Examine presenting problems in the larger societal and systems contexts.
3. Address negative consequences of gender bias.
4. Develop a collaborative, rather than directive, therapeutic relationship.
5. Encourage clients to develop their own understandings of their histories, behaviors, and emotions.

Sexual Identity

Doug began his outpatient group for gay men in 1993. To our knowledge, this is the longest continually running outpatient psychotherapy process group for gay men with OCSB in the country. The sociocultural, legal, political, health care, and dating landscapes have evolved in directions unimaginable when Doug first met with eight gay men on a Thursday night in October 1993. We continue to promote a separate sexual-identity OCSB group treatment despite the progress on all these fronts. For those clinicians interested in starting an OCSB men's group, we invite you to consider the following sociocultural and clinical factors when forming your selection criteria.

Establishing a long-term outpatient process group with men of all sexual identities may be relevant in some regions of the country. It is essential to gauge the clinical needs of the community in which clients are seeking treatment for OCSB. Equally important are the therapist's skills with navigating the complexities of OCSB treatment in conjunction with the fear, shame, stigma, and misinformation that surrounds homosexuality. Group leader's blind spots to contemporary sociocultural influences of gender and sexual identity may unwittingly recreate the same heteronormativity *and* reinforce gender norms that restrict emotional intimacy among men of all sexual identities. These influences run counter to the primary intentions for group psychotherapy. Although sociocultural stigmas have softened over the two decades since Doug started his gay/bisexual men's OCSB group, we caution against naïve optimism that a group therapist is capable of managing these forces without good training and ongoing supervision.

The negative health consequences associated with OCSB and men who have sex with men are well documented (see Panchankis et al., 2014 for current references). There are disproportional rates of gay-identified men seeking OCSB treatment. Stigma, social prejudice, rates of drug and alcohol abuse, the link between OCSB and HIV, and a history of sexual abuse and exploitation are frequently identified as significant factors related to sexual behavior problems and dysregulation (Parsons, Grov, & Golub, 2012). Gay and bisexual male research participants articulated internal sources and external circumstances when describing the origins of their sexual behavior problems (Parsons et al., 2008). The subjects in this study emphasized associations with mental illness, emotional dysregulation, attachment insecurity, and feeling inadequate or undesirable. External factors emphasized dynamics in current relationships, being single, family-of-origin rejection, emotional distance from family, managing easy availability for sex in large urban centers, and a history of sexual assault as children and adolescences. A study of gay male couples found high scores on sexual compulsivity or hypersexual disorder measures correlated with couples reporting interpersonal functional impairment as well as lower rates of condom use during anal sex with casual partners

(Starks, Grov, & Parsons, 2013; Yeagley, Hickok, & Bauemeister, 2014). To improve cultural competency for working with gay and bisexual clients, we briefly discuss in this section:

1. Influence of minority stress
2. Nonmonogamy as a sociocultural difference between gay/bisexual male couples and heterosexual couples

Minority Stress

Minority stress is a useful lens through which to understand the dispro-porte rates of gay and bisexual men seeking treatment for sexual behavior problems and OCSB. The term "minority stress" is used "to distinguish the excess stress to which individuals from stigmatized social categories are exposed as a result of their social, often a minority, position" (Meyer, 2013, p. 4). Meyer (2013) discussed three processes of minority stress relevant to the lesbian, gay, and bisexual (LGB) community:

1. Chronic or acute, stressful events or conditions
2. Expectations of such events and the subsequent vigilance this expectation requires
3. Internalized negative societal attitudes

Concealing one's sexual orientation has also been identified as a significant stress process (Cole, Kemeny, Taylor, & Visscher, 1996; DiPlacido, 1998).

Minority stress is correlated with behavioral health problems, including depressive symptoms, substance abuse, and suicidal ideation (S. D. Cochran & Mays, 1994; D'Augelli & Hershberger, 1993; Diaz, Ayala, Bein, Jenn, & Marin, 2001; Meyer, 1995; Rosario, Rotheram-Borus, & Reid, 1996; Waldo, 1999). Studies have found similar correlations between internalized homophobia and mental health issues, such as depression, anxiety, substance abuse, and suicidal ideation (DiPlacido, 1998; Meyer & Dean, 1998; Williamson, 2000). Various forms of self-harm (Williamson, 2000), HIV sexual risk taking (Meyer & Dean, 1998), and intimate relationship and sexual functioning difficulties (Dupras, 1994; Meyer & Dean, 1998; Rosser, Metz, Bockting, & Buroker, 1997) have been disproportionately found among lesbian/gay/bisexual (LGB) research subjects. Meyer (2013) urges caution in drawing conclusions about a higher prevalence of clinical disorders with LGB groups: "studies are few, methodologies and measurements are inconsistent, and trends in the findings are not always easy to interpret" (p. 13). However, Meyer (2013) acknowledges that whenever significant differences of mental disorder prevalence emerge, LGB groups consistently have higher rates of clinical disorders than heterosexual groups.

We do not discount that mixed sexual-orientation identity OCSB groups may offer ancillary benefits for men. For instance, the acceptance that nonheterosexual men receive from heterosexual men may aid in healing previous rejection wounds and minority stress previously experienced. Heterosexual men who are exposed to the sexual-minority experience may increase their empathy capacity and evaluate their heterosexual privilege. As important as these processes may be, the group composition must function in the service of treating OCSB and fostering sexual health. Group solidarity and cohesiveness is a mental health protective factor for gay and bisexual men coping with the strain of persistent interpersonal prejudice and discrimination (Meyer, 2013; Peterson, Folkman, & Bakeman, 1996). Gay men may be more responsive to sexual health change if they are not burdened by the prejudice and discrimination present in a mixed-identity group.

Nonmonogamy and Male Couples

Male couples report more open sexual agreements and less monogamous arrangements when compared with heterosexual and female couples (Hoff & Beougher, 2010; Parsons, Starks, DuBois, Grov, & Golub, 2013). *Monogamy* is an agreement in which both partners in a pair-bonded relationship have sexual contact only with each other. *Nonmonogamous* or *open relationships* are defined by one or both partners having sex with other people with or without the primary partner. The relationships with nonprimary sex partners range from anonymous or casual partners to regular partners that transform the original dyad into a triadic relationship. Furthermore, a large number of couple's sexual agreements do not fall into these simple monogamous/open categories. Sex advice columnist, Savage (2010) coined "monogamish" to describe couples who have made agreements that allow for some sexual contact with casual partners (either together or outside of the relationship) but are mostly monogamous.

Of course, not all gay male couples' relationships are open and not all heterosexual couples are monogamous. Sexual nonexclusivity, however, is generally more accepted among male couples than in heterosexual society in general (Shernoff, 2006). Rather than questioning whether sexual nonexclusivity is right or wrong, male couples commonly examine nonmonogamy in "morally neutral" terms. That is, will a version of nonmonogamy help or hurt the relationship (Bettinger, 2005)? Too often sex-negative judgments link nonmonogamy in male couples with the inability to maintain stable and enduring relationships. This generalization conflicts with studies that report male couples' relationship quality to be as high as that of heterosexual couples (Gottman et al., 2003; Kurdek, 2005). Research also does not support the perception that nonmonogamy is inherently destructive for couples. Although with some mixed conclusions, the most consistent findings about relationship and sexual satisfaction among male couples with differing monogamy agreements revealed no significant difference between monogamous and open arrangements (Bricker & Horne, 2007; LaSala, 2004a, 2004b; Parsons, Starks, Garamel, & Grov, 2012). Parsons, Starks, et al. (2012) defined "monogamish" as an agreement to have a third casual sexual partner join the couple for a sexual encounter. In this study, couples who engaged in this monogamy variation reported lower levels of depression and higher rates of life satisfaction compared with single gay men and more conventionally defined monogamous male couples.

GROUP LEADER PREPARATION

Ethics

It is incumbent upon OCSB group leaders to give considerable attention to the intent and context of their actions because the attempts of leaders to influence human behavior in general, and sexual behavior in particular, through group work always has ethical implications (Thomas & Pender, 2008). Several professional organizations that educate, research, and promote group psychotherapy practice have established group therapy ethical standards. As members of the American Group Psychotherapy Association (AGPA), we follow the ethical guidelines set for group clinicians (see AGPA website: www.agpa.org/home/practice-resources/ethics-in-group-therapy). The Association for Specialists in Group Work, a division of the American Counseling Association, distinguishes best practices in group therapy planning, practice, and process (see ASGW guidelines: www.asgw.org/pdf/Best_Practices.pdf).

As we discussed in Chapter 2, we chose to apply the sexual health principles to meet our ethical obligations to protect our client's sexual rights through providing the most effective but least restrictive care. OCSB groups are based on the explicit agreement between therapist and group members that the primary treatment outcome is aligning sexual behavior with the sexual health principles. The sexual health framework guides treatment planning and offers a foundation for evaluating individual and group treatment progress. When applied to group work, the principles frame interventions within public health standards of sexual health care and protect the clients from sociocultural sex negativity. When client sexual behavior is aligned with those principles, we only assert influence based on the client's motivation to change his sexual behavior.

OCSB group leaders have an ethical responsibility to respect diverse sexual expression among group members. Commonly, without leader guidance, group norms restrict specific sexual activity that is unconventional, problematic, or uncomfortable for one or more members. Group facilitation based on a principle-centered approach necessitates that leaders block the formation of restrictive sexual group norms that are based on act-centered values. OCSB groups frequently have members with diverse aspirations for sexual health behavior change. One man's vision of sexual health may include sexual behaviors that are considered unconventional or disgusting to other men in the group. The group leader is responsible for preventing group norms that restrict sexual expression simply because it differs from the majority of the group's sexual boundaries or interests. For one member, masturbation to sexual imagery is not a concern. At the same time, another group member may have viewing sexual images as an SHP boundary. OCSB group leaders are responsible for protecting client sexual rights and guiding group process with disparate sexual health visions among group members.

Group Leader Training

Facilitating long-term, outpatient psychotherapy process groups necessitates therapists investing in advanced study and practice beyond their group therapy graduate-course studies. Group leader training is intimately linked with group quality and effectiveness. Experience and specialization in OCSB individual therapy provides insufficient clinical training for facilitating OCSB psychotherapy groups. Group therapy training provides knowledge and experience for ethically and effectively employing group process to influence sexual health behavior change. The continued dispute among OCSB treatment models has perhaps limited the development of group leader training methods that differentiate themselves from individual psychotherapy methods linked with a specific treatment model for dysregulated sexual behavior. Group leader training specific for sexual addiction, impulsive–compulsive sexual behavior (ICSB), or hypersexual disorder is sparse. Therapists trained under Eli Coleman at his University of Minnesota ICSB program receive group facilitation training. Unfortunately, no manual or clinical publications describe these approaches. Being skilled in individual OCSB therapy does not translate into clinical proficiency as a group psychotherapist.

Fortunately, there is a well-established body of knowledge that can be used for developing group leadership competence. Trotzer (2013) organized group training into four specific areas:

1. Knowledge of group treatment as a professionally distinct modality with concentrated experience in group membership
2. Observation and leadership
3. Supervised practice throughout training and practice
4. A commitment to ongoing continuing education for group psychotherapy

Training specific to group work with OCSB, sexual addiction, ICSB, or hypersexual disorder is primarily obtained through on-the-job training in settings where therapists find themselves leading groups because of their content expertise, not their modality competence. Placing therapists who have extensive group therapy skills in sexual health psychotherapy groups, or pairing them with an experienced group therapist so they can learn clinical skills is rarely the practice.

The minimum requirement for the training of OCSB group leaders is graduate-training coursework in group therapy and a postgraduate internship/practicum leading or coleading groups under the supervision of a knowledgeable group therapy supervisor. Therapists greatly enhance their understanding of group psychotherapy when they concurrently participate in a group as a client or join an ongoing training group for a minimum of 1 year. Wagner and Ingersoll (2013) recommend an "apprenticeship model, in which practitioners build group skills over time with a more experienced colleague as a coleader" (p. 110). Participating in a professionally led group combines group experience with an explicit goal for explicating the multiple skills and tasks necessary for group leadership. There is no substitute for the empathy and insight experienced as a member of a professionally led therapy or supervision group. Too often this aspect of training is overlooked among OCSB group leaders.

Group therapy training plays an invaluable role in professionals developing an identity as a group psychotherapist. The lack of advanced group psychotherapy training for sexual dysregulation treatment is significant considering the central role group therapy plays in treatment of sexual behavior problems among all the leading treatment approaches. Given the development of basic skills, knowledge, and expertise in providing group therapy over the past few decades, current treatment programs risk becoming a clinical specialty with insufficiently trained group leaders. The foundations for group training are not specific to an OCSB clinical population. But it is much easier to bring group therapy principles into OCSB groups than it is to expect group psychotherapists to be informed about OCSB treatment. Knowledge about group work is widely available across various publications and professional organizations. Web sites for the American Counseling Association Specialist in Group Work, Division 49 of the American Psychological Association, and the American Group Psychotherapy Association describe processes for starting and maintaining ongoing group therapy.

REFERENCES

Addis, M. E., & Mahalik, J. R. (2003). Men, masculinity, and the contexts of help seeking. *American Psychologist, 58*(1), 5–14.

Baron-Cohen, S. (2003). *The essential difference: Men, women, and the extreme male brain.* Harmondsworth, UK: Penguin.

Baron-Cohen, S., & Wheelwright, S. (2004). The empathy quotient: An investigation of adults with Asperger syndrome or high functioning autism, and normal sex differences. *Journal of Autism and Developmental Disorders, 34*(2), 163–175.

Beck, R. (2008). When boundaries breathe. In S. Fehr (Ed.), *101 interventions in group therapy* (pp. 123–126). New York, NY: Haworth Press.

Bettinger, M. (2005). A family systems approach to working with sexually open gay male couples. *Journal of Couple & Relationship Therapy, 4*(2/3), 149–160.

Black, M. (2008). Creative use of the group contract in long-term psychotherapy groups. In S. Fehr (Ed.), *101 interventions in group therapy* (pp. 353–357). New York, NY: Haworth Press.

Bricker, M. E., & Horne, S. E. (2007). The impact of monogamy and non-monogamy on relational health. *Journal of Couple & Relationship Therapy, 6*, 27–47.

Brooks, G. R., & Good, G. E. (2005). A final word. In G. E. Good & G. R. Brooks (Eds.), *The new handbook of psychotherapy and counseling with men: A comprehensive guide to settings, problems, and treatment approaches.* San Francisco, CA: Jossey-Bass.

Cadwell, S. (2009). Shame, gender, and sexuality in gay men's group therapy. *Group, 33*(3),197–212.

Cochran, S. D., & Mays, V. M. (1994). Depressive distress among homosexually active African American men and women. *American Journal of Psychiatry, 151*, 524–529.

Cochran, S. V., & Rabinowitz, F. E. (1996). Men, loss, and psychotherapy. *Psychotherapy, 33*, 593–600.

Cole, S. W., Kemeny, M. E., Taylor, S. E., & Visscher, B. R. (1996). Elevated physical health risk among gay men who conceal their homosexual identity. *Health Psychology, 15*, 243–251.

D'Augelli, A. R., & Hershberger, S. L. (1993). Lesbian, gay, and bisexual youth in community settings: Personal challenges and mental health problems. *American Journal of Community Psychology, 21*, 1–28.

Diaz, R. M., Ayala, G., Bein, E., Jenne, J., & Marin, B. V. (2001). The impact of homophobia, poverty, and racism on the mental health of Latino gay men. *American Journal of Public Health, 91*, 927–932.

DiPlacido, J. (1998). Minority stress among lesbians, gay men, and bisexuals: A consequence of heterosexism, homophobia, and stigmatization. In G. M. Herek (Ed.), *Stigma and sexual orientation: Vol. 4. Understanding prejudice against lesbians, gay men, and bisexuals* (pp. 138–159). Thousand Oaks, CA: Sage.

Dugo, J. M., & Beck, A. P. (1997). Significance and complexity of early phases in the development of the co-therapy relationship. *Group Dynamics: Theory, Research, and Practice, 1*(4), 294.

Dupras, A. (1994). Internalized homophobia and psychosexual adjustment among gay men. *Psychological Reports, 75*, 23–28.

Gilbert, P. (2007). Evolved minds and compassion in the therapeutic relationship. In P. Gilbert & R. Leahy (Eds.), *The therapeutic relationship in the cognitive behavioural psychotherapies* (pp. 106–142). New York, NY: Routledge.

Goleman, D. (1996). *Emotional intelligence: Why it can matter more than IQ*. London, UK: Bloomsbury.

Good, G. E., Gilbert, L. A., & Scher, M. (1990). Gender aware therapy: A synthesis of feminist therapy and knowledge about gender. *Journal of Counseling & Development, 68*, 376–380.

Good, G. E., & Robertson, J. M., (2010). To accept a pilot? Addressing men's ambivalence and altering their expectancies about therapy. *Psychotherapy: Theory, Research, Practice, Training, 47*(3), 306.

Gottman, J., Katz, L., & Hooven, C. (1996). *Meta-emotion: How families communicate emotionally: Links to child-peer relations and other developmental outcomes*. Mahwah, NJ: Lawrence Erlbaum.

Gottman, J. M., Levenson, R. W., Gross, J., Fredrickson, B. L., McCoy, K., Rosenthal, L., Ruef, A., & Yoshimoto, D. (2003). Correlates of gay and lesbian couples' relationship satisfaction and relationship dissolution. *Journal of Homosexuality, 45*, 23–43.

Gresswell, D. M., & Hollin, C. R. (1994). Multifactorial model of serial killing. *British Journal of Criminology, 34*, 1–14.

Hoff, C. C., & Beougher, S. C. (2010). Sexual agreements among gay male couples. *Archives of Sexual Behavior, 39*, 774–787.

Kingerlee, R. (2012). Conceptualizing men: A transdiagnostic model of male distress. *Psychology and Psychotherapy: Theory, Research and Practice, 85*, 83–99.

Kolves, K., Ide, N., & De Leo, D. (2010). Suicidal ideation and behaviour in the aftermath of marital separation: Gender differences. *Journal of Affective Disorders, 120*(1), 48–53.

Kurdek, L. A. (2005). What do we know about gay and lesbian couples? *Current Directions in Psychological Science, 14*, 251–254.

LaSala, M. C. (2004a). Extradyadic sex and gay male couples: Comparing monogamous and nonmonogamous relationships. *Families in Society, 85*, 405–412.

LaSala, M. C. (2004b). Monogamy of the heart: Extradyadic sex and gay male couples. *Journal of Gay & Lesbian Social Services: Issues in Practice, Policy & Research, 17*(3), 1–24.

Levant, R. F., Hall, R. J., Williams, C. M., & Hasan, N. T. (2009). Gender differences in alexithymia. *Psychology of Men and Masculinity, 10*(3), 190–203.

Lucas, M. (2004). Introduction: Reflections on the therapeutic frame. In M. Lucas (Ed.), *The therapeutic frame in the clinical context: Integrative perspectives* (pp. 1–7). New York, NY: Routledge.

Meyer, I. H. (1995). Minority stress and mental health in gay men. *Journal of Health and Social Behavior, 36*, 38–56.

Meyer, I. H. (2013). Prejudice, social stress, and mental health in lesbian, gay, and bisexual populations: Conceptual issues and research evidence. *Psychology of Sexual Orientation and Gender Diversity, 1*(S), 3–26.

Meyer, I. H., & Dean, L. (1998). Internalized homophobia, intimacy, and sexual behavior among gay and bisexual men. In G. M. Herek (Ed.), *Stigma and sexual orientation: Vol. 4. Understanding prejudice against lesbians, gay men, and bisexuals* (pp. 160–186). Thousand Oaks, CA: Sage.

Pachankis, J. E., Rendina, H. J., Ventuneac, A., Grov, J. T., & Parsons, J. T. (2014). The role of maladaptive cognitions in hypersexuality among highly sexually active gay and bisexual men. *Archives of Sexual Behavior, 43*(4), 669–683.

Parsons, J. T., Grov, C., & Golub, S. A. (2012). Sexual compulsivity, co-occurring psychosocial health problems, and HIV risk among gay and bisexual men: Further evidence of a syndemic. *American Journal of Public Health, 102*, 156–162.

Parsons, J. T., Kelly, B. C., Bimbi, D. S., DiMaria, L., Wainberg, M. L., & Morgenstern, J. (2008). Explanations for the origins of sexual compulsivity in gay and bisexual men. *Archives of Sexual Behavior, 37*, 817–826.

Parsons, J. T., Starks, T. J., DuBois, S., Grov, C., & Golub, S. A. (2013). Alternatives to monogamy among gay male couples in a community survey: Implications for mental health and sexual risk. *Archives of Sexual Behavior, 42*, 303–312.

Parsons, J. T., Starks, T. J., Garamel, K. E., & Grov, C. (2012). Non-monogamy and relationship quality among same-sex male couples. *Journal of Family Psychology, 26*(5), 669–677.

Pearlman, L. A., & Courtois, C. A. (2005). Clinical applications of the attachment framework: Relational treatment of complex treatment. *Journal of Traumatic Stress, 18*(5), 449–459.

Peterson, J. L., Folkman, S., & Bakeman, R. (1996). Stress, coping, HIV status, psychosocial resources, and depressive mood in African American gay, bisexual, and heterosexual men. *American Journal of Community Psychology, 24*, 461–487.

Pollack, W. S. (2005). Masked men: New psychoanalytically oriented treatment models for adult and young adult men. In G. E. Good & G. R. Brooks (Eds.), *The new handbook of psychotherapy and counseling for men: A comprehensive guide to settings, problems, and treatment approaches* (pp. 203–216). San Francisco, CA: John Wiley & Sons.

Porter, K. (1993). Combined individual and group psychotherapy. In A. Alonso & H. I. Swiller (Eds.), *Group therapy in clinical practice* (pp. 309–341). Washington, DC: American Psychiatric Press.

Prochaska, J. O., & Velicer, W. F. (1997). The transtheoretical model of health behavior change. *American Journal of Health Promotion, 12*(1), 38–48.

Robertson, J. M., & Williams, B. W. (2010). "Gender aware therapy" for professional men in a day treatment center. *Psychotherapy: Theory, Research, Practice, Training, 47*(3), 316–326.

Roller, B., & Nelson, V. (1991). *The art of co-therapy: How therapists work together.* New York, NY: Guilford Press.

Rosario, M., Rotheram-Borus, M. J., & Reid, H. (1996). Gay-related stress and its correlates among gay and bisexual male adolescents of predominantly Black and Hispanic background. *Journal of Community Psychology, 24*, 136–159.

Rosser, B., Metz, M., Bockting, W., & Buroker, T. (1997). Sexual difficulties, concerns and satisfaction in homosexual men: An empirical study with implications for HIV prevention. *Journal of Sex and Marital Therapy, 23*, 61–73.

Savage, D. (2010). Monogamish. *The Stranger.* Retrieved August 17, 2015, from http://www.thestranger.com/seattle/SavageLove?oid=11412386

Sax, L. (2007). *Boys adrift: The five factors driving the growing epidemic of unmotivated boys and underachieving young men.* New York, NY: Basic Books.

Shernoff, M. (2006). Negotiated nonmonogamy and male couples. *Family Process, 45*(4), 407–418.

Starks, T., Grov, C., & Parsons, J. (2013). Sexual compulsivity and interpersonal functioning: Sexual relationship quality and sexual health in gay relationships. *Health Psychology, 32*(10), 1047–1056.

Symons, C., & Wheeler, S. (2005). Counselor conflict in managing the frame: Dilemmas and decisions. *Counseling and Psychotherapy Research, 5*(1), 19–26.

Thomas, R. V., & Pender, D. A. (2008). Association for Specialists in Group Work: Best practice guidelines 2007 revisions. *Journal for Specialists in Group Work, 33*(2), 111–117.

Trotzer, J. (2013). *The counselor and the group: Integrating theory, training and practice* (4th ed.). New York, NY: Taylor & Francis.

Wade, J. C., & Good, G. E. (2010). Moving toward mainstream: Perspectives on enhancing therapy with men. *Psychotherapy, 47*(3), 273–275.

Wagner, C. C., & Ingersoll, K. S. (2013). *Motivational interviewing in groups.* New York, NY: Guilford Press.

Waldo, C. R. (1999). Working in a majority context: A structural model of heterosexism as minority stress in the workplace. *Journal of Counseling Psychology, 46*, 218–232.

Wexler, D. (2009). *Men in therapy: New approaches for effective treatment.* New York, NY: W. W. Norton.

Wheelan, S. A. (1997). Co-therapists and the creation of a functional psychotherapy group; A group dynamics perspective. *Group Dynamics: Theory, Research & Practice, 1*(4), 306–310.

Williamson, I. (2000). Internalized homophobia and health issues affecting lesbians and gay men. *Health Education Research, 15*, 97–107.

Yalom, I. D. (1995). *The theory and practice of group psychotherapy* (4th ed.). New York, NY: Basic Books.

Yeagley, E., Hickok, A., & Bauermeister, J. A. (2014). Hypersexual behavior and HIV sex risk among young gay and bisexual Men. *Journal of Sex Research, 51*(8), 1–11.

CHAPTER TEN

OCSB GROUP TREATMENT—PRACTICES

The therapists' vision that guides and motivates the out of control sexual behavior (OCSB) group is comparable to the client's sexual health vision that guides his treatment for out of control sexual behavior. As Yalom (1995) eloquently stated, "your offer of professional help serves as the group's initial raison d'etre" (p. 107). Doug's motivation for beginning an OCSB group more than 20 years ago was sparked by his realization that no one was providing a culturally competent group for gay and bisexual men mandated to treatment for consensual sex with men in public spaces. Much has changed since the early 1990s, but the need for safe, respectful, and informed spaces for men to enhance their sexual health remains. In Chapter 9, we outlined principles used to guide the early formulation of an OCSB group. In this chapter, we discuss OCSB group leadership skills and structured events that foster the conditions for sexual health behavior change. For ease of reading group dialogues, the leaders' names are printed in bold.

OCSB GROUP LEADERSHIP SKILLS

OCSB group leadership skills are founded on general group psychotherapy practices (Corey, 2008; Luke, 2014). In this section, we highlight group leadership skills that we have found beneficial for facilitating a group process specific to men and sexual behavior problems. Maintaining a safe and productive therapeutic space in a sexuality-specific group is complicated by the negative sociocultural norms that influence sexual conversations in combination with the factors that contribute to out of control sexual experiences. We focus on eight group leadership competencies that facilitate sexual health conversations and create the therapeutic conditions to improve client sexual health. These competencies are intended to guide the choices of therapists in training, as well as provide a lens from which to self-evaluate leader practices.

Establish Psychological Safety

Our first leader skill is being able to establish group psychological safety. It goes without saying that psychotherapy process groups invite members to take personal and interpersonal risks. A process group that specifically addresses sexual health has the added complication of managing the shame, vulnerability, and rejection fears characteristic of men and their sexuality. Clients may be asked to share the precise details of their sexual behaviors and choices that may have injured them or people they love. Interventions will likely invite them to stretch their emotional and empathic capacities and learn to tolerate their discomfort with the affection of the other men. Clients may be asked to reveal shameful aspects of their erotic desires and sexual histories that have been hidden for years. Edmonson (2004) describes the intrapersonal process used for psychological safety as a person's "tacit calculus at behavioral micro-decision points" (p. 241). These decision points are how men momentarily assess the interpersonal risk of a specific sexual disclosure within the immediate or ongoing group climate. Members evaluate psychological safety by considering how the leader has mitigated previous hurt, pain, shame, criticism, or other emotional consequence of sexual health conversations. Attending to psychological safety is particularly important given the high prevalence of judgment, disapproval, or rejection OCSB treatment-seeking men have had directed toward them when discussing their sexual behavior problems in their personal lives.

Psychological safety begins with proper group screening, selection, and preparation (Wagner & Ingersoll, 2013). It is the leader's responsibility to prioritize the safety of the group when selecting new members. Establishing confidence in the client's fitness for group process is one of the many benefits of the methodical approach we take during an OCSB assessment. As such, we screen for manifestations of psychopathology (e.g., nonconsensual sex, perpetration of violence, etc.) to prevent admitting someone into the group who has a high propensity to harm others. The OCSB group leader's responses to sexual discussions that occurred during the screening and assessment represent the behaviors clients can expect from the leader when discussing their sexual lives with the group. These discussions can engender trust in the leader that the prospective group member later brings to his initial sessions. If group leaders implicitly transmit their own discomfort and negative judgment regarding particular sexual topics during pregroup individual sessions, then men may be less willing to risk being vulnerable in the group.

Once in group, leaders can learn how new members calculate their psychological safety through curious and targeted requests for them to articulate their microdecisions.

- "What made you choose to disclose this today?"
- "What tipped the scales for you when you thought about sharing this?"
- "When did you determine you were going to keep the agreement?"
- "What have you experienced in the group that helped you decide to be honest"?

Leader curiosity about the member's process prior to initiating a sexual health conversation is an opportunity for men to reveal their internal equation for psychological safety. From the onset of joining an OCSB group, members are invited to become increasingly aware of how their mind carries out the task of managing relationship risks. Members learn how they regulate emotional closeness or distance when leaders invite men to observe and describe their relationship choices. Members may not have seen their agency in regulating safety and these interventions can raise their awareness about how they manage interpersonal risks related to their sexual experiences.

Suspending Judgment About Sexual Practices

Earlier chapters review suspending judgment as an assessment skill needed by both therapist and client. We emphasize methods to avoid common sociocultural sex negativity in order to establish and maintain an empathetic and curious therapeutic space. Suspending judgment is an important process skill within OCSB groups as well. Man's ability to consciously observe and manage sexual judgments can improve group empathy, curiosity, and self-awareness. Group leader or member's judgmental thoughts will likely surface when certain sexual details are shared in group. Each group session calls on OCSB group leaders to regulate their own internal judgments while addressing group members who express their judgments in response to a sexual disclosure.

An OCSB group process can rapidly devolve into a whirlwind of opinions, comments, and ideas. One member may feel emboldened or entitled to share his opinion about another member's actions. He inadvertently launches a contentious idea about which the group can debate. This may lead to factions espousing forthright suggestions and opinions that solidify into subgroups. In the following example, Steve disclosed a sexual health plan (SHP) boundary crossing that involved not disclosing his HIV status with a new sex partner:

CARLOS: Steve, did you lie to him and tell him that you were negative?

STEPHEN: Well, I didn't lie. You know, if it doesn't come up, then he obviously didn't care if I was positive.

WILL: Wait, isn't one of your group goals to be more honest about your HIV status?

STEPHEN: Yeah, but sometimes, if he's really hot … and I don't top him, what does it matter if I don't tell him I'm positive?

CARLOS: Honesty matters a lot!

WILL: Don't you think that if you are not honest all the time with new partners, it just feeds your addiction?

STEPHEN: Well, lots of people aren't honest about their HIV status and they aren't all in a group for out of control sexual behavior.

It takes less time for a conversation like this to unfold in a group than it does to read it. OCSB group leaders may find it difficult to facilitate group process within real-time conflicts about sex. Their minds shift between content … process … content … process. Remember, most members do not bring developed sexual health conversations skills to an OCSB group and do not gracefully navigate highly charged sexual health conversations with other men. Men can climb a steep learning curve for managing their judgmental responses when trying to connect and discuss emotionally activating sexual topics. They tend to be more comfortable in an intellectualized debate than an emotional disclosure. Intellectualizing defenses allows the group members to avoid processing the feelings they experienced in response to sexual disclosures and provokes defensiveness in the other members who are being judged. The group will likely stay in that familiar judgmental space unless the OCSB group leader intervenes.

To move the group away from a debate, the leader (group leader's name appears in bold type) could respond to the devolving group dialogue about honesty by saying:

DOUG: Moments like this remind me how difficult it can be to live by the sexual health principles. We agree with them, but it can be hard to align with them. I found myself

> wondering how many times group members have left a sexual situation feeling disappointed with your honesty or openness and never spoke of it. It sounds like there are many unfinished conversations in the room right now.

The leader joins with the group in their collective distress while shifting the attention to processing the conflicting motivations inherent within principled sexual behavior. In heated moments, when the content is escalating into emotional reactivity, we recommend returning the group to the overall goal (i.e., living within the sexual health principles) by inviting group members to personalize their responses when proffering their thoughts about another member's sexual choices.

- What did you feel when you heard Steve talk about his honesty conflict with his sex partner?
- I noticed people had strong reactions to Steve's decision not to be honest. What feelings came up?
- How can you relate to Steve's conflict about honesty and HIV during a sexual situation?
- What are you trying to say to Steve that is behind your advice?

The leader can invite members to describe their internal experience in response to Steve rather than their opinions and judgments. Judgmental statements or advice giving do not reveal the group member's underlying intention. Was the group member attempting to communicate concern for Stephen's sex partner? Was he feeling angry and wanting to express his disapproval? Did he feel the hurt he imagined Steve's sex partner's might feel if he knew about Steve's choice? Suspending judgments encourage men to directly verbalize what motivated them to speak up without creating emotional distance.

Group judgments may also take the form of negative self-talk. The following was a conversation between Carlos and Doug:

CARLOS: I have to report a sexual health boundary crossing to the group. I can't believe I am still doing this. I imagine you're all just sick of me telling you this. I am sick of it, too.

DOUG: Carlos, before you go further, can you slow down a bit. Look around the room. See if what you are saying matches the men's faces. Are the judgments you are making coming from your mind or from the group?

Doug addressed Carlos's projective defenses before focusing on his sexual health plan boundary crossing. He wanted Carlos to observe his automatic negative self-talk to increase his self-monitoring capacity and study his disowned self-judgments.

Members' judgmental thinking patterns can be subtly revealed through the sequence men choose to disclose their sexual health plan boundary crossings. Frequently, they give the group their opinion or conclusion about the SHP boundary crossing before they describe or deconstruct their behavior. When OCSB group leaders listen closely for this pattern, they may hear how men bring conclusions that explain the boundary crossing while marginalizing the details of their sexual urges, thoughts, behaviors, and consequences. This pattern can be linked with men's motivation to keep the group agreement, but not more fully explore the situation and subsequent uncomfortable affect. Group members are often unaware of the defensive function served by their explanatory summary. Simply redirecting him to recollect his thoughts, urges, and competing motivations associated with the sexual situation may increase group awareness of this defense.

For example, the following is an exchange among group members Jackson, Michael, and Simon. Jackson had been in the group for several months. He was fired from his job for using company equipment to visit sex sites.

JACKSON: I know I should have known better. I was being stubborn, I fooled myself. I thought I could bring my phone with me to Starbucks and I would be just fine. I thought I would not look at sex sites sitting in a public space.

MICHAEL: Jackson, I wonder if you can try again. You started by telling us your conclusions and your take-away lesson. Can you walk the group though what happened without jumping ahead to tell us your opinion about what happened?

SIMON: I used to do exactly what you're doing right now. I would come to group knowing I had to talk about my sexual health plan and I would start by telling the group all the mistakes I made and what I learned. What I had a real hard time doing was telling the group what I was thinking in my mind. I remember when I had to really stop and describe what I was doing. I had to see a couple things about me that I really didn't want to know, like the times I thought "Fuck it, I don't care, I'm going to just go to the strip club." I didn't want to see

> that I actually made a choice. I never really saw what
> was going on inside me before I crossed my boundar-
> ies. I didn't think that I actually had any control.

OCSB group leaders model an important sexual health conversation skill when they help clients to suspend their own immediate judgments and find a compassionate inner dialogue for reporting an SHP boundary crossing. Like other mindfulness interventions, this provides opportunities for men to increase their self-awareness of automatic negative self-talk and to remain connected to others while experiencing a wide range of emotions.

Process Sexual Health Moments in the Here/Now

Much of the content discussed during group psychotherapy sessions consists of historical and current life events. Leaders balance the group's focus on external there/then issues with here/now group dynamics and introspection. The group must "recognize, examine and understand process. It must examine itself; study its own transactions; it must transcend pure experience and apply itself to the integration of that experience" (Yalom, 1995, pp. 129–130). When OCSB group leaders successfully move groups beyond reporting what happens between sessions, members can improve their self-observation skills and involve the other group members in their change process. Developing member familiarity and acceptance of group process takes time, but it is an important investment. Here/now interventions promote awareness of group process and maintenance of OCSB treatment frame boundaries. The following examples are common here/now interventions we regularly use during OCSB group work.

Welcome Sexual Health Conversations

OCSB group therapists implement a range of here/now interventions to welcome client curiosity about sexual health.

- A group member describes his success in walking away from an automatic teller machine before withdrawing cash to pay for sex and the leader responds, "Something changed in your face just now, your eyes looked away and you shrugged. What did you just feel?"
- A man reports the satisfying process of negotiating a new masturbation agreement with his spouse. The leader is curious about the group's nonverbal behavior. "The group all seemed to laugh

together just now, as I looked around there seemed to be a smile on everyone's faces. What were people feeling?"

Welcoming sexual health conversations is especially important for new group members unaccustomed to informed, safe, and respectful sexual conversations among men. New members commonly depend on the leader to guide early adaptation to the sexual health language in the group. Sexual terms, body parts, sexual acts, orgasms, erections, lubrication, ejaculation, kissing, nudity, breast size, penis size, paying for sex, and unconventional sexual interests are all possible topics when attending an OCSB group. The leader asks members to clarify their language by interjecting brief questions such as: "When you said 'it' did you mean 'penis'?" or "What kind of sex are you referring to?" If this is a new skill for the group, a follow-up question may include, "What did it feel like to have me ask you to be more specific and precise about your language?"

Invite Feelings and Thoughts in Response to Member's Sexual Disclosures

- "How did the group feel listening to Hector describe having sex with a partner he was not attracted to?"
- "What did you feel listening to Hector describe his thoughts when he was in a high-risk sexual situation?"

Here, the leader moves the group from content and invites them to focus on their here/now emotional responses to the group member's story. Depending on the context, a leader could also ask about the group members' thoughts as they listened to Hector. The OCSB group leader subjectively determines when to focus the group on deliberative or affective processes, especially when the sexual behavior is socially controversial or unconventional. These here/now interventions are especially important when a client reveals a sexual or erotic detail for the first time. Members disclosing new sexual activity or erotic interests to the group may have anticipated a range of reactions from the group or themselves. Whether anticipated or unexpected feelings unfold, either occurrence is valuable for the group to process. The disclosing group member will need to pause and explore his thoughts and emotions related to his disclosure as well as any irrational beliefs generated in his mind leading up to this moment. Taking the time to discuss both anticipatory anxiety and here/now emotions is an opportunity to increase men's awareness of avoidant coping strategies that may be common patterns in their relationships in the group and their sexual/erotic-identity development.

Elevate Attachment and Relational Consequences

- "Are people feeling closer or more distant to Jay right now?"
- "David, you made quite a sigh just now, is there something you want to say in response to Jay?"
- "How is Jay doing with being clear and specific about his sexual concern?"
- "What is happening with the group that so many questions are being asked of Jay? Is there something someone wants to say to Jay that is behind these questions?"

Here, the leader suggests that the group engage in a direct interaction between members by verbalizing unspoken or nonverbally expressed thoughts and feelings. These interventions help raise the group member's awareness about how others experience him in interpersonal moments. The leader can draw immediate attention to the one of two effects of his behavior: emotional closeness or distance. The leader is looking to identify when the member's dismissive, preoccupied, or fearful attachment patterns are present in group interactions. This process moment provides an opportunity for group members to evaluate their attachment style pattern and connect it with similar relationship patterns outside of the group.

To Stay Attuned

Here/now leader interventions can enhance therapist attunement when a group member discloses sexual behavior problems. This can be done through an empathic inquiry about unspoken self-appraisals, opinions, or feelings concerning a vulnerable sexual decision.

- "What was it like to decline her sexual advance and leave the work party? You had previously said to the group that you thought you would not be able to set this kind of boundary in future sexually exciting situations. How are you feeling as you share this SHP boundary success with the group?"
- "Carl, you just went into so much detail about all the thinking that goes through your mind prior to having intercourse with a man when neither you nor your partner have discussed your current

HIV status. Can you take a moment with us and just focus on what it is like to let us all in on these thoughts?"

Process Pleasure

It is easy for an OCSB group to fall into a pattern of focusing on sexual problems and neglect the experience of pleasure. When OCSB groups remain overly focused on their problems with sex, it dismisses the dynamic role played by their sexual desire, excitement, pleasure, and fulfillment. After all, sexual pleasure is likely one of the primary motivations that compel the client to desire and seek out the sexual behaviors he wants to stop. Balancing group focus on sexual problems with sexual pleasure is essential to promoting sexual health. The *mutual pleasure* sexual health principle prioritizes pleasure as fundamental to sexual health. Men improve their understanding of this sexual health principle through group conversation that first assists men in becoming more comfortable and capable of communicating what they find sexually pleasurable. Men will be more motivated to change sexual behavior when their sexual health plans include a focus on mutual pleasure.

Leaders are encouraged to explore the pleasurable aspects of all sexual behaviors, but especially the problematic ones. It helps to identity the components of the member's sexuality that he has been highly invested in preserving. They may represent elements of his sexual/erotic orientation that he was willing to engage in despite significant negative intra- or interpersonal consequences. For those with shame-based sexuality narratives, talk about sexual excitement and pleasure can support positive sexual/erotic-identity development. The OCSB group leader can focus on the group-as-a-whole to assist each man in finding compassion for these conflicts. By acknowledging the struggle associated with accepting one's sexual and erotic orientation, the group member can build self-compassion and the other members can build their empathy capacities. Men in OCSB group therapy benefit from experiencing the relief felt by ending their sexual problems combined with the joy of a fun, exciting sex life. Discussing their sexual pleasures and processing the here/now thoughts and feelings provides opportunities to celebrate sexual enjoyment and the fundamental importance of pleasure to men's sexual health.

- "Will, how did you feel telling the group about the really intense orgasm you shared with your husband?"
- "How did the group react to Will's description about what it was like to have such an intense orgasm with his husband?

- "Evan, your eyes were tearing just now when you were telling the group about how excited your wife looked when she used restraints during sex last weekend. Did you have a feeling just now when telling the group about this?"
- "Carl, what about the sexual videos you were watching really turned you on? What really captured your attention?"

Frame Content Within Sexual Health Principles

Applying the sexual health principles to daily life takes time and practice for which group is an excellent modality. Group provides the space for members to reflect on their sexual behaviors, evaluate their choices, and develop new modes of sexual expression. At any point in this process, the sexual health principles provide the framework to critically think about the changes under consideration. For example, Pedro, in treatment to stop paying for sex, disclosed a recent encounter with a sex worker who was high on heroin. His "sustain talk" remained focused on the political and moral argument that sex work should be legal between two consenting adults. The group was more interested in how his sexual behavior aligned with the sexual health principles. In this situation, the leaders chose to focus on Pedro's boundary crossing as a misalignment with the nonexploitive sexual health principle. Because Pedro's stage of readiness seemed contemplative, our intervention needed to avoid triggering his defenses while raising his self-awareness about his choices.

- "What was the role of heroin in the interaction?"
- "Was her sex work a means to support her drug addiction?"

If a client has not previously considered the exploitative nature of his choices, we might introduce the concept without specifically using the word *exploitation* to give the client an opportunity to identify it himself. If he does not make the connection, the leader can also rely on the group, who are also aware of the principles: "What sexual health principle do you hear me inviting Pedro to think about?"

The leaders can also choose to link the behavior with protection from STI/HIV.

- "How did you protect yourself from an STI/HIV?"
- "What is your relationship with HIV now?"

Leader follow-up questions can focus on the activated emotions stemming from a focus on sexual health principles.

- "What does it feel like to consider that paying for sex with a heroin user may be exploiting her drug addiction for your sexual pleasure?"
- "What did it feel like to hear that you may have exposed yourself to HIV?"

The sexual health principles are important frameworks for maintaining sexual health when previously partnered group members become single. As men begin disclose dating experiences with women, leaders can inquire about how they are preventing an unintended pregnancy:

- What is your vision of sexual health now that you are single?
- What is your contraception plan with your new partners?"

Newly dating members or those recovering from a breakup might prematurely engage in sex without having a new sexual health plan in place. Having this conversation could prevent an unintended pregnancy in the near future. The sexual health principle of honesty is frequently a topic for newly single group members living with a viral STI (e.g., genital herpes, hepatitis B, human papillomavirus HIV). Group members may need to talk openly with the group to clarify their disclosure expectations when becoming sexual with a new partner: "What level of honesty about living with herpes is sufficient for you when beginning a sexual relationship?" Process questions invite the group to function as the sanctuary for men to evaluate sexual health-based interactions. The group is also a space for the leader or other members to address sexual health knowledge gaps or misinformation about sexually transmitted infections.

Revisiting the sexual health principles helps group members determine whether to change a specific sexual behavior pattern or add a new behavior to their sexual repertoire. Men in OCSB groups have experience focusing on eliminating negative sexual consequences and may find intentional sexual health decisions both essential and intimidating. For instance, Christopher was distressed about the regularity with which he and his husband were having sex with a third partner. He was worried that he was engaging in sexual behaviors that were "unhealthy." During group, Doug suggested, "It sounds like you are not sure you should continue this sexual relationship because you think that it's unhealthy. Let's compare this sexual behavior with the sexual health principles and then see what you think." Together, the group reviewed the nonmonogamous arrangement through the six principles. They determined it was *consensual, nonexploitive,* and *protected against STI/HIV and unintended pregnancies.* The member reported that he and his partner were *honest* about the arrangement with each other and with the third partner, they all were enjoying the experiences (*mutual pleasure*) and shared in the meaning of the encounter (*shared values*).

After reviewing the principles, we returned to Christopher's concern. "From your description, your behavior seems to fall within the sexual health principles. Rather than try to determine whether this behavior is healthy or unhealthy, can you share how you are feeling when you think about your behavior now?" In general, members are motivated to align their behaviors with the sexual health principles. However, men (and many therapists) frequently confuse unconventional sexual practices with "unhealthy" sex. The group evaluated Christopher's worries through the lens of the sexual health principles in order to tease apart his conflated notions of healthy relationship practices from conventional relationship behaviors. If there is nothing inherently unethical about your sexual behavior, what is creating this self-discrepancy? Refocusing the dialogue to the client's internal conflict provided an opportunity to explore the unprocessed emotions that prompted Christopher's question. In this situation, Christopher was troubled by the affection developing between him and his new sex partner. He assumed that his husband's feelings toward the new partner meant that his husband felt less affection for him. Christopher was also worried that his friends and family would judge him as deviant or careless. He assumed that his unconventional sexual relationship agreement would be pathologized as a symptom of OCSB. He was in unfamiliar territory and feeling insecure with his primary relationship. Understandably, Christopher's inexperience with honest exploration of his erotic desires and managing relationship insecurities contributed to his distress. The group process offered an opportunity to evaluate his beliefs about relationships and intimacy, his vision of his marriage, and how the nonmonogamous sexual arrangement fit within that vision.

Prioritize Sexual Health Plan Boundary Crossings

Leaders prioritize the group's attention on a member's disclosure of an SHP boundary crossing. Every group member agrees to self-initiate disclosing SHP boundary crossings with the group. These disclosure events are a pivotal leadership moment to focus the entire group process on a central thesis of OCSB group work: honoring agreements. Leaders accomplish this function by fluidly working between content and process interventions. They can re-emphasize the importance of honoring the group agreement. Leaders can help group members deconstruct and examine their cognitive and emotional processes as they prepared to tell the group about their sexual behavior. They can also invite the group to reflect on specific content of the client's sexual behavior or invite them to reflect on the first few times they came to group to discuss an SHP boundary crossing. Although members self-initiate disclosures, they often deploy a range of defenses that influence the direction of the conversation. Defenses, such as fleeing to hopelessness/helplessness, deflecting, blaming others, and other strategies, move the group focus away from examining his actions. Regardless of the defenses enacted, it is the leader's role to facilitate a sexual health conversation that examines the contradiction between a member's sexual commitments and his sexual behaviors.

- "How did you benefit from crossing your boundaries? What did you like about it?"
- "How ready are you to return to following your sexual health plan?"
- "What do you think prevented you from maintaining your boundaries?"
- "What would need to change for you to be more willing to maintain your boundaries?"

The leader may have the members focus on the aspects of their SHP that they are following despite the recent boundary crossing.

- "Let's look at the boundaries you are keeping. How do you keep some of your boundaries but not others? Perhaps we can learn something by focusing on the boundaries you are keeping to find clues to help you to better regulate areas you continue to have difficulty regulating."

Men are less likely to progress with other clinical areas until they begin to have success with maintaining their SHP boundaries. It is incumbent upon group leaders to reinforce this basic premise in response to a pattern of SHP boundary crossings.

- "As a group leader, I have not seen any member meet his sexual health goals without first maintaining his sexual health plan boundaries."

Because we prioritize treatment frame interventions, it is important to remember that boundary crossing may indicate an issue with group facilitation. Leaders might identify group functions that need to be improved or added when they invite the entire group to talk about current group dynamics. For example, to avoid upsetting the leader, the group has been actively avoiding talking about its dissatisfaction with the group process.

- "If the group and I were functioning in a manner that improved the likelihood of maintaining your boundaries this week, what would we be doing?"

This can remind everyone in the group that sexual health is a collaborative process. The leader welcomes group discussion that may lead to a course correction in the current group process. Leaders can model that facilitating group is a constant learning process, just like maintaining one's sexual health.

Block Interference With Sexual Health Conversations

It is the leader's role to stop counterproductive behaviors within the group (Corey, 2008). One common counterproductive behavior seen in an OCSB group is a member diverting the group from meaningful sexual health conversations. It falls on the group leader to collaboratively redirect behaviors and comments that interfere with maintaining the focus on emotionally activating sexual topics. OCSB group leaders protect the group space for sexual health conversations by blocking members' defensive delays or monopolizing behavior that disrupts intimate dialogue or detailed sexual disclosures. Group leaders who feel ambivalent about blocking interventions or lack confidence in interpersonal and group facilitation skills may fail to assert this level of authority and directness. Finding an approach that works to block interference of sexual health conversations in a manner that avoids a shaming or dismissive exchange (especially when the topic is sexuality) is an important leader process skill. Sexual health conversations among group members flourish when leaders protect the space.

Blocking is a particularly important skill to master considering standard social etiquette. The most uncomfortable person in the room often regulates the sexuality-related conversations. Social and cultural deference is learned early in families, school, church, and neighborhoods, and often bestows the gatekeeping authority to the loudest voice of discomfort. When it comes to talking about sexuality, children learn at an early age to monitor their questions and comments based on the perceived or explicit displeasure exhibited by the adults with whom they are talking about sex. It is the OCSB group leader's responsibility to balance the need for a member to share his discomfort while not shutting down sexual health discussions. Members are welcome to express personal discomfort regarding the content of the discussion, but the leader is accountable for preventing uncomfortable members from stopping the sexual health conversations. For instance, the blocking member may attempt to change the subject. The group might take responsibility for avoiding the member's emotional discomfort by self-censoring sexual topics. Either way, the group loses a valuable opportunity to explore the many underlying concerns causing the member's discomfort.

Blocking works on the individual and whole-group levels. The leader protects the group functioning as a space for sexual health while empathically addressing individual member's defenses. In the following dialogue, Truman disclosed his strong feelings of guilt and disappointment in giving oral sex to his wife. Arturo responded with a deflective comment on the prevalence of oral sex in the general population. Potential leadership interventions include:

- Premature movement to content by a member may benefit from the leader redirecting back toward the affective process. "Arturo, I am interested in the group focusing on Truman's feeling. Is there a feeling you can find that is behind your statement?"
- The leader may direct the member away from the thought about a sexual story of a group member to the activated emotions in the room. "That is an opinion, can you try again and tell us what you are feeling right now?"
- Another blocking intervention is to direct a group member to suspend his focus on a judgment and focus the group members on remaining curious. "That sounds like a judgment. Can you set that aside for right now and find your feeling?"

Interrupting is also a form of blocking. The leader may choose to interrupt a member who is avoiding direct sexual health dialogue. Interrupting with a here/now intervention brings the conversation back to the present moment.

- "I'm sorry to interrupt. I understand you have many disappointments about your wife's sexual desire. Can you focus on what you are wanting to address with the group?"
- "Alex, let me interrupt for a second. Can you let the group know what you want from this discussion?"

Encourage Sexual Health-Based Feedback

When the leader is not focused on managing defenses that block discussions pertaining to the sexual health principles, he or she can promote sexual health feedback among members. It is reasonable to expect that men will enter an OCSB group with low proficiency in providing feedback to men about their sexual lives. This may be especially prominent among men who have attended 12-step fellowships where crosstalk is prohibited. How do men learn to give constructive feedback in an OCSB group? The simple answer is they observe the leader, who is usually the first to model and promote feedback among members. We recommend the leader demonstrate how to ask men for their permission to give feedback. This is different from the judgmental statements that we discussed earlier. Although both judgments and feedback involve one group member's viewpoint about another group member, feedback is invited in which judgments are typically given without the person's permission.

- "Before we move on to another topic, Frank, I was wondering whether you are interested in hearing how the group experienced you sharing about your boundary crossing?"
- "Jeff, let me interrupt. Carlos, did you want to hear feedback from Jeff right now?"
- "Carlos, are you interested in hearing what the group thinks you could do to avoid this problem in the future?"

Leadership Transparency

OCSB group members often present with a complex clinical picture. Leadership transparency is a valuable intervention facilitating groups in which the clinical issues that surface may need a personal anchoring perspective directly stated by the leader. Wagner and Ingersoll (2013) identified four components of leader transparency: self-disclosure, feedback, meta-communication, and openness regarding internal processes. *Disclosing personal information* is valuable when judiciously shared to help clients feel comfortable about their own self-disclosures. *Feedback* involves sharing thoughts about the client's circumstance, actions, or decisions. *Meta-communication* involves a discussion about the client's communication style and its impact on his relationships. *Openness about internal processes* includes reflections about the group processes, deliberations between the cotherapists, and the proposed direction taken for group dialogues. These four components can produce positive outcomes when used in any process group. Over the life of OCSB groups, openness interventions are helpful when preparing members for changes in leadership involvement, orienting members to unsettling group dynamics, or to taking responsibility for group events.

For instance, sometimes therapist disclosure serves an administrative function:

- "We [the two leaders] want to spend some time tonight discussing something with the group."

- "We have a group guideline concern we would like to discuss."
- "There is a problem about processing payments and we would like to get the group's input."

Other times, therapist transparency is a process observation used between the leaders.

- "Michael, I wonder whether we are more concerned about Xavier's sexual health plan than he and the group are?"
- "Doug, it occurs to me that Troy was hoping you would have listened to his frustration rather than correct his sexual health language. I felt some tension during the conversation."

Demystifying the process through leader transparency promotes a collaborative endeavor for OCSB group work. Openness about the leaders' internal process is a helpful strategy to welcome members' unexpressed idealization about the leaders' competencies. As much as we recommend that therapists receive specialized group psychotherapy training, a leader can never be fully prepared for every situation to faultlessly facilitate every session. Developing an approach that includes transparency about professional limitations is a helpful strategy in response to emotionally intense yet unprecedented group moments. In these moments, it is common to hear one of the following transparency interventions:

- "That's never happened before."
- "We need time to reflect on your request, let us get back to you next group."
- "We could have handled that better."

Novel group moments that activate high-energy group responses provide the leader with an opportunity to balance the emotional activation with a deliberative perspective. First, the leader acknowledges the unprecedented nature of the current situation. This can enjoin the group in a shared moment, a time to be present together to address the situation and perhaps find a new way of interacting. Some situations demand immediate decisions (e.g., building evacuations during a power outage or fire alarm). Other circumstances are not as urgent, but benefit from acknowledging the novelty without an immediate expectation for decisive action. It is important for leaders to remember that not all unusual group situations can be addressed within one group session (e.g., former sex partner joins group, online sexual encounter occurred with two group members between sessions, medical emergencies that prevent a member from attending group unexpectedly). OCSB group leaders must keep in mind that unexpected situations are not emergencies and may be best resolved over time.

Eventually, OCSB group leaders will experience regret about certain group interactions, ill-timed comments, or clinical observations that were not attuned with a group member or the entire group. Sometimes group leaders create distance, hurt, or anger with a stage-incongruent intervention or an injurious interpersonal group interaction. OCSB group leaders will disappoint themselves, their coleader, individual group members, as well as the group-as-a-whole. OCSB group work is difficult at times, especially when learning to treat out of control sexual behavior in combination with learning OCSB group psychotherapy skills. Recurrent leader misattunement that is not eventually processed in a manner that reconnects the leader and members will likely have negative repercussions for both the individual and the group.

Roback (2000) summarizes leadership factors that contribute to adverse group therapy outcomes. They include: "negativistic" interventions (e.g., rejecting comments or behaviors), misapplied technical skills, maintaining overly distant or technically rigid clinical models of group facilitation, not helping members understand their intense feelings generated by the group process, or severe boundary violations. Linden (2013) proposes a model for defining, classifying, and assessing negative side effects from psychotherapy that range from unwanted events caused by incorrect, improperly applied, or even correct treatment. Group therapy can lead to no improvement, worsening, or limitations in a member's treatment outcome resulting from his individual circumstance. Group leaders have a responsibility to monitor the group progress and the effects of their interventions. When leaders conclude that they could have done better and see that a regrettable outcome has transpired, a relationship repair is recommended. Leaders model the very accountability we ask of our clients when their internal investigation, "Could I have done better?" is revealed to the group.

STRUCTURED OCSB GROUP EVENTS

OCSB group treatment is a series of planned or predictable group events. The planned events are the individual or group sessions with structured agendas and clear objectives. The predictable events are occurrences in the life of the OCSB group for which the therapist also has clear objectives, but are not preplanned by the leaders. Establishing and maintaining leader skills to facilitate both planned and unplanned group events is essential for OCSB group effectiveness. The remainder of this chapter addresses structured events that are expected components for leading OCSB groups.

Group Orientation Meeting

We begin with the group orientation meeting. This one-time meeting occurs at the completion of the OCSB assessment and after the client has completed his written SHP. In this section, we review the group orientation meeting objectives. When the group is co-led, the orientation meeting provides an opportunity to meet with both leaders prior to meeting the entire OCSB group. During the group orientation appointment, the client reviews his SHP and goals for group treatment. The group orientation meeting is the final step before a prospective group member commits to entering group. The client reviews and signs the OCSB group guidelines, which function as both the informed consent for treatment and the acknowledgment of OCSB group treatment commitments and expectations. It is only at this point in the orientation meeting that the candidate agrees to enter group and is formally enrolled in the OCSB combined treatment program.

Meeting the Group Coleader

OCSB group leaders meet with prospective members to establish the group leadership team, which includes the therapist who performed his assessment and the group's other coleader. In many circumstances, the therapist who conducted the OCSB assessment process will continue as the client's individual therapist. The orientation meeting is the beginning of the client relationship with the OCSB group leadership team. Meeting both leaders prior to starting the group can ease anxiety about the first session and the new member can focus his attention on meeting the other members. The new member will know both leaders and can focus on meeting the members. Barring an extraordinary event, the orientation meeting is the only time the member meets with the group coleaders separate from the OCSB group. Before the group orientation meeting, we recommend the therapist obtain written authorization from the client to exchange protected health information between the coleaders. This authorization allows the coleaders to discuss the client's assessment information, Unique Clinical Picture, sexual health goals, and the conjoint session (if completed) prior to the orientation meeting.

Frank

Frank was eager to join one of the two sexual health groups for heterosexual men. Doug noticed that Frank's face looked more tense and muted as he greeted Michael, his soon-to-be group cotherapist. Michael congratulated Frank on reaching this point in the OCSB assessment process. We planned for Michael to begin the meeting by reviewing the objectives for the hour. This was designed as an early opportunity for he and Frank to engage with each other. Michael's agenda for the meeting was:

1. To meet the coleader
2. To discuss his assessment experience
3. To review his sexual health plan
4. To discuss overall group process and the events of his first session
5. To review and sign the group guidelines

The group orientation meeting juxtaposed Frank's established connection with Doug and his new relationship with Michael. This context provided leaders and Frank with a glimpse into his defenses and interpersonal approach to discussing his out of control sexual behavior beyond the dyadic assessment process. After Michael reviewed the agenda, Doug facilitated the initial focus of the meeting.

> **DOUG:** What would you like Michael to know about your situation and your assessment?

Frank began with his online sexual behavior workplace crisis. He discussed his generalized anxiety condition, and ended with describing his history of paying for sex. Other than with Doug, this was the first time Frank disclosed that he had paid women for sex.

> **MICHAEL:** How has it been for you to talk more openly about paying for sex with someone you've never met?

The orientation meeting is a place for men to practice disclosing their SHP and the details of their Unique Clinical Pictures. Michael's question reflected an intention to provide Frank with an in vivo experience of the first group session. When Frank joins the group, he will re-experience a similar moment with the new group members. We hoped to prepare Frank by eliciting some of the feelings and thoughts he may experience during his first group in the safety of the orientation meeting. Michael's question focused Frank on processing his potentially shame-activating disclosure of his out of control sexual behavior. Inviting Frank to observe and describe his internal thoughts and feelings when discussing paying for sex was also an opportunity to experience Michael interacting with Frank in preparation for similar exchanges in the group meetings. The coleaders commented to Frank about the similarities between this conversation and the task of self-disclosure with the ongoing OCSB group.

Reviewing the Sexual Health Plan and Treatment Goals

After Frank discussed his personal history, Michael and Doug focused the conversation on Frank's SHP and asked him to read it aloud. This is also a practice exercise for the new member to prepare reading his SHP aloud on the first night of group. It is unrealistic to expect members to accurately describe the specifics of their plan by memory, especially given the emotional activation surrounding the first night of group.

DOUG: Tell us about your decision to list "paying for sex" in the Ambivalence column.

FRANK: I have been doing this for so long, it was really a big problem in my marriage. I lied all the time about it. But I'm not married anymore so I guess, I wasn't ready to make a decision either way. Is that going to be a problem?

MICHAEL: Can you say more about "going to be a problem"?

FRANK: Well, I just imagine all the men in the group being, well, pretty hard on me for this, wanting me to write it to my Boundary column. I don't know, maybe they'll think I am not right for the group if I can't make up my mind about this.

MICHAEL: I appreciate your honesty about your ambivalence. We don't believe that it is always helpful to make every sexual health change all at once. Group is a place to explore your thoughts and feelings about paying for sex and to use the group to contemplate how this or other aspects of your plan fit into your vision of sexual health. Do you have any thoughts about how you might feel or what you might say should the group respond in the way you are imagining? Perhaps some preparation will be helpful?

At this point in the orientation meeting, we focused on building coleader rapport with Frank. He will have many group therapy sessions in which to explore his ambivalent feelings about his sexual behaviors. Frank envisioned group judgments in response to his current sexual health plan. His fears provided an opening to orient Frank to OCSB group feedback. We acknowledged that members might ask questions about his SHP and emphasized our role as coleaders to manage unsolicited advice giving between members, especially on their first night in the group. It is not uncommon for group members to give unsolicited advice with a sincere interest in helping others. Similar to the assessment process, however, protecting client sexual autonomy is a valued function of the coleaders. Reflecting on our previous discussion about the spirit of motivational interviewing (MI), groups that integrate MI "encourage individuals to sort through conflicting ideas, feelings, and values to achieve an owned, if fallible, plan" (Wagner & Ingersoll, 2013, p. 65). Frank's anxiety about group member's response to his current sexual health plan is an excellent opportunity to remind him that his sexual health plan is grounded in his vision for his life.

Review Group Process

It is important to prepare OCSB clients for the experience of psychotherapy group process. We first distinguish process group psychotherapy from psychoeducational group work. OCSB groups are not classrooms—there are no lesson plans, homework assignments, or routine tasks. Instead, groups are more like relationship laboratories that raise their awareness about how they interact with others. When group interactions manifest in common client interpersonal patterns or emotional activating defenses, the leaders slow the group process to create time and space for observing and describing these patterns. An important weekly imprimatur for engaging in group process is when each group member influences the group flow in order to request the group's attention within the 90-minute session time frame. We believe each man's response to this group process will have similar relationship patterns found within the regulation and attachment aspects of the OCSB Unique Clinical Picture. When here/now moments reflect their clinical pictures, the door opens to individual members and the group-as-a-whole to engage in introspection. We explicitly remind the group that every symptom is welcome into the group space. It may sound counterintuitive to welcome member's OCSB symptoms into the group, but we want to see these patterns firsthand so we can assist the client in developing new ways of coping.

Inpatient or intensive outpatient sexual addiction treatment programs, which rely heavily on group treatment, regularly refer clients to outpatient OCSB treatment. These men may have been in psychoeducational groups, peer-support groups, or group sessions with rapidly changing memberships. When men from these residential or intensive outpatient programs enter the OCSB group, they will need clarification during the orientation meeting to review how the OCSB group structure differs from the groups they have experienced. Distinctions to review with prospective group members who first went to sex addictions intensive treatment programs or are immersed in 12-step fellowships groups include:

- The recovery philosophy or messages from their sexual addiction program may contrast with the approach taken in a sexual health group.
- They will not hear the treatment language of sexual addiction programs from the leaders.
- Crosstalk is welcome.
- There are no expectations that group members concurrently participate in a 12-step fellowship.

Will

Will seemed unaware of the faraway look on his face when Michael was describing a process group.

MICHAEL: You seem to be looking away just now, as if you are thinking about something.

WILL: Well, I was trying to think about what it would be like to be in a group where I just tell people what I think. I usually get into a lot of trouble when I do this. People tend to not want to hear what I have to say. They just roll their eyes like they will put up with it if they have to.

MICHAEL: If this happened in the group, we would encourage you to say what you just said to us. This is what a process group is like, we are interested in you letting the group know what goes on in your body, what you are thinking and feeling during the group. We find when group members choose to be vulnerable and share what's going on inside, it is a chance to understand yourself. And you may find that you're not alone. Group members often share similar experiences and would likely tell you that they prefer getting to know you. We find that most of the time the group wants to feel more connected with each other.

WILL: Well, that's just the thing. I get pretty anxious and my mind speeds up and I start thinking all sorts of things.

I guess, I just worry that no one will want to put up with hearing what goes on in my head.

DOUG: What you're doing right now is an example of why we think you will be a welcome addition to the group. I like how you told us what you were thinking in response to Michael's observation. You did a nice job of explaining to us what happens when you feel worried. You withdraw and start wondering if other people will dismiss you. We encourage you to be as open as you are now with the group.

Review Group Guidelines and Agreements

As we discussed in previous chapters, the OCSB group treatment agreements often elicit defenses and emotions that replicate behavior patterns associated with men's out of control sexual experiences. Conscious and unconscious challenges to the group agreement are expected during OCSB groups. OCSB group leaders look for parallels between the behavior members report outside of the group session and similar patterns seen during group sessions. A clear treatment frame establishes an expectation that the leaders, and eventually group members, will discuss members' patterns of managing competing motivations that are observed in OCSB group events. Allowing plenty of time to clarify the group agreement is important. This provides an accountability framework for future groups when leaders implement here/now interventions to address behavior that crosses group agreements. The orientation meeting is the anchor that leaders can reference in future groups when a member crosses any one of the many OCSB group agreements.

New Members Joining the Group

Groups are often curious about membership changes. "When will we have a new member? The group has been the same for a while, I feel ready to have some new perspectives." "I like the group the way it is. I wouldn't mind having the group stay as we are for a while. I like this group." Or "I am worried about a new member joining the group, it seems like we are in a rocky spot, he might get here and wonder what he has gotten into." Announcing a new member may evoke anxious or ambivalent feelings about the anticipated loss of the current group dynamic. Introducing a new member brings a shared vulnerability to each man in the OCSB group. The new person represents the vulnerable work of forming another new attachment, as well as managing feelings associated with reforming the group. New members will often activate each member's defenses, which reflect some aspects of how they regulate emotions and form new attachments.

We introduce new members with the following structure. Current group members introduce themselves first. They disclose their SHP, treatment goals, treatment progress, and anything else about themselves they would like to share. Then the new member introduces himself by disclosing the same things (minus the group experience) as well as confirming his initial 6-month commitment to group membership. We advise the new member that he does not need to provide a comprehensive life disclosure in the first session; the group has plenty of time to get to know him.

Adding a new group member presents an opportunity for leaders to assess the current group dynamic and developmental stage. Leaders may comment on a member's treatment progress or note how the men chose to represent themselves at this point in their treatment. How specific are their descriptions of their sexual behavior? What tone, mood, and sense of openness does each member and the group-as-a-whole seem to convey? Some long-term members may use welcoming a new member as a moment to discuss their progress toward completing group treatment. The leader may need to transition the group from introductions when the group's curiosity about the new member outpaces his desire to disclose additional information. "Is the group ready to move from introductions toward what is on people's minds for tonight's group?" "There will be plenty of time to learn more about each other in future group meetings, how is this for a start?" "What was it like for the group to hear everyone's introduction?"

New members are vital to the overall group stability. Managing group composition and size communicates the leader's investment in maintaining the ongoing life of the group. The longer the group goes without new members or the size of the group stagnates at six (even though group size can be up to eight), the greater the potential risk of a rapid departure when several members complete their treatment goals at similar times.

OCSB group will likely have new members who fail to complete their 6-month commitment. Over the course of our OCSB groups, we have had members leave before 6 months as a result of life circumstances outside of their control (e.g., unexpected work transfer, loss of job), some of whom left abruptly. Some men were poorly matched for group therapy and chose to leave despite their 6-month agreement. These false starts can disrupt group cohesion and present an interesting challenge for the leader. We encourage OCSB group therapists to be transparent about their responsibility in selecting members who left before completing 6 months of group work. Group leaders can make use of an early termination to invite group members to express any disappointment they may feel toward the group leader or historically abrupt attachment ruptures they have experienced either in the group or other relationships.

6-Month Review

Group members agree to several membership-related commitments. The first commitment is to remain in the group for 6 months. The 6-month review was not an original structured process in our groups. It started with a group member's request. He was a member of the heterosexual men's OCSB group and he asked whether he could get some feedback about his progress in therapy. He had just completed his initial 6-month group commitment. The client found it very useful to hear group members' perceptions of him and how they differed from his own self-observations of his treatment progress. He was able to reflect on the changes in his sexual health since beginning the assessment. The experience led to other group members asking for similar feedback. Michael and Doug noted the many benefits expressed in this intentional sexual health conversation. Several weeks later, we proposed making this an ongoing group procedure.

The 6-month review is now a routine element of the OCSB groups. The member has an opportunity to discuss his progress since he started group and the direction he would like to see his treatment go from this point. The other members can provide feedback about his treatment progress, their experience of him during the group or whatever else they would like to express related to their shared time in group. In addition to the formal feedback process, the leaders can remind the member that their group participation shifts from the time-oriented agreement to his subjective satisfaction with meeting his treatment goals. He can stay in the group until he feels he has met his sexual health goals.

Higher Level of Care

An unplanned yet common group event is a member's change in symptom acuity that requires a higher level of care. Some group member's sexual symptoms continue to escalate in frequency and severity. Clients may have an emerging or acute relapse of major depression, bipolar disorder, or substance addiction for which they would benefit from an intensive outpatient or inpatient treatment program. The leader will need to explain to the group why a member's undertreated psychiatric disorder or return to substance abuse must be stabilized in order to successfully address his sexual health problems. The treatment planning revolves around whether concurrent services are sufficient to address the symptoms or whether OCSB treatment needs to stop until the symptoms are addressed at a higher level of care. Group members can contribute to this process. They have witnessed the group member's deteriorating functioning and their perspective provides important reality-based feedback for the member in question. The leader can support the group member and the whole group to have honest and genuine discussions about possible levels of intervention. Ultimately, the leader must decide whether outpatient individual and group OCSB treatment remain a viable treatment plan. Besides the ethical responsibility to refer the group member to the most effective treatment, a member's deteriorating behavioral health will dominate the group's attention and undermine the overall effectiveness of the group process.

Sexual/Erotic Orientation Disclosures

In Chapter 4, we discuss the role of shame defenses as obstacles in sexual/erotic-identity development and in fostering intimacy in romantic relationships. In Chapter 9, we identify shame reduction as one of the many benefits of conjoint and combined treatment. A common sequence in OCSB treatment is processing sexual shame first in individual therapy and then disclosing the sexual/erotic conflict in group. Specific details of a man's sexual interest, unconventional turn-on, a sexually transmitted infection, infidelity, unplanned pregnancy, abortion, and sexual abuse histories are often a source of shame for men in OCSB groups.

Shame plays an essential role in forming and maintaining one's conscience, identity, dignity, and intimate relationships (Kaufman & Raphael, 1996). In relation to sexual health, shame may be activated when a person realizes that he has acted contrary to his values of acceptable behavior based on personal ethics or interpersonal relationships (Deonna, Rodogno, & Teroni, 2012). Shame often emerges when clients experience motivations that conflict with their sexual health principles and personal visions of sexual health.

Most people have an inherent capacity to experience shame, although they may generate shame feelings in a variety of ways. In moderation, shame is adaptive and often motivate clients toward changing their sexual behavior patterns. However, shame is detrimental if experienced intensely or internalized over time. Shame is internalized through its interconnection with other emotions, drives, and motivational states. When people learn to generate shame through repetitive shaming events (e.g., repeatedly being told as a child that touching one's penis is disgusting), the affective experiences associated with that event (e.g., sexual desire, arousal, or pleasure) become tied with shame. Over time, the subsequent activation of those affective experiences might spontaneously generate shame without the external shaming event (Kaufman & Raphael, 1996). In other words, the child may feel ashamed the next time he touches his penis even without being scolded. People defend against feeling the pain of shame by avoiding the shame-inducing stimulus or mentally disowning shameful aspects of the self. These defenses can lead to a generalized forestalling of the emotion, drive, or motivational states connected to shame. Through these shame-binds, shame exerts a powerful and eventually constricting force in sexual expression, attachment regulation, and sexual/erotic-identity development.

To transform shame-binds, Kaufman and Raphael (1996) recommend a strategy wherein people carefully and consciously endure shame, rather than banish it. Group process provides an opportunity for men to improve their affect tolerance and decouple shame from other affective states. The goal for clients is to see how their undifferentiated shame manifests in their bodies, relationships, and their sexual choices. When clients describe the details of their sexual urges, thoughts, and behaviors, they may for the first time slow down to describe the micro-moments within these experiences. It is this verbalizing of their mental and emotional experiences within the safety of group that provides an opportunity for curiosity and dialogue. What exactly generated the shame? How does the client defend against his shame (i.e., use of humor, deflection, vague language, etc.)? What was it like for the client to identify, label, and express his shame?

Preparing men to face shame in the group is often first cultivated within individual therapy. For example, members project sociocultural sex-negative norms onto the group. This replication of societal rejection generates shame defenses that often significantly inhibit honest exploration of group members' erotic-identity development. Men build confidence within individual therapy to bring highly vulnerable and shame-activating sexual content to the group. Considering the greater emotional and interpersonal risks for disclosing unconventional or commonly judged sexual activities in group, individual therapy prepares the client to know his own mind and shame before he navigates the group's reaction to his sexual/erotic disclosure. The time between individual therapy processing and group therapy disclosure depends on the client's ability to discuss his erotic urges, thoughts, and behaviors in the cultural context that generated so much shame and identify the other factors that inhibited an integrated erotic self. Much of the individual work focuses on the client familiarizing himself with his own shaming narratives, in part by voicing his projections about group disclosure. What does he fear will happen? How does he think he will be judged? Does he think he will be rejected? Identifying a mental image of his internalized shame and thought distortions in individual therapy develops confidence in mitigating potential flooding or dissociation while disclosing erotic conflicts to the group. In turn, we predict that clients will be better prepared to enter into direct sexual health conversations about their erotic needs and their partner's sexual desires through the practice of bringing their erotic conflicts to a sexual health-based OCSB group.

Completing Group Treatment

Completing OCSB group treatment is often bittersweet. Group members are usually ready to leave group when they express satisfaction with maintaining behavior changes or they realize they have accomplished as much as they can. It is a rare experience for men in OCSB groups to chose to end meaningful and successful relationships. As part of the preparation for leaving the group, we ask members to reflect on their experience preparing and actually saying goodbye as part of the process of leaving important relationships. Frequently, group members are unfamiliar and unprepared for intentional and direct goodbyes. Traditional male socialization and conformity with gender-role expectations often restrict emotional expression and intimacy that limit men's exposure to deeply expressed and meaningful goodbyes. Group members will reflect the same pluralistic society without shared perspectives on rituals or observances intended to deal with endings like death or loss (Mangione, FortI, & Iacuzzi, 2007). Group members may also bring a complicated history of unprocessed relationship disruptions and endings that shape their reactions to group termination. In the OCSB group, we provide safe and structured terminations for men to be able to honor their accomplishments, join in a ritualized farewell, and process past relationship ruptures.

Each goodbye represents the culmination of the client's investment in his sexual health. He chose to schedule the consultation appointment with an OCSB specialist and participate in a lengthy OCSB assessment. He attended weekly OCSB group meetings and regular individual psychotherapy sessions. Some members also attended additional meetings to address co-occurring psychiatric disorders, substance addiction, medical issues, and relationship problems. The farewell session presents an opportunity to review the progress achieved since that consultation appointment and to celebrate all the achievements of treatment.

Each member agreed to give a minimum 3-week notice after he decides to leave OCSB group therapy. We suggest members approach leaving as a relational dialogue and encourage open contemplation of the decision with the group and the leaders. This circumstance presents an opportunity for a candid discussion, an appraisal of group treatment goals, and a redirection toward couple therapy or another specific specialized treatment. The three sessions between the termination announcement and the last session provide the group with time to review the member's detailed plans for maintaining his sexual health. This often leads to meaningful group discussions about the departing member's specific skills and behavioral changes observed by the group about the departing member. The interim weeks allow an opportunity to explore each group member's anticipated feelings and experiences about the group when the departing member is no longer in group. Leaders can encourage the group to air their history of conflicts, disappointments, and hurt feelings along with the cherished moments of appreciation, joy, and respect.

Men preparing to leave group may have increased worries about sexual health plan boundary crossings. "Do I wait to leave group until all my sexual problems have remitted?" "If so, how long do I maintain my sexual health plan boundaries before I entertain the idea of leaving group?" "I feel ready to leave group but my wife is afraid if I leave group I will go back to my behavior." "My life is going well, but I am not sure whether things will stay that way without group." It is important to normalize uncertainty about maintaining sexual health when ending combined individual and group therapy. We often say to group members that the skills for *maintaining change* are different from deciding *to change*. Some group members, when given this distinction between the action stage and maintenance stage, refocus their group treatment goals and remain for a time to develop confidence in their maintenance skills before leaving the group.

Group members often use the departure announcement to revisit feelings and memories of a lifetime of goodbyes. Many previous losses that are associated with grief and sadness (death, divorce, children leaving home, ending military careers, or lost hopes for finding enduring love and companionship) may temporarily move to the forefront for the departing member and within the entire group. Each group member may ponder his own eventual goodbye as he says farewell to the graduating group member. After all, leaving the group is the intended outcome for each group member.

The group response to a departure may reflect the level of attachment and closeness that developed between the group and the departing member.

Leaders can encourage the men to honor the different relationships that exist between each group member by soliciting honest feedback. Leaders can also facilitate an exchange between group members that links their level of investment in the group relationships and the emotions experienced during their farewells.

- "You have been who I have felt closest to in the group. I am going to miss you more than anyone else who has left the group."
- "I know we were not that close, but I learned so much from you as you went through really difficult struggles to maintain your sexual health plan boundaries. I would often think about the consequences you had to endure when I was in a vulnerable emotional place. I don't think I ever told you that, but it was a help to me. Thank you."
- "I remember when you first came to group, you were so judgmental and always had an opinion. I didn't really like you that much. But you also worked hard, I have come to really like you and appreciated all of the times you were so vulnerable and honest about your feelings. You helped me learn that I can change how I feel about somebody that I initially don't like."

The departing member can benefit from taking the time to review his experience with the group-as-a-whole, each individual member, and the leader(s). For men to express their honest feelings toward authority, mentors, or caregivers is traditionally a rare experience. In group, men can express their gratitude or disappointment, which, in previous relationships, was avoided, feared, or went unspoken. The departing member often shares his thoughts about treatment and his observations and feelings about depending on the group leader(s). Saying farewell to the group leader relationship is important, even when the group member will continue individual therapy with the leader. Lastly, be prepared for the departing member to express different things to each coleader. Differentiated feedback is a welcomed expression that allows the client to sincerely reflect on the meaningful yet different impact each leader had on his life and group work.

REFERENCES

Corey, G. (2008). *Theory and practice of group counseling* (7th ed.). Belmont, CA: Thomson Brooks/Cole.

Deonna, J., Rodogno, R., & Teroni, F. (2012). *In defense of shame: The faces of an emotion.* New York, NY: Oxford University Press.

Edmonson, A. C. (2004). Psychological safety, trust, and learning in organizations: A group-level lens. In R. M. Kramer & K. S. Cook (Eds.), *Trust and distrust in organizations: Dilemmas and approaches* (pp. 239–272). New York, NY: Russell Sage Foundation.

Kaufman, G., & Raphael, L. (1996). *Coming out of shame: Transforming gay and lesbian lives* (p. 7). New York, NY: Doubleday.

Linden, M. (2013). How to define, find and classify side effects in psychotherapy: From unwanted events to adverse treatment reactions. *Clinical Psychology & Psychotherapy, 20*(4), 286–296.

Luke, M. (2014). Effective group leader skills. In J. DeLucia-Waack, C. Kalonader, & M. Riva (Eds.), *Handbook of group counseling and psychotherapy* (pp. 107–119). Thousand Oaks, CA: Sage.

Mangione, L., Forti, R., & Iacuzzi, C. M. (2007). Ethics and endings in group psychotherapy: Saying good-bye and saying it well. *International Journal of Group Psychotherapy, 57*(1), 25–40.

Roback, H. (2000). Adverse outcomes in group psychotherapy: Risk factors, prevention, and research directions. *Journal of Psychotherapy Practice and Research, 9,* 113–122.

Wagner, C. C., & Ingersoll, K. S. (2013). *Motivational interviewing in groups.* New York, NY: Guilford Press.

Yalom, I. D. (1995). *The theory and practice of group psychotherapy* (4th Ed.). New York, NY: Basic Books.

CHAPTER ELEVEN

OCSB TREATMENT:
CLINICAL CASE STUDIES

Our overall mission in writing this book was to share our combined individual and group psychotherapy approach for out of control sexual behavior (OCSB) treatment. We began by exploring the current treatment models for OCSB and the evolving definitions of sexual health. We adapted the dual-process theory of human behavior as the conceptualization for problematic and out of control sexual behavior (Loewenstein & O'Donoghue, 2007). Men changing their behavior to live in alignment with sexual health principles and their personal vision of sexual health is the template for treatment planning and to measure treatment outcomes. We explained the OCSB protocol and outlined clinical interventions for the Screening Procedure, Assessment Plan, Unique Clinical Picture, and the sexual health plan. We now weave these components through clinical case examples based on the men we introduced in the opening chapters—Jay, Hector, Frank, and Will.

The case examples focus on specific OCSB interventions implemented over the course of each man's treatment. The many years of sexual conversations in Doug's Sexual Health Group for Gay and Bisexual Men and the two sexual health groups for heterosexual men that Doug and Michael co-led during their San Diego collaboration are imbedded in these clinical narratives. Each client is in group treatment and sees either Doug or Michael or the initial referring therapist for individual therapy. The clinical dialogues offer glimpses into individual psychotherapy interventions, group processes, and sexual health conversations that correspond with each man's Unique Clinical Picture and his respective treatment interventions. The subheadings within each case identify the clinical area that is described within either the assessment, individual therapy, or group therapy session. The clinical dialogues are meant as examples of OCSB treatment intervention options, not "the" prescribed approach.

As you read the final chapter of this book, we invite you to imagine how you might address each man's OCSB Unique Clinical Picture. How would your clinical work address imbalances between the affective and deliberative systems of the mind? What vulnerability factors, regulation issues, or sexual conflicts are central to the psychotherapy dialogue? When is it necessary to elucidate a specific sexual health principle? We encourage you to stay interested in the application of the OCSB protocol elements and remain curious about how you would envision sexual health-based psychotherapy with these men in treatment for OCSB.

JAY

We met Jay in a moment of crisis, while he was waiting for a couple therapy session following his wife, Veronique's, discovery of his secret online sexual activity. Married, with two children under 7 years old, they were not prepared to end their marriage yet were ambivalent about a future together. Veronique was angry, hurt, and disillusioned. She began her own individual therapy and the couple continued working with David. Jay completed the OCSB assessment (see the full Assessment, sexual health plan [SHP], and clinical notes in Chapter 8), entered Michael and Doug's outpatient OCSB group, and chose to continue his individual therapy with Michael.

Motivation for Change: Normalizing Ambivalence

Jay read his sexual health plan at his first group meeting after listening to each current member's introduction. Roger is an 18-month group veteran with 8 years in recovery from alcoholism. He asked Jay to clarify some SHP details.

> ROGER: You mentioned drinking alcohol in your Ambivalence column. Can you say more about that?

> JAY: I am worried about how much my wife and I fight. Sometimes it gets really bad. We are in couple therapy for that. I don't want to stop drinking so Michael suggested that I put "drinking" in the middle column.

> ROGER: I was just wondering whether you were doing something about it. Fred has talked about how he would have never made the progress in his sexual health plan without deciding to stop drinking. He said he never

planned to stop drinking when he started group, but he eventually did. Are you trying to decide whether you are going to stop drinking, is that why it is in your Ambivalence column?

JAY: Well, I am not really sure. I did agree with Michael to monitor it for 3 months and see what I learn. I am not sure how this works with the group, but I know I will be talking with Michael about it.

MICHAEL: Jay, until now you have only talked about your relationship with alcohol with me during the assessment. What is it like to have the group interested in this part of your sexual health plan?

JAY: I guess things get started right away in here. I feel a bit awkward, not sure what to say. I appreciate Roger asking me. Michael told me this might happen, that people would probably have questions about my plan. I'm just not used to talking like this. I did agree with Michael to give it 3 months and see what I learn.

ROGER: So, in 3 months you may have more to tell us?

JAY: Well, yes, I guess so.

SIMON: (*the most recent addition to the group after Jay*) I remember my first night. I was so scared. I didn't know what to expect. So glad you're being honest with us. I remember having to tell the group I pay for sex. I couldn't believe I was talking about that on my first night in the group. I never told anyone that before. It was really hard. So, it's great that you're being honest with us. And it's kind of nice not to be the new guy anymore.

The stage was now set. Jay introduced his ambivalence about changing his relationship with alcohol and invited the group to engage with him in an ongoing conversation about his drinking. Jay and Michael predicted that Jay's contemplative stage of readiness for alcohol abstinence would be a subject of interest, probably from the first group meeting. We focused on a stage-wise intervention that respected his ambivalence and connected him with the other members. Jay was encouraged to share any feelings of shame or embarrassment connected with disclosing his relationship with alcohol. Drawing attention to Jay's emotional response in revealing his ambivalence about his drinking is an attempt to join with other men who can empathize with his competing motivations. Jay continued to have urges to avoid the topic in group, but whenever he chose to honestly share his ambivalence, we affirmed that his choice did not create distance in the group. Talking about a self-discrepant relationship with alcohol is an important moment for any OCSB group member's first session. Jay benefited from the group honoring and welcoming his ambivalence rather than judging or moving to a premature commitment to change.

Attachment Regulation: Honoring Agreements

Later that month in his individual therapy session, Jay told Michael he got drunk watching hockey with some friends and had a heated argument with Veronique afterward. Despite his intoxication, he left before Veronique escalated into uncontrollable rage.

JAY: I don't know what to do. It was such a mess. She was out of control. I know I had been drinking, but not nearly as much as I was before I started seeing you. I followed the safety plan we discussed in the couple therapy. But, I still ended up going online after she went to bed. Now I have to tell her about crossing my boundaries. She is going to just hit the roof.

MICHAEL: What made you decide to be honest with me about what happened?

JAY: I am just tired of living this way. I sat in the parking lot and thought about not telling you that I had been drinking. Then I thought, why did I start group if I was just going to lie to you? So I just said to myself, "Your going to tell him what happened." It felt kind of good to know I could come in and tell you. It just seemed like you would be able to handle it.

MICHAEL: This is the first time you crossed your SHP boundary since you started group.

JAY: I know. I have to tell the group. Roger is going to be all over me because I had been drinking. The whole group is going to focus on that. But I am still more worried about the fighting.

> **MICHAEL:** It sounds like you are going to keep the agreement with the group.
>
> **JAY:** Do I have a choice? I have to tell the group.
>
> **MICHAEL:** Of course, you have a choice. What you disclose is always up to you. Just like you choose to attend a group knowing this commitment; it is your choice to keep it. I'm not at liberty to disclose this to the group. Only you can do that. And, the good news is that it sounds like you are preparing to honor your agreement with the group.

The early phase of OCSB combined treatment often stabilizes client vulnerability factors. Jay's physical safety and his problematic relationship with alcohol needed to be discussed in individual, group, and couple therapy. Michael focused Jay on his choices when he was in a highly activated state. Jay's language revealed his disempowering beliefs about his agency, especially when under duress. Michael slowed down his conversation with Jay to examine "I had to" or "she made me" statements. Jay expressed feeling resentful when Jay perceived that he had no freedom of choice in his marriage and breaking his sexual agreements freed him from his fallacious restraints. Clients discover their specious notions of self-efficacy when we direct them to reflect on their choices during heightened emotional states. For example, we remind clients that they demonstrate a capacity for decision making when disclosing an SHP boundary crossing knowing it will activate intense feelings. In this example, Jay defended against seeing his SHP boundary crossing disclosure as his choice and believed Michael was forcing him to disclose his crossing to the group. This individual therapy dialogue prepared Jay to explore the larger themes of accountability in his marriage (e.g., not honoring his relationship commitments when feeling resentful toward his wife) and the role alcohol played in their conflicts (e.g., not acknowledging how his drinking contributes to the intimate partner violence).

Self-Regulation: Self-Monitoring Defenses

Jay discussed his physical safety, drinking, and SHP boundary crossing at the next group.

> **JAY:** I had a real knock-down-drag-out fight with my wife the other night. I had a couple of drinks

watching the game and we got into this silly argument. I almost threw a beer bottle at the wall, but instead I remembered the safety plan and left the room to calm down. But, I did go online after my wife was asleep and watched porn. I knew I would have to come here and talk about it. I was thinking about you, Roger, and how you would want to talk about my drinking. I don't know, I just felt so upset, but at least I didn't throw things like I used to do.

SIMON: I'm glad you came and told us.

ROGER: Well, as long as you thought I'd ask, I might as well be the one to ask. How much did you drink?

JAY: I had about a six-pack over the whole game. I had a good buzz, but I wasn't as drunk as I would have been before I came into therapy.

ROGER: Well, I guess it was progress that you were at least thinking about how much you drank. Do you think drinking had anything to do with what happened with your wife or going online?

JAY: I don't know, I hadn't really thought about it. It all seems so silly now, like what was all the big deal?

CHRISTOPHER: (*a group member for 9 months, in treatment for online OCSB and generalized anxiety disorder, single, 38 years old, divorced, no children*) What do you mean by "silly"? Isn't this one of the issues in your marriage, how you and your wife get into big fights?

DEAN: (*a group member for 15 months, in treatment for seeking sexual massages and affairs with coworkers, recently divorced, 52 years old, three children*) Yeah, I agree, you make it sound like you're almost making fun of it, like it was funny.

JAY: Well, I don't know, it seems like I just made a big deal out of nothing, seems like sitting here, I wish I could have just realized that she was getting all out of control again and I need to just chill.

DEAN: But, it's not that easy. You had been drinking, and you told us that this situation has been going on for a long time in your marriage. And then, you crossed your sexual health plan that night. And, you're talking about all of this in such a casual way.

DOUG: Jay, what do you hear the group saying to you?

JAY: I am not sure. I thought I did the right thing by coming to group and being honest, but it seems like I am doing something wrong and I am not sure what it is. I'm frustrated. This is what it is like at home. I try to do the right thing and then it just seems I get criticized.

DOUG: Let's slow things down a bit and talk about what is happening in the group. Jay, can you tell us what are you feeling right now? (*A silent moment in the group; Jay appears uncertain of what to say.*)

ROGER: Man, this looks so familiar. I remember when I did what you're doing. Doug would do the same thing. He would stop me and have me talk about what I was feeling. I had no idea other than it bugged the shit out of me. It was like, what do you mean what am I feeling? I would get so flooded with feelings and thoughts, I couldn't even think about how to answer the question. What I did learn was that I was deflecting, I didn't want to look at what I was doing. I just wanted to talk about what everyone else was doing. I thought it was always someone else's fault. When I thought it was someone else's fault, it was almost a sure thing that I would cross my sexual health plan. I would go online and look at sex massage ads. I would start planning my next massage. I would just check out.

MICHAEL: Jay, how are you doing now, can you say anything about what you are feeling?

> JAY: I feel like I screwed up, I don't know. Like I'm not doing this right.

> DOUG: See if you can let go of that judgment and focus on your body. What does your body feel like right now?

> JAY: I feel tense. I don't know why, but I feel kind of afraid right now, like something really bad could happen. When you asked me to talk about what happened, I just felt scared, and kind of mad. I didn't want to talk about me, I wanted to talk about what happened over the weekend.

> DOUG: OK. Tense. Afraid and mad. Those are feelings. Great.

Self-monitoring, as we discuss in Chapter 3, is when a person observes the self by comparing the actual state of the self with his or her standards and expectations (Baumeister & Vohn, 2007). To enhance motivation for change, the group can assist a member by raising his awareness of how an action meets or falls short of his standards. Becoming aware that actions do not match standards may sprout from exploring an uncomfortable interaction. Jay minimized his drinking and subsequent altercation with his wife through his word "silly." Group members evaluated the events differently. This difference in perspective brought conflict and the concomitant feelings stemming from Jay's defenses. Jay's defenses were provoked in response to the group's feedback about their here/now experiences of his contradictory statements. The leaders shifted the group from the content of Jay's situation to here/now process observations. We were interested in developing Jay's nascent emotional awareness when his behavior falls short of his expectations and less interested in the group getting sidetracked in his defensive posture.

Jay needed to learn how to identify and monitor his affect regulation defenses. OCSB groups provide practice in developing monitoring skills when leaders ask men to move between the content of their behavior and the here/now group processes. We invited Jay to describe his feelings in the moment, such as the embodied experience and reaction to his group disclosure. With guidance, Jay let go of his judgment and identified his fear and anger. The here/now group interaction interrupted Jay's "there and then" focus, which had distanced him from his internal feelings. Doug redirected Jay from his misconstrued judgmental thoughts ("screwed up" and "not doing this right") to focus on his immediate embodied feelings. He guided Jay to eventually find his feelings in the moment ("tense," "afraid," and "mad"). This assist served as a useful building block for improving his own capacity for self-monitoring, which is an essential component of activation regulation. In Jay's case, increasing his self-monitoring abilities was an important aspect needed to improve his regulation of alcohol, interrupting the cycle of intimate partner violence, and maintaining his SHP boundaries.

Group members initiating disclosure of an SHP boundary-crossing with the group is an important movement from contemplation to preparation/action stages of change. This level of honesty provides a necessary space for the group to contemplate Jay's sexual behavior with him. We encouraged the men to focus on the value of Jay keeping his group agreement. The group spent time deconstructing the details of Jay's deliberative process leading up to his disclosure. After this debriefing, we invited the group as a whole to describe times they felt closeness and distance during the discussion. The group expressed feeling closer to Jay when he moved away from his automatic defenses to a more vulnerable and embodied awareness.

Vulnerability Factor: A Changing Relationship With Drugs and Alcohol

Jay kept a record of his drinking during his first 3 months of combined treatment. Michael and Jay discussed the frequency of his drinking; the amount consumed; and the effects on his physical safety, relationship with Veronique, and his vision of sexual health. Jay continued to report middle-of-the-night online sexual imagery viewing and masturbation. His Sexual Symptom Assessment Scale (SSAS) score fluctuated between 21 and 33. Elevated SSAS scores correlated with drinking larger quantities. Jay became increasingly conflicted about his relationship with alcohol and his fears about "being an alcoholic." In individual therapy, Michael and Jay contemplated the benefits of Jay scheduling an assessment for entering drug and alcohol treatment. Jay was not ready to take that step. He wanted more time to monitor his drinking.

Over time, Jay began connecting his drinking with feeling anxiety and shame about his sexual behavior. He told the group he drank in his car at the end of the work day before walking into the house to face his wife. Three months of monitoring his relationship with alcohol produced a clear picture about his drinking pattern. In the following group dialogue, Jay acknowledged his dependency on alcohol.

ROGER: I am so glad that you are starting to see that you need help to stop drinking. That was one of the hardest things for me to admit. I had thought alcoholics were derelicts who were weak willed and pitiful. That's not how I thought of myself.

JAY: That's what I thought too. My dad was a drunk. He never got help. He drank until the day he died. I told myself I would never be like him. He was an embarrassment.

CHRISTOPHER: So, what does this mean? You have been pretty sure you could change your drinking on your own. What made you change your mind?

JAY: I was so ashamed that I had once again crossed my sexual health plan even though Veronique and I had actually been getting along better. I was really confused and upset. I told Michael about crossing my boundaries but I couldn't blame it on having a fight with my wife. I don't know what got into me, but I bought a little bottle of scotch and drank it in my car before my appointment with Michael. He could smell the alcohol and asked me about it. I thought about lying, but, well, I... (*Jay pauses, tearing up. The group sits quietly and waits for him to continue.*) I'm sorry. (*His voice trails off.*)

ROGER: Jay, it takes a lot of courage to face the fact that you can't stop drinking on your own. There's nothing to be sorry about. I think you are being really honest with yourself and with us.

DEAN: I agree with Roger. You said when you started the group that you knew your drinking had to be looked at. It sounds like you have been doing that in your sessions with Michael and you have been telling us about your drinking. I don't think you have anything to be ashamed of. When I started group, I wasn't reporting crossing my sexual health plan boundaries. I acted like I was fine, but I felt so sick to my stomach the day I finally told the group, after being here like 2 months. It was such a weight off my back. I was so relieved to be telling the truth.

MICHAEL: Jay, the group seems to have a lot to say to you, what are you hearing?

JAY: I don't know, it's hard to pay attention right now. I am so freaked out I might be an alcoholic. Shit, sorry, but man, I just never thought I would be like him.

DOUG: Who is "him"?

JAY: My dad, I just didn't think I would be a drunk like him.

ROGER: Didn't you say he never got help? You're not like your dad, he never sat in a group and said what you just said to us. You're talking about getting help. You may do something for your kids that your own dad didn't do for you.

By slowing the pace of group feedback and asking Jay to describe his immediate experience, we helped Jay regulate his affect and reflect on the associations that stimulated his emotional reaction. Jay "left the room" and remembered his childhood promise not to be like his alcoholic father. Michael sensed Jay needed guidance to regulate his activation and asked Jay to describe his here/now experience in the room: "What are you hearing?" Michael spoke to Jay's deliberative system during a highly activated moment. Jay may not have retained any of the thoughtful interaction with the group had he remained flooded with emotions. Jay was able to provide a description of his internal experience and regulate his affective system. Finally, Doug asked for Jay to clarify the word "him." Removing the vague pronoun clarified the competing motivations between Jay's promise to himself and his investment in drinking. Ultimately, Jay changed his treatment plan to include an abstinence commitment. He started attending Alcoholics Anonymous (AA) meetings and decided that, if he did not stay sober, he would admit himself into an alcohol treatment program. He made this agreement with Michael, Veronique, and the group and remained sober through his 6-month review.

Physical Safety: The Blame Game

Jay was unsatisfied with his inability to regulate his threatening behavior. He understood that his aggression served a purpose in moments of distress (e.g., to create distance with his wife). With Jay no longer drinking, he was disappointed that he still resorted to threatening his wife.

Jay was practiced at articulating the fine details of his wife's escalating reactivity. He mimicked the sound of her voice, repeated her words and phrases, and explained how she would "push his buttons." He was particularly skilled at fixating on the minutiae of her emotional escalation. Jay was unknowingly maintaining a precontemplative stance about how he responded to his wife's distress. As we often see within groups, precontemplation is evident when a group member is invested in educating the group about the details of his spouse's patterns of reactivity, which serves to deflect the group's attention away from his responsibility in the relationship.

In his individual therapy, Jay explained to Michael how he felt "less of a man" when he "tolerated" Veronique's escalating rage. It occurred to Michael that Jay's masculinity might be challenged by an unspoken belief that a "wife" is more blameworthy for her rage because it transgresses expected female gender roles (see Lamb, 1996). Fixed in his narrative about Veronique's perceived character failure ("She can be such a bitch") or mental illness ("I think she is crazy"), Jay deflected a focus on his contribution to the cocreated relationship dynamics.

Eight months after joining the OCSB group, Jay discussed another incident of escalating rage with the group.

> JAY: It happened again. I lost it with Veronique. She was driving and started telling me how tired she was of having to check the computer to make sure I didn't go online. She was sick of looking at my text messages. She was yelling about how she wasn't sure how long she could put up with this. I couldn't just walk away. We were in the car. So, I did something really stupid. We were at a stop light, waiting for the light to change and I just grabbed the steering wheel

and told her to get out, "I was going to drive." She had that look in her eyes like I knew she was just going to blow up. Cars were all around us. I noticed this other driver staring at us as Veronique raised her voice. She was screaming, "Get out of the car!" So I got out and stood in front of the car so she couldn't drive away. It was a mess. I eventually moved out of the way and she drove off. I called my sponsor and he picked me up and took me home. Veronique was crying and upset. I wouldn't talk to her. I told myself I was not going to cross my sexual health plan boundaries, but I was really hopeless about our marriage. She just keeps exploding like this.

(Jay stops talking and there is a brief pause. It is the kind of moment when the group catches its collective breath.)

SIMON: I am exhausted just listening to you. I don't mean to sound uncaring, but it sounds kind of strange. I hadn't heard this in your stories about your marriage before, but this time, you said she was crying when you got home. Usually you only talk about how angry and mean she gets. It seemed strange for me to picture her crying.

MICHAEL: Can you say more about what seems strange to you about picturing Veronique crying?

SIMON: I don't know, it just seems like all the times he talks about . . .

MICHAEL: *(interrupts Simon)* You can say this directly to Jay.

SIMON: Oh, that's right. Jay, you talk about her like she is a scary monster or something. But, when you said she was crying, it was like seeing her as more of a person. I started wondering what she was crying about.

MICHAEL: Can you say more to Jay about what you have experienced in his stories about this pattern of threatening between he and his wife?

SIMON: Well, I am realizing right now, that I have only seen her as a, well, I hadn't thought of this word before, but like a perpetrator and Jay is like a victim.

CHRISTOPHER: (*interjecting immediately after Simon*) Wow, it's funny you say that, I was having the same experience. I was beginning to think that Jay's story was too simple. I know for me, with my sexual behavior, I would get so mad at being seen as if it was my entire fault; I was the only one who had to change. I was the one who had done all these bad sexual things to hurt people, like I was a perpetrator and they were just passive victims. It's kind of weird, but when I was listening to you just now, Jay, I thought you sounded a bit like my wife. She wanted to blame me for everything that was happening in the marriage because of my sexual behavior. You sounded just like you were blaming Veronique for your behavior. I mean, you stood in front of the car at an intersection! What was that about? Are you blaming her for that?

JAY: I don't know. She pissed me off. And when that guy looked at me and saw my wife was screaming at me . . . I am so tired of all of this. I just didn't know what to do.

SIMON: Did you ever slow down to think that maybe she was scared of you? You keep talking about what you're going through. That is kind of what we keep, or I keep doing. I just keep listening to how hard this is for you. For the first time, I was thinking about how hard this must be for her too. Do you ever think

> about that? Like when you saw her crying.
> You stood in front of the car. She must have
> been really scared of you. Do you ever think
> that what you do is scary?

At this point in the group process, a readiness discrepancy among group members was emerging. Some members felt empathy for Veronique, whereas Jay was not ready to feel empathy toward her. We managed this stage discrepancy by checking in with the precontemplative group member, but we did not block the stage-discrepant group feedback.

> DOUG: Jay, the group seems to be seeing something about
> your situation that is new for them. They seem
> interested in knowing whether you have had
> similar ideas cross your mind. Thoughts about
> how your wife was feeling in response to your
> behavior. Am I hearing the group accurately?

(Group members confirm their earlier statements and the remaining members are open to seeing both Jay and Veronique as feeling scared and anxious. The leaders facilitate this discussion and return to Jay.)

> MICHAEL: How are you doing, Jay? The group had a lot
> come up in response to what you shared.

> JAY: Christopher, when you said I sounded like
> your wife, what did you mean? What did you
> mean by "blame"?

> CHRISTOPHER: Thanks for asking. Well, I just pictured you in
> front of the car, blocking the intersection and
> I was wondering whether you looked at her
> face. I just imagined she must have been pretty
> scared, even if she couldn't show it. You tell
> us you're scared of her, but not about how she
> might have been feeling. You seem to think
> it's her fault that you lost your temper. Maybe
> there's a different way to look at this? You got
> mad and threatened her.

Asking Christopher to elaborate on his feedback was a signal from Jay that he was curious about how he is contributing to the marital conflict. We perceived this as Jay shifting toward a more contemplative stage of readiness to change. Indeed it was. In the ensuing months, Jay was increasingly curious about his blaming defenses and began monitoring his blaming thoughts and judgments. He started to understand Veronique's anxiety and her hostility as a coping mechanism for her fear. Jay's judgmental thoughts toward himself and his wife noticeably decreased in his group discussions. Jay developed an alternative narrative that shifted away from his wife's anger as emasculating to a camouflaged expression of her being afraid of him. This differentiated perspective increased his ability to remain present during his wife's heightened emotionally activated states.

Jay's pattern of escalating threats with his wife diminished as he continued to maintain his sobriety. Each incident was less intense and occurred less frequency. His SSAS scores were routinely below 15 and he was maintaining his sexual health plan as he continued to focus on keeping his agreement to not engage in threatening behavior. He was surprised to find an increased connection with his wife. He enjoyed the day-to-day home life with his family as the hostility with his wife diminished. He felt closer to his children and an unexpected parenting collaboration between he and Veronique emerged. Much to their surprise, it turned out that they made a good parenting team.

Erotic Conflict: Unconventional Turn-On

Unresolved erotic conflicts are a significant source of imbalance between the affective and deliberative systems of the mind. This imbalance is evidenced by client awkward mumbles during the first verbalizations of unconventional sexual interests. Jay often fantasized about having anal sex and feared rejection from each new premarital sexual partner if he revealed his desire. He avoided this disclosure his entire sexual life. Until now Jay's fear of rejection competed with asserting his interest in anal play.

As he maintained his sexual health plan boundaries, remained sober, and changed his pattern of intimate partner violence, Jay began to feel ready to look more honestly at his unspoken sexual desires. He read *Anal Pleasure & Health* (Morin, 2010) and used individual therapy to understand his barriers to talking about anal sex with his wife. Jay recalled his wife's previous passing comments that revealed her belief that anal sex degrades women. Jay (and to a lesser degree, his wife) identified an unspoken worry that his interest in anal sex was an unexamined sexual interest in men. Most of his online sexual imagines were anal sex videos. In his mind, Jay had merged his OCSB with his secret erotic desires.

After a year of OCSB treatment, Jay and Veronique recommitted to their marriage. Veronique had begun her own individual therapy and they continued couple therapy with David. Jay told Michael he felt ready to talk directly with Veronique about his interest in anal sex. His goal was to integrate anal pleasure into his marriage. Jay agreed to first disclose his erotic interest with the group as part of preparation for talking with his wife.

> JAY: I have something I want to bring up tonight that I've been talking about with Michael. Ever since I can remember, I have had a certain sexual interest that I've always kept secret. I like anal sex. It's something that I want to do with any woman I'm sexual with. But, not only as the person who is doing the penetrating. I also like receiving it. That's the really tough part to say. I guess I have always worried about all the judgments that women would make about me. That they would tell their friends and I would get branded a pervert or a guy into strange things. I have only talked with Michael about this up to now, so this is really new to me. I think a big part of my out of control sexual behavior has been that I have always kept this a secret. I always liked it, but I was afraid of my partner's reaction. I want to tell my wife, but I'm really worried that she thinks it's disgusting or won't want to do it. Anyway, I'm thinking about bringing it up in couple counseling and wanted to let you all know before I brought it up.

(The leaders pause, leting the group take in what Jay has discussed.)

> **DOUG:** How are you feeling right now, Jay?
>
> JAY: Well, I'm a little shaky, but I'm glad that I started talking about it.
>
> **DOUG:** What feeling goes with your body feeling shaky?
>
> JAY: I was very nervous before I started, but I'm feeling more relieved; it feels like a weight has been lifted. I knew at some point I was going to talk about this. I felt guilty about talking about it with Michael and not bringing it to group. But, I needed time to get comfortable with it myself.

MICHAEL: Just so we're sure, Jay, what is "it"? The group will need language from you to be clear about what you are referring to.

JAY: I know, I meant that I am relieved that I can talk about my interest in anal sex.

MICHAEL: How did you feel just now saying "anal sex," using those words with the group?

JAY: It was easier than the first time; this is why I wanted to talk about it.... I mean this is why I wanted to talk about anal sex in the group, to practice just making it a more normal part of me. I want to stop feeling so ashamed about it.

DEAN: Exactly, that's what you sounded like you were feeling. You sounded like you feel so much shame about it. I hear the shame in your voice. Even though you were telling us about anal sex, you looked like you were embarrassed to say how much you enjoy it. Especially when you said you like it when you're on the receiving end.

JAY: Well, what's funny about that is I actually never told anyone about that before. Not even Michael. I'm sorry, I didn't mean to spring this on you.

MICHAEL: It was new to me. But, it's your information to share whenever you feel comfortable. How did you decide to say it today?

JAY: I was debating in my head about it all day. But, once I got started, I figured I shouldn't hold anything back.

ROGER: You do look more relaxed, even right now. What was it that made you so ashamed to talk about anal sex with us?

JAY: Well, I thought the group would think I was trying to change my sexual health goals. Like I was trying to go back on my sexual health boundaries or you would judge this as being out of control. That the group would only want to talk about the dangers of getting out of control again. I guess that this would be like seen as my addiction talking.

ROGER: I get it. When I talked with my sponsor about my turn-on with women's panties he immediately thought it was my addict bargaining. He was really adamant that panties could not be part of sexual recovery. It was really tough to sort out. Was I in denial about my addiction or was this part of my sexual health? Sometimes it is not always so clear. But, as long as it was consensual and gave me pleasure, I thought that there wasn't a reason it couldn't be a part of my sex life. And now that I have honestly disclosed this to my wife and I don't hide it or take people's underwear, it's still a turn-on, but it isn't as important as it once was. I don't feel ashamed about it anymore.

In the next few months, the group continued to discuss Jay's disclosure as well as his vision of integrating anal pleasure into his sexual repertoire with his wife in an honest and open way. The group helped Jay distinguish between his shame-based behavior and his vision of sexual health. Anal sex was not the source of his out of control behavior. The tension from keeping sexual secrets, avoiding erotic expression, and the real relational consequences of disclosing his erotic interests all contributed to his out of control online sexual behavior. Jay eventually learned that maintaining his sexual health plan boundaries was linked with an honest and vulnerable exploration of his sexual life with his wife.

Michael coordinated with the couple therapist about Jay's goal to reduce his shame and integrate his erotic identity within his marriage. Ultimately, Jay "came out" to Veronique about his erotic interest. Jay told the group that she was not immediately rejecting, but had some reservations. She thought she might enjoy it from time to time, but did not want their sexual expression restricted only to anal sex. She worried she might feel obligated to have anal sex or that Jay would get frustrated and resume his online sex chatting.

As combined treatment was coming to an end, Jay was enjoying anal pleasure solo and through intercourse with his wife. His arousal and attraction were no longer fraught with the tension and fear that was present prior to treatment. Their unexpected parenting teamwork and differentiation as a couple created a newfound sexual excitement and connection. Jay completed OCSB group therapy a little more than 2 years after his first session. He continued his recovery in AA, reduced his individual therapy to once a monthly, and couple therapy became the primary treatment focus. Jay ended individual OCSB treatment more than 3 years after his initial consultation appointment.

HECTOR

We met Hector the day he disclosed to his outpatient drug and alcohol treatment program that he had contracted gonorrhea from oral sex with an anonymous sex partner he met in a masturbation booth. Earlier that day, his partner, Phil, demanded Hector move out after once again violating their relationship agreement. This event caused Hector to wonder whether he needed help to change his sexual behavior. His rehab counselor suggested that Hector make an appointment with Letty, a bilingual Spanish-speaking outpatient addictions therapist. Letty's first recommendation was a psychiatric medication evaluation for his newly diagnosed generalized anxiety disorder and postraumatic stress disorder (PTSD). Although Hector maintained abstinence from drugs and alcohol, he did not stop his anonymous sex in adult video stores. During their work together, Letty recommended that Hector consider adding an OCSB group to his treatment program. Hector agreed and initiated the assessment process with Doug. Hector agreed to enter the OCSB sexual health group for gay men and fulfill the individual therapy agreement with Letty. Doug spoke several times with Letty and Hector's psychiatrist to coordinate treatment. Hector's work with Letty and his psychiatrist would primarily address his ongoing recovery, anxiety, and trauma-related symptoms. The OCSB group would focus on his sexual health. Doug oriented Letty to the group agreements, structure, and purpose and explained how Hector would agree to disclose his SHP boundary crossings to the group and his individual therapist. Letty confirmed that Hector had been forthcoming about his sexual behavior since beginning individual therapy and that she would reinforce the accountability agreement with the group.

Relationship Agreements: Group Accountability

Before entering the OCSB group, Hector had agreed to a monogamous sexual arrangement with Phil. The OCSB group would be the place where Hector would learn how to be accountable for his sexual behavior agreements. When Hector told the group how difficult it would be for him to keep his sexual boundaries and disclosure agreements, they joined with his struggle by discussing how important it had been for them to keep the OCSB group accountability agreement.

Four weeks later, Hector crossed his SHP boundary, but did not tell the group at his next OCSB group session. He did tell Letty about his boundary crossing and not keeping the group agreement in his next individual therapy appointment. Letty and Hector explored his avoidant defenses with the group, which prepared Hector for disclosing his boundary crossing in the next group.

HECTOR: I am really scared and anxious. I told my therapist I would tell the group that I went to a bookstore a week ago last Friday and had sex with two guys. I knew last session that I was supposed to say that I crossed my boundary, but I just felt so anxious. The longer I waited the worse it got. At some point, I just checked out and didn't really pay that much attention in the group.

BRENT: (*Interrupting; 39-year-old, single, White, gay-identified, HIV-positive man who has been in group for over 2 years and has maintained his SHP boundaries for the past year. He is 3 years into recovery from crystal meth addiction. He has a history of childhood sexual abuse.*) I remember last week looking across the room at you toward the end of group. You looked far away. I thought about saying something, but I didn't quite know what to say. Now it makes sense. You were checked out.

MANISH: (*A 46-year-old, single, South Asian Indian who moved to the United States for work at the age of 27. An out gay man since early 30s, he has never been in a partnered relationship. He has been in the group for 11 months, the past 5 months of which he has maintained his SHP boundaries. He is being treated for bipolar disorder that was diagnosed during his OCSB assessment.*) I agree, you were really quiet last week. I'm really glad you told us. I did the same thing in group when I crossed my boundaries for the first time. I didn't tell the group, but I told Doug in our individual session. I don't know what was worse, crossing the boundary or not telling the group. Do you want to say more about what happened?

HECTOR: I'm not sure where to start. I have never done this before.

DOUG: Hector, you made a really important decision to talk with your therapist about your boundary crossing and prepared to tell the group. We can discuss the details about your sexual boundary crossing later. I think a good place to start is to talk to the group about what you went through last week in the group session. Can you tell us what was going through your mind?

Hector told the group about how tense he felt when he was sitting in the waiting room before last week's group meeting. He had difficulty making eye contact and wished he had waited in the car so he could walk in just as the group was starting. He described how his thoughts went back and forth between telling the group and trying to forget what happened. Hector made a connection between his anxious indecision in the previous group and similar feelings he had after he returns home from having anonymous sex at an adult bookstore. He called it "this mental thing" in which he convinces himself that something he did that he is scared to talk about didn't actually happen.

> **DOUG:** How are you feeling right now? I thought I would just check in with you and have you let the group know what you're feeling.
>
> HECTOR: I am kind of surprised by what Brent said, that he noticed I was checked out. It never occurred to me that someone might notice that. No one has ever said that to me before. I felt kind of relieved when he said it. It made it easier to talk just now about what was going on in my head. I feel strange talking about what I am thinking. Especially to talk about what I am thinking and saying it in English. I mostly think in Spanish.
>
> BRENT: Well, I kind of saw myself when I noticed you staring off. I did that a lot when I first started group. In my therapy with Doug, I learned that I would dissociate when I was feeling too much. My body shuts down when I am flooded with feelings. I decided to asked the group to tell me if I looked dissociated. I didn't know whether you knew about dissociation so I didn't know what to do last week. I avoided looking at you the rest of the group.
>
> HECTOR: Thanks. I do it so much, I am not even aware when I do it.

> **DOUG:** Just so you are clear with the group, what is the "it" that you are not aware of that you would like the group to point out to you?
>
> **HECTOR:** I get really quiet, sit still, and don't make eye contact. Especially not looking. I stared at the carpet a lot last week. I guess I would want someone in the group to ask what is going on to pull me back from being checked out.
>
> **DOUG:** Thanks. What does the group think about Hector's request for help him when he dissociates in group?

Hector's request was an important step forward in improving self-regulation. Over the next few months, the group told him when he looked dissociated. Hector responded by telling the group what he was thinking or feeling. The group was interested in understanding the function of his defensive reactions. Hector noticed a pattern of dissociating during periods of group closeness and intimacy. When group members were sharing honestly and empathizing without judgment, Hector became more aware of an anxiety spike. As he "zoned out," he escaped the group's emotional intensity. His thoughts were about things unrelated to the moment at hand. It was an effective strategy used to regulate his flooding sensations and create distance from the group. Over time, group members shared their childhood histories of chronic sexual abuse, violence in their homes, and rejection for being perceived to be gay as situations in which they developed their dissociation defenses. The group found common ground with Hector by linking their diverse adverse childhood experiences with similar dissociative defenses. The group's interruption of his dissociative pattern increased his self-awareness during heightened emotional states. Hector began to improve his affect tolerance, which helped him stay present in the group. This awareness provided an opportunity for Hector to mindfully choose how to regulate his internal experience and stay connected during periods of emotional activation. It would become an important skill in his relationship with Phil.

We chose to first emphasize the here/now group dynamics when Hector disclosed his failure to keep the group agreement. By first describing his thoughts, feelings, and behaviors when avoiding his commitment to the group, Hector was able to educate the group about his competing motivations in an emotionally present and honest discussion. What was previously unknown to the group could become explicit material for many future group meetings. Bringing Hector's avoidant and fearful defensive behaviors into the here/now increased his awareness of the interpersonal consequences of breaking relationship commitments. Group members dishonoring the SHP disclosure group agreement provides the entire group an experience of being on the receiving end of a broken relationship agreement. This group process is an opportunity for group leaders to identify and build empathy among the men in group for the many people they have wounded through broken sexual agreements.

Physical Health: What Is Your Relationship With HIV?

GIL: (*A 57-year-old, married, White gay-identified male in a 20-year partnered relationship. He has an interest in sex involving urination and other unconventional sexual behaviors. He struggled to integrate this erotic interest into intimate relationships. Recently married, his husband read an online chat history with another man in which Gil tried to arrange a sex date. Gil was attending group to address his relationship erotic conflict, dismissive attachment style, and symptoms related to a previously untreated anxiety disorder.*) I still want to get back to your boundary crossing. I can't remember all the boundaries in your plan. What boundary did you cross?

HECTOR: I had anal sex with two guys. One of them didn't wear a condom. So, I had sex outside my relationship agreement, sex in a public place, and didn't use a condom during anal sex. I crossed three boundaries.

GIL: I think you mentioned that you got an HIV test before starting group. Didn't you say you were getting tested again? I was just wondering, now what are you going to do? Does Phil know this happened?

DOUG: Gil, you asked several questions. I want to slow down a bit here and focus on what you are interested in having Hector respond to first. You talked about Hector's plan to determine his HIV status. You were interested in what his sexual agreement is with his partner. Where do you want Hector to start?

GIL: Well, I guess I was really focusing on your relationship with HIV. I jumped to focus on your relationship with Phil because I always get a bit paranoid when I hear stories like yours. I lied to my husband for so long about everything I was doing sexually. I was really out of control. If he hadn't found my online chat site on my phone, I don't know what it would have taken for me to stop. But, I also remember how important it was for me to start somewhere, and I felt really good about knowing my HIV status. I had just assumed I was positive. When I got tested and then re-tested, I knew for the first time in my entire adult life that I was negative. It was amazing. I had no idea what a burden it was to walk around thinking I was positive, or at least thinking it was inevitable. Between getting my anxiety treated and then knowing I was negative, I felt so relieved. So, here's my question. Since you just put yourself at risk for HIV, is your treatment goal to know your relationship with HIV? How much extra energy are you spending just not knowing whether you're negative or positive?

HECTOR: Wow, I wasn't expecting you to say that. I was expecting you to say that I have to go home tonight and tell Phil. I was ready to argue with you. I mean, we're not having sex right now and I haven't agreed to disclose every boundary crossing right now. I guess I thought I was supposed to put all my attention on him. I was surprised to hear you were thinking about whether I may need some... (*Hector's voice changes, his eyes tear. He stops talking and looks down. The group sits quietly.*)

DOUG: Hector, your voice changed and you looked down. You looked like you were feeling something. I haven't seen you look quite this way before. Can you put words to what is happening for you right now?

HECTOR: I have lived with anxiety my whole life. I was always afraid, always working hard to not show how afraid I was. It never occurred to me that I could talk about being afraid. I am thinking about how hard I worked to not let anyone know what I was going thr... (*Hector begins to cry softly with his head down. He takes a deep breath, looks up momentarily, then experiences a wave of tears and sobs for about 30 seconds. The group sits attentively. Hector looks up again, covers his eyes with his hands.*)

DOUG: How are you feeling? You cried, looked up, and then covered your face.

HECTOR: I don't know, I guess I just felt so sad, then, when I looked up, I thought the group was thinking I was being a crybaby. Like that all happened so long ago and I was just using this as an excuse to cross my boundaries.

ELLIOT: (*A 29-year-old, first-generation Vietnamese American gay-identified male, single, HIV positive. He joined the group 2 months ago. Sexual health concerns involved online sexual behavior, such as meeting men through sexual apps during the workday; missing sleep; and having public sex in bathrooms, parks, and his gym. He wanted to form a long-term partnered relationship. His parents and extended family have a rejecting attitude toward his sexual identity.*) What did you think we were going say?

HECTOR: Like I said, I thought the group would think I was just making excuses, trying to justify what I did.

ELLIOT: I worry about the same thing in the group. I haven't crossed my boundaries. I can't stand the thought of coming to group and having to tell everyone. I worry more about disappointing the group. Like I would be letting everyone down. I didn't think there could be a different reason why someone would fear telling the group about their boundary crossing. I'm positive, so I don't have that worry about becoming positive. Listening to you makes me remember when I didn't know my status. It's been 4 years now, I guess, I'm a little envious of you that you still have a chance to be negative. I didn't have any place like this to talk about worrying if I was positive.

DOUG: (*speaking to Elliot*) It seems like Hector's description of his thoughts and feelings has given you a moment to reflect on your own thoughts about the group agreement and your past and current relationship with HIV.

GIL: So... Hector. Do you still want to know for sure?

HECTOR: Sitting here makes me more upset with myself. It felt good to know that my first test was negative. I just have to start over again, which means I need to get tested again.

The University of California San Diego, Antiviral Research Center (http://avrc.ucsd.edu) provides a free viral load blood test for people who have engaged in behavior that places them at high risk for HIV infection. The test detects the presence of the virus, not antibodies developed in response to an HIV infection. It is part of a study to examine the trajectory of viral growth within newly HIV-infected men and women. To find study participants, they provide testing when someone fits specific criteria for this early form of testing. It has been a useful intervention for men with OCSB to take immediate responsibility for sexual behavior that is high risk for HIV infection and several members of the group have used this free service. They suggested Hector contact the university for a test. They talked about how having access to treatment at the onset of an infection is really important (see Le et al., 2013). Hector left group that night with the goal of clarifying his relationship with HIV.

The group process moved Hector beyond fear of group rejection or judgment. The group deepened their relationship with a new member and prioritized his OCSB vulnerability factor (i.e., physical health). Hector's disrupted vulnerability factor (change in relationship with HIV) was a more significant starting place than prematurely focusing on his self- and attachment regulation deficits.

Self-Regulation: Willpower

Hector wanted to talk about the specifics of his sexual health boundary crossing in the next group. He was feeling more motivated to maintain his sexual health plan and reported having followed his sexual health plan all week.

ELLIOT: (*noticing Hector's quietness; only 30 minutes remained for tonight's group*) I wanted to just check in with you, Hector. You said if we thought you might be dissociating to ask. You've been pretty quiet.

HECTOR: Well, I was just waiting for a pause. As I was listening to Gil talk about having sex with his partner, I was just trying to imagine having sex with Phil again. But, I didn't want to start talking until Gil was done.

GIL: No, I have been talking about this stuff for a while, so I don't have anything that I need to decide tonight. I feel relieved now that my husband and I can talk about kink without it immediately being connected to fears about crossing my boundaries. My husband and I have really come a long way since starting group. But, I'm done.

DOUG: Hector, what you just saw is how the group transitions from one focus to another. One of the tools in being a member of the group is to say either "that's enough" when you feel ready to move on or "I need to talk" or some variation on that. What do you think would have happened if Elliot had not asked you about being quiet?

HECTOR: I'd like to think I would've interrupted and eventually said something. But, as the group kept getting closer to the end, I was getting more anxious about how to start talking. I probably would have waited until there was only a couple of minutes left and maybe mentioned about being disappointed for not speaking up. I would have been pretty hard on myself for waiting so long.

DOUG: What would you like to do now?

HECTOR: Well, I really want to talk about my boundary crossing. It was about 2 weeks ago, on a Friday. I was on my way home from work. Wait, I guess I should back up. I had been chatting on Grindr all day [*a mobile app men use to meet other men for dates or sex*]. I know I'm not supposed to be on Grindr. I feel so bad, that was another boundary I broke. I just realized that now. Man, that's fucked up.

DOUG: Hector, try to set aside your judgments right now and continue telling us what happened without judgment. For right now, see what it is like to describe your behavior and decisions without evaluation or commentary.

HECTOR: OK. I was on Grindr all day. There was this guy I had been messaging on and off for a year. He knew I was into him. He asked to come over, but I said no. I couldn't have anyone at my house. And neither could he. He suggested we meet at the bookstore so I drove there. While I waited, I played around with another guy for a little bit. Eventually he showed up. He told me he wanted to fuck; we never talked about condoms or anything. I was afraid if I said anything about condoms he would just leave. So, we had sex and when he was close to coming I pulled away so he wouldn't cum in me. I had never done that before. Someone in rehab told me that's what he did. I remembered that and gave it a try. He looked a little disappointed. He pulled up his pants and it was over. I went home and felt terrible. I thought about drinking briefly, but didn't want to ruin everything just because of this. After dinner I told Phil I had to go to a meeting. He was in bed when I got home. The next day we kind of just had our usual Saturday. (*Hector stops. Looks around. Looks at the leader.*) What do I do now?

DOUG: Are you asking the group?

HECTOR: I am not sure where to go from here.

(*The group asks for clarification on a couple items. Hector adds how he was chatting on Grindr at work and had downloaded Grindr the day before. He isn't sure why he downloaded the app.*)

HECTOR: I can't believe I forgot this. The day before, my brother, the one who, uh, molested me, sent me a text to remind me about our grandmother's birthday party next month. I didn't know what to do. I had decided to keep some distance from my family, but I hadn't thought about birthday parties and that kind of stuff. I remember I just kind of froze when I read his text. I didn't tell Phil, and, come to think of it, I didn't even tell my therapist.

DOUG: Do you remember what you felt?

HECTOR: I just kind of zoned out. I didn't know what to do. It wore me out to even think about it. I didn't return the text. I just wanted the whole thing to just go away. I did tell my sponsor on Sunday, but I had forgotten about the text before going to the bookstore. It was kind of a blur on Sunday. My sponsor was really focused on what a good job I did staying sober after my brother's text. I didn't want to disappoint him by telling him about hooking up.

(*Group members are curious about Hector not wanting to disappoint his sponsor. They ask how often he was not honest so as to manage what others think about him. Before the group ended this discussion, they invited Hector to evaluate his expectations to internally self-regulate his sexual behavior when he was cruising with his smartphone.*)

MANISH: You keep thinking that you have to have a smartphone with you. I know you charge your phone in another room at night so it is not right next to you in bed. Is there something else you can do to break your habit? It sounds like you just go on autopilot. I remember during periods of mania when my meds were being adjusted, I had to change things. I couldn't do everything the same way. I had to protect myself from some impulsive decisions that could harm me. The group helped me with this. I decided to put a filter on my home computer and I gave the password to my friend. I could have worked around the code, but just knowing my friend knew kept me from that. I knew I needed some external help.

Hector valued his independence and self-reliance and was determined to change sexual behavior patterns. To achieve the latter, he relied on environmental and structural boundaries to avoid situations in which he was not ready to rely on willpower to maintain SHP boundaries. His pattern of inadequate internal regulation when sexually excited led Hector to more honestly evaluate his need for external controls.

Men in OCSB groups often feel ambivalent about implementing environmental controls to keep their sexual health boundaries. Male gender norms commonly link masculinity to self-reliance and a capacity for internal regulation. Men may experience competing motivations between fulfilling their masculine ideal and their personal vision of sexual health. Relying on external controls may evoke feelings like that of a young boy who is learning to ride his bicycle with training wheels and the older boys on the street call them "sissy wheels." OCSB group leaders often hear masculinity narratives that trigger shame and embarrassment and obstruct implementing external controls. Members are encouraged to view external regulation as important energy conservation skills that prevent unnecessary willpower demands that contribute to ego depletion. Reducing unlimited access to sex meet-up apps conserved Hector's energy for managing his anxiety, trauma symptoms, and his daily emotional life with his partner.

Hector listened to group members describe how they came to accept various external controls as part of their early behavior change for establishing their sexual health boundaries. He said he would research buying a temporary cell phone with basic features. To improve his sexual and nonsexual activation regulation he added "daily 10-minute meditation at work" to his Health column. Six months into OCSB group treatment, he was maintaining his self-implemented recovery program through AA, treating his anxiety and PTSD with medication and individual psychotherapy. Hector also, for the first time in his life, knew for certain he was HIV negative. A group member also suggested he talk with his doctor about PrEP (pre-exposure prophylaxis). Hector agreed to consider taking PrEP as an added measure to prevent HIV infection and possibly infecting his partner. He wanted to talk with his partner about PrEP and agreed he would initiate discussions about future SHP boundary crossings. Hector and Phil began to meet with a therapist who specializes in working with male couples.

Attachment Regulation: Attachment-Related Avoidance

As Hector's self-regulation capacity improved and he treated his OCSB vulnerability factors, his avoidant attachment style moved to the forefront of his group psychotherapy. Despite engendering warm group relationships and continued positive feedback about his sexual behavior changes, Hector's group relationships vacillated between too distant (passive quiet observing) or too close (anxiety, fear, withdrawal, dissociation).

Doug phoned Hector's therapists to discuss the emerging group attachment pattern to see whether similar patterns were present in his individual and couple therapy. His individual therapist described how Hector had begun to link his avoidant patterns with his history of sibling incest, family violence, and immigration trauma. All therapists agreed on a clinical focus to develop more secure attachment skills in Hector's current relationships. In group, we used here/now group interactions for Hector to improve his insight into his defenses and emotion regulation patterns associated with his adverse childhood experiences. Could Hector develop more secure attachment patterns as he learned to observe his trauma-related interpersonal patterns? The group provided an experimental space for Hector to learn and practice interpersonal skills that he could bring to his relationships with his partner, friends, and recovery community.

When the following dialogue occurred, Hector had completed his first year of OCSB group. He had continuously maintained his SHP boundaries for the past 3 months and was approaching 2 years of alcohol sobriety. His anxiety symptoms had reduced and he continued his anxiety medications, regular meditation, and body-focused relaxation tools. Despite this progress, Hector had sex three times with a man he met online and did not tell the group, Phil, or any of his therapists. After his third boundary crossing, he decided to tell the group. This return to early treatment behavior and his passive avoidance in maintaining relational agreements greatly interested the group.

BRENT: So, I want to make sure I have this straight. You came to group the last few weeks and had crossed your boundaries and didn't tell us?

HECTOR: I wanted to, I sat here and thought about it. After all this time in the group and doing so well for the last few months, I just didn't want to deal with what happened. I know it sounds strange, but I can't believe I did it either.

DOUG: What part of your behavior do you find hard to believe?

HECTOR: Well, I guess, I found it hard to believe that after all this time, I would come to group and not disclose a boundary crossing. I have been doing this a while. I didn't think about drinking and I really wasn't all that interested in the sex. In fact, it was kind of boring. I don't know, it just doesn't make sense.

DOUG: You told the group a few months back that you were working through some of the past traumatic events in individual therapy. You have been intentionally looking at the consequences of being raped by your brother, witnessing your father assault your mother, and how your mother fled from Mexico to the United States with you to escape your father. Rather than be surprised by your not keeping the agreement with the group, what if you thought about this behavior as having something to do with the trauma work you are doing?

HECTOR: I am not sure what you mean.

DOUG: Does anyone in the group have any thoughts about my invitation to Hector? What might I be inviting him to think about?

BRENT: I guess that's why I was so interested in making sure I was clear about your story. I totally understand. One of the things I learned how to do when I came home after we did it again was to not say anything.

DOUG: After "we did what," Brent?

BRENT: I know, I need to say it. After my brother had sex with me, I had to pretend like nothing happened. There were times I came home and I thought for sure my parents would know, but they all acted like nothing happened. Sometimes I wanted to scream, "How can you not tell what just happened?" But, I learned in therapy that I was really good at acting like I was fine. It took me a while to realize how good I still am at this. I've had to learn how to let people know what I am feeling. So maybe Doug is wondering whether what you did with us is sort of like what you did when you were a kid?

ELLIOT: I had no idea you had broken your boundaries the last few weeks. I am kind of shocked that you hid it so well. I am glad you told us now, but I really get a sense of how good you are at this.

DOUG: Elliot, what is it that Hector might be really good at, just so you are being clear with the group?

ELLIOT: Well, I mean your ability to be feeling something inside and not show it on the outside, especially with people who know you pretty well.

HECTOR: I really did want to tell you. I didn't want to break the group rules. I was so upset when I didn't say anything the last two groups.

DOUG: Did you ever have a time when you really wanted to tell your Mom what your brother was doing to you?

HECTOR: (*Sits quietly. A familiar faraway look appears on his face.*)

GIL: Did you just go away? You looked like you just checked out.

HECTOR: (*remaining quiet for a few more seconds*) I was remembering one day, it was the last time it happened. I told him I was not going to do it again. That was it. He made his usual threat about keeping it a secret; he had always told me that Mom would throw us out if she knew.

LOUIS: (*Joined the group 7 months after Hector, 44 years old, second-generation Mexican American; in a 6-year relationship that* *ended when his partner discovered his online sexual behavior. Louis had infected his partner with syphilis, which he contracted by using crystal meth and meeting anonymous men for sex.*) I had the same fear growing up. I assumed I would be kicked out if my dad ever found out I was gay. Funny though, I didn't think my Mom would kick me out, but my Dad was in charge. He was like my grandfather, he would yell "pinche joto" at the TV when news stories about AIDS came on. That would be like someone saying "fucking faggots" in English. But, I wasn't molested like you were, Hector. I didn't have to worry about covering that up on top of being gay.

DOUG: Tell us more, Hector. What were you remembering just now?

HECTOR: That is what my brother called me right after he was done. He would push me away, kind of with this look of hate in his eyes. He said it every time. "Punte joto," then he wouldn't say another word. He just got up and left. Later, when I would see him in the house it was like nothing happened. So, when Louis said the same words, I was just flooded with feelings. I never told my mom because she would think I was just a faggot. She wouldn't care. Like I would not be her son anymore, I would just be a faggot. Like all the other faggots. (*He paused, his eyes rested on Louis, they share a knowing glance and smile. He took a deep breath and an emotional wave came over him. He sobbed, placing his head in his hands. The group sat quietly. Doug scanned the room.*)

DOUG: Hector, can you take some deep soothing breaths? (*On the last of several deep breaths, Hector looks up at the group. He glances around looking for tissues. A group member hands him the tissue box and he blows his nose. He takes several more breaths. Then much to his surprise, he begins to cry again. He looks a bit startled.*)

DOUG: It's OK; just let your body feel what it needs to feel. Remember, you can stop at any time.

(*Hector's tears flow, the group remains attentive.*)

HECTOR: I haven't cried like that since I was in rehab. I don't think I ever really felt that before.

MANISH: What were you feeling that made you cry so much? I know what it was like when I cried like that one night in group, but what were you feeling?

HECTOR: I just really felt how awful he was to me. He had a look of hate in his eyes. I never really felt that before. How could he hate me that much and be my brother? I felt really scared and hurt and confused. Then I remembered he left his cum on me. I always had to clean up after him. It made me sick. I always had to go clean up before I could go back to the family. That's what I remembered when I cried again. I thought that was really sad. I saw me at 14 trying to clean his cum off of me and then acting like nothing happened.

DOUG: Perhaps this is what you wanted the group to learn about you? How well you did this. How skilled you were at hiding really painful experiences from people you were close to, even loved. Because even if they loved you, if they learned about this "disgusting" part of you—joto, faggot, or gay—that no matter how much you felt love for them, they could just discard you.

HECTOR: Exactly, it wasn't until I was 16 that I realized my brother just said that to keep me quiet, to control me. When I figured out my mom wouldn't throw me out because I was gay, then I knew I didn't have to do it anymore. I am not sure exactly how it happened, but it turned out that that was the last time. We never spoke about it, and he never tried to make me do it again. (*pauses*) I'm not sure about all this; it kind of over-whelms me to think about it right now.

DOUG: That's good you know that. You don't need to do any-thing with that thought right now. You just released a lot of emotional energy. Want to take a break or continue?

The group learned how Hector brought his trauma symptoms to the group through his actions before he could tell them with his words. He unwittingly demonstrated to the group his defense for hiding pain, dis-tress, and conflict. As a new group member, when Hector did not keep the group agreement, he was avoiding the uncomfortable emotional consequences of disclosing his SHP boundary crossing (e.g., shame and anxiety). A year later, violating the agreement served a different function. He was unintentionally recreating a familiar emotional tension related to his childhood sexual abuse. Doug was not distracted by the perception that Hector's sexual behavior indicated a treatment failure or relapse. He remained curious about the contradiction in Hector's behavior. Why was Hector so distressed when he has been through similar group agreement violations before? Hector told the group that he actually wanted to honor the agreement and was conflicted about not keeping the agreement. Hector's distress was from *not connecting* rather than the anticipated distress of actually connecting. He was ready to be seen by others. However, that desire competed against his primary coping strategy: remain on the periphery to avoid being seen. As a child, his passive stance functioned to preserve the attachment with his mother. He did not make a scene, disappearing during tense moments between his parents, and never disclosed the sexual assaults. The childhood solution of withholding information and relational passivity minimized the threat of rejection for being gay or being accused of instigating the sibling incest. By remaining curious and empathetic, the group provided an opportunity to reveal the underlying trauma defenses that contributed to his withholding behaviors.

In the succeeding months, Hector developed greater compassion for himself when he understood his behavioral contradictions through the additional lens of his childhood trauma (mental health vulnerability factor). Rather than unintentionally stay on the periphery, Hector mindfully chose how to manage his interpersonal insecurities in group. He was honest about his sexual behavior with the group, his therapists, and his partner. He began to assert himself by requesting group time. When he felt hurt in response to something that happened in the group, he expressed it. When Hector was open and honest with the group, it reflected his newfound motivation to be seen and known by the other members. He had learned that his fears about the group's rejection were unfounded. He routinely reached out to his therapist and husband despite his anticipatory anxiety of being negatively judged. He followed the boundaries of his sexual health plan for a year before leaving group, 2½ years after he first attended. After leaving group, he continued his individual therapy, AA program, and couple therapy.

His group departure was his first goodbye with people who really knew Hector. His goodbye proved to be another trauma-processing point. He never said goodbye to his father. When Hector was age 12, his mother fled with her two children to the United States. During one of his last OCSB groups, Hector emotionally processed his unsaid goodbye to his father, which was prompted by his intentional farewell to the group. Hector's vulnerability was a generous gift that touched everyone.

FRANK

Frank was caught. His boss told him to stop looking at online sex sites at work or he would be fired. Humiliated by the ultimatum, he turned to his psychiatrist for help. His medication helped with his anxiety, but it didn't change his out of control sexual experiences. Frank felt disappointed when his psychiatrist suggested OCSB outpatient therapy rather than simply changing his medication. Although hesitant to call Doug, Frank was invested in keeping his job.

Self-Regulation: Monitoring

Each assessment appointment began with Frank taking his seat, sighing heavily, and silently gazing out the window. He would scrunch his nose, constrict the muscles around his mouth, and slightly curl his lip. His face relaxed as soon as he made eye contact with Doug. Frank's facial expression of disgust appeared to be an automatic behavior that dissipated when he looked at Doug. In the first three assessment sessions, Doug observed this pattern without comment. He wanted to collect more information and establish rapport before discussing his observation. When Frank described his online sexual behavior, the familiar nose scrunch immediately appeared. At times, the intensity of Frank's disgust seemed to merge with his anger and self-contempt about his lifelong struggle with anxiety. His throat clenched and his neck muscles tightened. This state subsided when he stopped discussing his anxiety and became immersed in detailed stories about his behavior.

The process for building Frank's monitoring capacity as part of improving his self-regulation began during the fourth assessment appointment. Frank sat down as usual and paused briefly for what Doug now privately thought of as Frank's "self-disgust pause."

> DOUG: Frank, I want to start the appointment a bit differently today. I want to first start by talking about something I have observed in our appointments. Remember I said that part of the assessment would be completing

a range of measures and that we would also prepare you for entering group treatment? Part of group and individual therapy involves discussing experiences that happen between us during a session or between members of the group. Do you remember us talking about this?

FRANK: (*with a smirk on his face*) Yes.

DOUG: I notice at times you get a look on your face that I am not sure you are aware of. Your nose scrunches up a bit, your lip curls up, and sometimes even your neck looks tense. It looks like the kind of face a person makes when he smells something really awful. (*Doug makes the face.*) It looks a little like this. I was wondering whether you are aware when you have this look on your face. I can't tell if you are.

FRANK: You look like my Mom. (*laughing and smiling*)

DOUG: Can you say more?

FRANK: That's how my mom looked all the time. When she was mad or upset at one of us kids, or my dad did something to piss her off, she would get what we called "the look" and you knew to get out of her way. She didn't have to say anything. She could just be stone silent, look over at you, and give you that look.

DOUG: So, I am interested in talking with you about when your face may look a bit like that. I have noticed that there are times you have a look similar to what you just described. You may not look as intense as your mom was when you were a child, but I would like to talk more openly with you when I notice this look on your face. Can you tell me what you're feeling when your face has "the look"?

FRANK: Well, it seems strange to be talking about this. I am not really sure what is going on with me. Sometimes I just talk about myself in here and I think I can't believe my life has come to this. I got anxiety. I looked at porn at work and could lose my job. I'm single and now I have to take meds for anxiety and be in a group with a bunch of wackjobs like myself. Is that what you're wondering? I think about this all the time. I just can't believe things got this bad.

DOUG: Well, you said a lot, but yes, this is what I am interested in talking about when I see that look on your face. You told me what you think, what goes through your mind and the judgments you have toward yourself. What emotions or feelings do you have when you're thinking like this?

FRANK: Well, I guess I am just sick of myself. It just seems so pathetic. Is "pathetic" a feeling? (*His nose scrunches, his lip curls.*)

DOUG: Just now, did you notice how your face changed? Your nose scrunched, your lips curled. What are you feeling right now?

FRANK: Hmmm, well, I don't know, I get so sick of this. It's like something isn't right and I can't stand it.

DOUG: OK, I didn't want to assume you had language for this feeling. Most of the men who begin therapy for out of control sexual behavior do not have language for what they are feeling. When I see this on your face, you look like you're feeling disgusted. For many people, disgust is expressed in the face when the nose scrunches up and the eyes get a little more closed, the mouth gets tense, lips may curl up. It is a pretty universal face. We don't really have to think about it, our face knows how to do this. Perhaps you feel disgust? You may not be aware that you are feeling it or aware that your face is showing disgust. Knowing when you are feeling disgust might be important for understanding and changing your sexual behavior. That's why I wanted to establish that we would talk about it together in both individual and group therapy.

It is not uncommon to find a subset of men in OCSB treatment that has high disgust sensitivity or low disgust tolerance. Disgust is a feeling of strong aversion to an object or situation that motivates the individual to avoid the stimulus. This is different from sexual excitement, which motivates one to approach the stimulus. Tybur, Lieberman, and Griskevicius (2009) propose three domains of disgust that "evolved to motivate behavioral solutions to multiple distinct problems" (p. 105): (1) *Pathogen disgust* evolved to prevent contact and ingestion of pathogens. (2) *Sexual disgust* developed to avoid sex partners or behaviors that jeopardize reproductive success. (3) Finally, *moral disgust* moves people to avoid those who inflict a social cost to oneself or others in one's social network. Sexual activity can elicit disgust in all three domains, not just the second. Pathogen disgust is elicited by stimuli likely to contain infectious agents (e.g., bodily substances: blood, mucus, feces, vomit, urine, and semen) and relies on sensory cues (e.g., foul odors, distaste, and visual associations). Dynamics that elicit moral disgust pertain to broad social transgressions, including behaviors seen as non-normative or antisocial. Sexual experiences may intentionally or unintentionally involve all aforementioned bodily substances or involve unconventional sexual thoughts, urges, and behaviors that are contrary to one's moral upbringing in a manner that is repellent to the individual (Tybur et al., 2009).

The language of men's disgust appears in words or phrases that allude to physical illness or distaste when describing their sexual behaviors: "It was gross." "I'm so sick for thinking like this." "It made me nauseous." How one generates disgust influences one's sexual choices and behaviors. Disgust has been identified as a sexual arousal inhibitor (Koukounas & McCabe, 1997; Vonderheide & Mosher, 1988) and sexual thoughts, urges, and behaviors may elicit any combination of pathogen, sexual, or moral disgust. Commonly, people minimize their exposure to disgust-triggering objects or situations when wanting to maximize sexual pleasure-inducing activities. A troublesome bind develops when one's disgust overlaps with one's sexual object. Similar to shame defenses, regulating disgust by avoiding sexual triggers restricts the range of available pleasurable sexual activities. Because disgust inhibits against another formidable drive, men with OCSB may have developed remedies that defend against their disgust while at the same time engaging in pleasurable sexual activity. This persistent tension between disgust sensitivity and sexual drive is a situation that *feels* out of a man's control and his solution may be the sexual behavioral symptoms whose consequences motivated him for OCSB treatment.

Frank complained about his pattern of losing sexual desire and attraction with his romantic partners. Although not an uncommon development for long-term intimate relationships, Frank's dilemma did not revolve around more common themes of sexual boredom or domestic time constraints that befuddle many long-term couples. Frank described painful, stomach-clenching experiences that obstructed his earnest wish to have pleasurable and connected sex. He made statements like, "It just grosses me out when I think about going down on her" and "even though she has a beautiful body, I can't get aroused." Frank wanted his long-term relationships to include regular, satisfying sex, but his sexual revulsion eventually replaced his limerant lust. To his frustration and bewilderment, his sexual drive persisted. He masturbated, watched sexual videos and, which precipitated his crisis, paid for sex. It was a curious contradiction. He wanted sexual satisfaction with a long-term partner, he had an intact sex drive, and was sexually active with himself and sex workers, but not with his partner.

Through continued dialogue, Frank's sexual pattern emerged over the course of therapy. He learned that he felt disgusted by bodily substances expelled through urination, defecation, and menstruation. As is common with cohabiting relationships, he was exposed to the bathroom habits and menstruation cycles of his partners. Once that human dimension was added, his disgust started competing with his sexual desire. He lost his ability to objectify his partner, to access his lusty self once he experienced a pathogenic disgust with her. Unaware of this bind, his unintentional solution was to restrict his sexual pursuits to "clean" erotic objects. In other words, women whom he did not know and who had yet to elicit his pathogenic disgust reaction. Paying for sex allowed him to maintain an illusion of cleanliness and defend against his disgust. He was sexual with women whom he did not know or with whom he did not share a living space and found a way to enjoy his sexual expression without the intrusion of disgust.

Sexual Health Principles: Nonexploitation

Frank was in the process of completing his sexual health plan and discussing his ambivalence about including "no paying for sex" on his sexual health plan.

> FRANK: I know I should put "no paying for sex" in my Boundaries column. What is the group going to say to me when I say I want to stop going online at work, but I can still pay for sex? What do you think?

> DOUG: You sound anxious about your decision. How about we focus on how you feel first and then talk about your health plan and the groups response?

(Frank takes some breaths and closes his eyes for minute.)

DOUG: What is going through your mind now that you have taken a moment to regulate your anxiety?

FRANK: Well, I was picturing the guys rolling their eyes, shaking their heads, thinking that I don't know what I am talking about.

DOUG: What do you imagine that group members will be feeling when they behave this way?

FRANK: Funny, I knew you were going to ask that. I think they will look like me when I feel disgusted. They will look at me and feel disgusted that I still want to pay for sex.

DOUG: I am not proposing you prepare for any particular group response to your plan, but I am wondering what it is like for you sitting here and imagining being on the receiving end of group members' disgust?

FRANK: It's not like I haven't lived with this my whole life, but I guess I was imagining the guys in the group would be less judgmental, that I wouldn't have to deal with the stuff I had to deal with growing up. My mom was always looking at me with "that look."

DOUG: What is it that you want the group to know about your motivation for paying for sex? We have talked about this, so what do you want them to know?

FRANK: Well, I have not really ever felt disgust or really much conflict in paying for sex. I have done it for so long, the women seem to enjoy being with me. I really like their company. I can afford it. I like being with women who like sex. It just seems like two adults making a decision. It has not been out of control. I only pay for sex about six times a year, usually with the same few women. It's only when I think about telling others about it that I get so anxious. I learned in the assessment that one of the sources of my anxiety is anticipating disapproval, judgment, and disgust. I guess I imagine the group thinking there must be something suspicious about me because I am not conflicted about paying for sex.

DOUG: It looks like your sexual health plan will be a good opportunity for you to start being honest with the group instead of avoiding them because you are imagining their disapproval. What do you want the group to know about your decision to put "paying for sex" in the sexual health plan Ambivalence column?

FRANK: Well, like we talked about before, I have not really given much thought to the part about paying for sex being exploitive. That was a whole new concept for me to think about. It is different to think about paying for sex as exploitive rather than just wrong or illegal or disgusting. I really want to talk to the group more about this idea. I am not convinced paying for sex is necessarily exploitive, but I still want to talk about it.

The purpose of this sexual health conversation was to understand Frank's anticipatory anxiety, which competed with his motivations for considering a "no paying for sex" sexual health plan boundary. The focus of this assessment discussion was Frank's discrepancy, not the group's or Doug's conflict about the behavior. Frank agreed with nonexploitation as a sexual health principle and was open to evaluating his behavior for exploitation. He was not ready to stop paying for sex, nor was he interested in changing his behavior simply to avoid disapproval and judgment. It was a new sexual health priority for Frank to be honest about his sexual activity even though the group might hold different opinions and attitudes about paying for sex. Frank was practicing being open and honest about his sexual desires as well as preparing to engage in a values discussion to explore his curiosity about how sexual exploitation manifests in his erotic life.

Attachment Regulation: Sexual Narcissism

OCSB therapy provided a safe, informed, and respectful space for Frank to determine the compatibility of paid sex with his personal vision of sexual health. The group was less reactive to his ambivalence about paying for sex than Frank anticipated. It was important for the group to know Frank was interested in whether paid sex met his expectation for nonexploitive sex. As a result, Frank was encouraged to remain honest and open with the group about his paid sexual activity. Group members suspended their negative judgments about paid sex and allowed Frank the space to clarify his sexual values. It also created the conditions necessary to process another dimension of Frank's Unique Clinical Picture that was influenced by his sexual choices.

SIMON: (*coughing*) Well, I just wanted the group to know I that I'm getting over a cold. I may cough a bit tonight.

FRANK: (*Sitting in the seat next to Simon, Frank stands up quickly. He looks around, but immediately sits down again.*) Why did you come to group? You could infect us.

ROGER: Wow, that was a little rough.

FRANK: What do you mean? When someone in the group is sick shouldn't they just stay home? Do you think he should be able to come here when he is sick?

MICHAEL: Frank, before we answer your questions, can we back up a moment?, What happened after Simon said he had a cold? You stood up.

FRANK: Well, I don't want to catch his cold and here I am sitting right next to him. I stood up to change seats, but there's nowhere else to sit. Can I change spots?

MICHAEL: Pay attention to your body, and tell us what is happening?

FRANK: I can't right now, I'm mad, I don't want to get sick.

DOUG: Simon, how are you doing right now?

SIMON: I'm surprised. I didn't think having a cold would make people so upset. I washed my hands before group.

DOUG: Can you describe to Frank what you felt when he reacted to what you said?

SIMON: Well, I already said I was surprised, but even more I guess I felt angry and a bit hurt. It seemed he . . .

DOUG: You can talk directly with Frank.

SIMON: Well, (*turning to look at Frank as he speaks*) it just seemed like you were concerned about yourself and you didn't think about how I was feeling. It just seemed like everything became about you.

(*The group is quiet, the leaders let the process between Simon and Frank unfold. Frank continues expressing his displeasure. The other group members offer their feedback, which is consistent with Simon's.*)

MICHAEL: How familiar is the group's feedback?

FRANK: I've heard that before. It's funny. My ex-wife always said I had a way of making things about me. I get now what she meant. I didn't really understand or really care at the time; it just made me anxious to hear it.

MICHAEL: What is the "it" Frank?

FRANK: I don't think it's all that important how someone else feels when I am anxious or upset. When Simon ... when you said that you had a cold, I just got so nervous about getting sick that it never occurred to me to think about how you feel. In fact, I was annoyed with Doug when he asked you to tell me how you felt. (*Frank pauses, puts his chin toward his chest, looks far away, then quickly looks up, yet he seems unaware he has just gone into his thoughts.*)

MICHAEL: Frank, where did you just go now in your mind? It looked like you may have had a thought that took your mind away for a brief moment.

FRANK: I was just thinking about one of the reasons I like to pay for sex. I like just showing up and not having to think about what she is feeling, what her day is like. I like the attention on me. When Simon said, "it just seemed liked everything was about me," I can actually remember times looking forward to meeting up with a woman and I would feel more relaxed knowing that I wasn't going to have to think so much about her to have sex. It's kind of a relief for me, I like it.

DOUG: Can you say more about how you felt annoyed when I asked Simon about his feelings?

FRANK: I don't know what else to say, I just felt mad, like why are you so concerned about how he feels? He didn't seem to think very much about how I would feel.

CHRISTOPHER: Isn't that just like what you said you liked about paying for sex? You don't like to think about how someone else feels. Maybe the women you pay to have sex with feel like you just did? I know I had to look at this when I began to think about my online sex and looking at porn. I just didn't want to think about how others may feel about what I was doing. Maybe they get tired of it always being about you.

DEAN: Exactly. When I was paying for sexual massages, I never had to think about her or what she was feeling. I began to see that she was really good at playing a role, making it all about me, but I got used to this. Even the affairs I had, when the woman became too needy, I wanted out. It has been a real eye-opener to me to see how little I would think about my sex partners and what they felt.

MICHAEL: Frank, what are you hearing from the group right now?

FRANK: I'm not sure; I guess I am not the only one who likes sex without having to think about what the other person feels or what's going on with her. I know I wanted to learn more about exploitation as part of paying for sex. Is this part of that?

DOUG: Great question, Frank. Before we discuss that, I want to get back with you about your request to change chairs.

FRANK: No, it's OK, I am fine with sitting here. I just needed to calm down a bit.

A range of personality patterns are common among men in treatment for OCSB. Personality traits are specifically addressed in two areas within the OCSB Unique Clinical Picture. The mental health vulnerability factor includes screening for personality disorders and integrating their treatment throughout the combined OCSB treatment model. Second, in the attachment clinical area, sexual narcissism is assessed as a potential contributing factor in both group and individual treatment. McNulty and Widman (2013) study narcissistic personality patterns as a factor in lower sexual relationship satisfaction and their research suggests that people's elevated sense of entitlement, tendency toward exploiting others, lack of empathy, and a grandiose confidence in sexual prowess are associated with decreased relationship satisfaction. OCSB treatment examines the role of situation-specific narcissistic traits that are activated in client's sexual relationships or activities. It is important for men to understand how narcissistic traits can influence their out of control sexual experiences in general and the role of sexual narcissism domain traits in particular.

After hearing themes of low empathy in his relationship history and witnessing entitled behavior in the therapeutic setting, we were curious about whether sexual narcissism was a factor in Frank's OCSB. Treating narcissistic tendencies is complex, slow work, especially when trying to form an alliance with the client without fatally triggering his hostility and relationship-severing defenses. Our approach with Frank was to establish a therapeutic alliance in which he could hear feedback about his behavior. We then waited for him to display a narcissistic trait during group. We invited his curiosity with here/now interventions to introduce common themes within sexual narcissism. His low empathy response to Simon's cold was an access point for the group to explore his narcissism.

Frank's empathic gaps in sexual situations meant he had one less restrictive system among his competing motivations and sexual health behavior. Frank felt impatient when sexually excited. He thought he should not invest the time and energy needed to cultivate a relationship with a woman who may or may not want to have sex him. Paid sex allowed him to bypass his social anxiety and rejection fears in a sexual relationship in which the partner was focused exclusively on his needs. Over time, Frank's awareness of his limited capacity to understand the internal world of his sexual partners increased his ambivalence with paid sex. Was paid sex keeping him from learning how to consider a sex partner's emotional well-being or pleasure?

Frank experienced increased self-discrepancy with paid sex as he was more honest about his motivations. To re-enter a long-term intimate relationship, he believed it was important to find relational solutions to his low empathy, disgust–lust bind, and social anxiety. Paying for sex allowed him to avoid the relational opportunities he needed to stretch his empathy capacity, improve his sexual satisfaction with romantic partners, and remain emotionally present during anxious states. After more than a year in the group, Frank decided to move paid sex to his Boundary column.

Frank began to see how he chose isolation and loneliness as a strategy for living with his anger, disgust, and, at times, contemptuous feelings. He observed how anxious he was about people being exposed to his hostility and began to self-monitor this hostility when he felt it in group. He listened to the men describe their experiences of him after he directed his impatient wrath at someone in the group. This feedback triggered high anxiety for Frank. Gradually, he expressed interest in the idea that he might have paid for sex to avoid the consequences of interpersonal limitations.

The group was a place where Frank learned to regulate his anxious feelings and stay present when group members were sharing. The group frequently provided feedback whenever he turned the conversation away from an emotional process, which usually meant something intellectualized or advice focused. When Frank decided to try online dating, the group gave him suggestions on how to practice being interested in his partner's emotions. As leaders, we drew attention to here/now behaviors that demonstrated Frank's emotional concern for another member's well-being. After low-empathy or entitled interactions, we commonly asked the group, "Are you feeling closer to Frank now, or more distant?" These moments helped Frank observe his contribution to relationship conflicts and stretch into new interaction patterns.

His distancing interactions and anxiety management remained a focus of Frank's ongoing individual therapy. He had not crossed his sexual health plan boundary at work for over a year. He had not paid for sex since he moved this to the Boundary column of his sexual health plan. Feeling confident in regulating his sexual behavior, he decided to end his group work. Frank knew expanding his interpersonal skills and improving his disgust tolerance would be a slow, prolonged focus. The group was disappointed that Frank chose to not continue group therapy to further address his interpersonal patterns associated with his sexual narcissism and openly expressed their disappointment. Frank was satisfied that he had stopped his online workplace sexual behavior, paying for sex, and begun anxiety management. The group was faced with balancing Frank's treatment gains with their disappointment that he chose not to engage the group in treatment beyond resolving his OCSB. Frank left group after 18 months.

WILL

Will's wife divorced him after finding out she acquired a syphilis infection from him. He was sure this would be enough to get him to change his sexual behavior. He also thought his anonymous online hookups with men would stop after he came out. He was an attractive, newly single, gay Black man in his twenties. Will soon learned he could have as much sex with men as he wanted and divided his work day between processing insurance claims and checking mobile sex and dating apps. He met men for quick sex during lunch breaks. He had sex with men on his way home from work or the gym. Much to his disappointment, most of the men he encountered wanted a "black top." Sometimes, after a night out drinking, Will would "let a guy top him." Will wasn't interested in using condoms. He would only wear one if the other guy insisted. He knew guys taking HIV medications were likely undetectable and posed little risk for infection, but assumed most guys were negative. And, because he rarely was the receiver during anal sex, he figured he might as well enjoy himself when it happened. Now almost 30 years old, Will told Danny, his therapist at an HIV mental health clinic, that he wanted to make some life changes. He missed being married and wanted to meet someone and fall in love again. After taking a sex history. Danny suggested he find a "sex addiction" group and gave him Michael's number.

OCSB Screening Procedure: Motivation for Change

In his phone conversation with Michael, Will disclosed his recent HIV-positive test results and how Danny recommended the appointment. They agreed to meet for a one-time consultation to discuss his situation and determine whether an OCSB assessment was indicated.

MICHAEL: I know Danny suggested you call for an appointment, but I was curious about what interested you in meeting with me.

WILL: Well, Danny thought it would be a good idea. He thought I might be a sex addict and said you could talk with me and decide whether I needed some help with stopping my sexual behavior.

MICHAEL: How is your health, how are you doing?

WILL: I started my HIV meds. All of my test results are moving in the right direction. But, I have no interest in sex. I can't imagine having sex right now. I feel like I put sex away for a while.

MICHAEL: So, you started HIV meds and your health is improving, but you have lost interest in sex. I'm curious, if you are not interested in sex, why meet a specialist in out of control sexual behavior?

WILL: Danny said I might be a sex addict and that this would be a good time to check that out.

MICHAEL: Well, what do you think? What concerns you about your sexual behavior?

(*Will reviews his sex history, his patterns of anonymous intercourse with men, condomless receptive anal sex after drinking, and his belief that his behavior would stop after his divorce and coming out. He indicates that he is motivated to fall in love and find a long-term relationship. They also review the remaining screening criteria. Michael has initial concerns about depressive symptoms and alcohol abuse.*)

MICHAEL: Let's go back to the question we started with. I hear what concerned you before you tested positive, what is it that concerns you now?

WILL: Well, nothing right now. I am not on Grindr anymore. I am a little worried I'll start going back on again. But, for right now, I can't even think about sex. My mind starts racing at the thought of telling guys that I am positive, or using condoms, or whatever. So, I'm taking a break and I'm okay with that. I guess I'm not sure what concerns me right now. I mainly came to talk because Danny suggested it.

MICHAEL: OK, what I'm hearing you say is that currently, you don't feel sexually out of control? You are already working with Danny who can help you adjust to living with HIV and depression. I'm concerned that I'd be duplicating services if we proceeded with OCSB assessment and/or treatment. Let's hold off on scheduling the first assessment appointment until I talk with your therapist. I'll let him know about the OCSB assessment process and talk with him about his reasons for recommending a screening appointment.

Michael reviewed Will's screening appointment with Danny. He described the OCSB assessment process and the combined group and individual outpatient treatment program. Danny discussed Will's adjustment to living with HIV and the emerging loss of interest in sex. They both agreed Will did not have sufficient motivation or current symptoms to begin an OCSB assessment.

Eighteen months later, Will called Michael to schedule an appointment. Will felt his sexual behavior was out of control and reported to

Danny that he was once again having frequent and anonymous sex with other men. He was beginning to put together in his own mind that becoming positive was not going to change his sexual behavior and decided he wanted help.

OCSB Assessment Plan: Minority Stress

Will endorsed five of the 10 items on the Adverse Childhood Experiences (ACE) Study questionnaire. His weekly SSAS scores fluctuated between the high 20s and low 30s (out of a possible 48) throughout the 8-week assessment. Will felt daily intense urge states between appointments that were accompanied by high anticipatory excitement when imagining sex or just prior to an anonymous encounter. His pleasure during the actual sexual behavior/situation decreased with each passing week. Will spoke of his increasing dissatisfaction with the limited role of being the object for a stranger. His sexual life was a disappointing cycle and he remained unsettled about condomless anal sex.

> WILL: I gave myself a one on item 10. ("On average, how much excitement and pleasure did you feel when you engaged in problematic sexual behaviors? If you did not actually engage in such behaviors, please estimate how much excitement and pleasure you would have experienced, if you had.") I have this idea in my head that somehow this time it will really be hot, but more and more, when I actually meet up with a guy, it is almost boring. I play the role of this masculine Black top, but it doesn't do much for me.

> MICHAEL: You scored a "3" in anticipatory excitement, but your actual excitement and pleasure is decreasing. How do you understand the decrease?

> WILL: It isn't until I am actually with a guy that I kind of get that this is more about him than me. I guess I'm hoping someone will be interested in what gets me off, but it just seems like the guys I hook up with are pretty much into the scene we set up. Then I just go ahead with it even though I am not into it.

> MICHAEL: What is the "it" you go ahead with?

> WILL: Being the top. And, I still only put a condom on if they want me to. I tell them that I'm positive and

undetectable, but I'm still not sure I am OK with barebacking. I just don't know.

MICHAEL: It sounds like things are starting to change for you. You sound more present, a bit more self-aware in these sexual situations. Can you tell me more about what you it's like for you to continue having sex even though you're not into it?

WILL: I feel too guilty to just leave. I just can't imagine ending it without giving him what he wants. So I get him off as soon as possible so I can get out of there. (*pauses, sits quietly for a moment*)

MICHAEL: Your voice got a bit louder just now and your face looked like you were starting to feel something.

WILL: I was feeling embarrassed that I have to get a guy to cum in order to stop sex I'm not into. It sounds pretty pathetic.

MICHAEL: What does your body feel like when you're embarrassed?

WILL: My face is warm. As soon as I said it, all I could think about was what this might sound like to you. Then I told myself that you have heard it all, but I still felt embarrassed. I remembered I hooked up with this guy and I could not get hard. He was not going to cum until I fucked him. I stayed for like an hour or more. I didn't think I could just leave. Finally, he said he was done. I felt so embarrassed. Man, I don't want to do that anymore.

MICHAEL: What don't you want anymore?

WILL: I don't want to stay and have sex with someone just because I don't know how to leave. I guess I never really thought about what this does to me.

MICHAEL: What does it do to you?

WILL: Well, I don't know how to say it...

MICHAEL: Take your time. Take a breath if that will help.

WILL: (*He takes a breath and looks up at Michael.*) I don't want to start a confrontation, to deal with their shit about a

Black guy looking upset or mad. I have to deal with that all the time. I know the look, when all of a sudden they see me as this scary Black guy. (*voice raised, eyes watering, fists clenched, looking away at the wall*) I hate that, and I hate it when I have to deal with that from a guy I'm having sex with. I just go through with it and get out of there. (*pauses, he looks down*) That's what it does to me.

MICHAEL: What are you feeling now?

WILL: Tired. And angry. Having to always take care of White guys so they don't get worried about some angry Black man. I was always worried about being the target of the guys I grew up around. Worried they would know I was gay. I thought it would be better when I was around other gay guys. But, instead of being able to relax, I have to worry about them being scared of me.

MICHAEL: What is it like for you to show your anger with me right now?

WILL: You know, I was wondering about that. I guess I didn't see that look on your face that I was going to have to calm down.

Race-related distress may be an important assessment topic to consider as a factor to recognize and explore as an influence on sexual behavior. "Examining the immediate distress elicited by racial microaggression experiences may allow health researchers and health professionals to more fully understand the distress evoked by these seemingly mild, but recurrent forms of racism" (Torres-Harding & Turner, 2014, p. 23). Within the Racial Microaggression Scale, Torres-Harding and Turner (2014) examined six distress microaggression experiences subscales. They include:

1. Perceived as foreigner
2. Likely to engage in criminal activity
3. Low achieving or undesirable
4. Sexually stereotyped by race
5. Absence of people from their racial heritage in environments
6. Being invisible, overlooked, or contributions dismissed based on racial heritage

Clients may be unaware of the interplay between their race-related distress and their sexual behavior. Motivations to manage this distress may have sexual expressions that influence their self- and attachment regulation or generate erotic conflicts. Michael postulated that managing chronic racial microagressions was connected to Will's ego depletion and subsequent willpower failures. As Will became more open and aware of the energy spent managing minority stress, he clarified his vision of sexual health and started asserting his sexual interests more with his partners.

Attachment Regulation: Needs Assertion

WILL: I crossed one of my boundaries. I wanted to say it before group got into something and before I would talk myself out of saying it. We can talk about it later in the group.

DOUG: How is it for the group to have Will let us know what he needs from us?

HECTOR: Wow, I am impressed. I crossed my boundaries when I was first in the group and came for a few sessions before I was honest. I am glad you told us.

BRENT: I agree. Why did you want to tell us right away?

DOUG: Will, I know you asked to not start the group with talking about your boundary crossing. Brent is interested in your decision to follow the group agreement. How will it be for you to talk about your choice to keep the group agreement now and we can return to the details of your sexual behavior later?

WILL: I didn't really think about not telling the group. I just don't want to jump right into talking about what happened.

BRENT: So, what made you decide to want to tell us right away?

WILL: I just thought I better get it over with.

DOUG: (interrupting) That's the same sentence you told us that you say to yourself when you are having sex with a guy you are not into.

WILL: What?

DOUG: I just noticed that the same thought you had about keeping the group agreement is the same thought you have when you want to leave a sexual situation that you're not sexually excited about. "I just want to get it over with."

GIL: It's funny to hear Doug say that, I thought the same thing. I thought maybe the group is like one of your tricks; you just want to get out of here. (*The group shares a laugh.*)

WILL: It's a phrase I use a lot. When I want to do something, it helps me get motivated. Just hurry up and do it, get it over with.

DOUG: What was the "it" you were trying to get over by telling the group right away about your boundary crossing?

WILL: Well, I wanted to tell the group. But, sometimes I get tired and didn't want to change my mind.

BRENT: Now you're answering my question. You told us about your sexual health plan boundary crossing before you got tired.

WILL: I guess that's it. Sounds different when you say it. It sounds kind of pathetic.

BRENT: Ouch, that was harsh.

WILL: I don't know, I do get tired, but it seems like a cop out. Like I'm complaining.

DOUG: What's your objection to telling the group you get tired?

WILL: It sounds weak.

ELLIOT: I think the same way. I have a hard time saying I get tired. It might mean something about my HIV, like my drugs aren't working and I might have to change them. Or that people might think I was having sex all night and lying about it. I've been keeping my boundaries for a while, but I think people won't believe me.

MANISH: If I mention I'm tired, I worry my bipolar meds aren't working. Sometimes I don't tell my psychiatrist about it because I don't want him to mess with my meds.

DOUG: The group seems to identify with what Will is saying about himself. There seems to be common worries about how others will perceive you if you express feeling tired.

WILL: I just flashed on something I haven't thought about for a long time. Oh, man, I am not sure I want to say it . . .

DOUG: Will, like earlier, whatever you share is up to you. You're not obligated to tell us what you thought right now.

WILL: It's OK. It was about my mom's boyfriend Ralph. The guy who molested me in middle school. When I came home from school. I was in sixth grade in a new school. I was one of the only Black kids enrolled. I came home and told him about how a couple of White kids called me names and pushed me. I told Ralph about it when I got home. He asked me if I needed a hug. He asked me to follow him into the basement, which we had done before. But, this time he took his clothes off.

DOUG: Help me understand what happened in group right now that triggered this memory?

WILL: I was just thinking about what I said earlier. "To get it over with." I had that same thought when I was in the basement. (*His voice sounds angry and his fists are clenched.*)

DOUG: You had had a difficult day at school. You went home to an adult whom you thought would understand, which is what we encourage adolescents to do when they are being harassed. And, you were being targeted because of your race and went to a Black adult for support. But, he exploited and assaulted you. I image that would make talking about your needs more difficult in the future. Sounds like you have been dealing with this bind since you were a teenager.

WILL: It's true. I was looking for someone who had been through it. Then he just went and made it worse than I could ever imagine.

In OCSB groups, much can be learned through processing men's choice to keep the group agreement before prematurely focusing on the specifics of their sexual behaviors. The group supported Will in directing what he wanted to talk about by asserting a relationship boundary. The leader focused on Will keeping the group agreement while inviting exploration of his strength in keeping the agreement. The there/then discussion of the SHP boundary crossing could wait until Will had sufficient energy to discuss the details of this behavior. Out of control sexual symptoms are not assumed to be a crisis in an OCSB group; not keeping the group agreement is a more urgent matter.

In this early group interaction, Will set the stage to address several key aspects of his treatment plan. The group was a space where race and race-based microaggressions (both past and present) were met with empathy and curiosity. Will began to identify how he developed defenses that restricted his impulse to reach out to others for comfort when faced with racism. In the group, Will practiced needs assertion within nonsexual relationships and slowly developed less avoidant patterns for self-soothing. His incremental improvement in needs assertion with the group transferred into assertiveness with his sexual partners. Will frequently discussed the minority stress he experienced related to race, sexual identity, and HIV status. The group expanded their empathy for how minority microaggression experiences impacted sexual health and wellness.

Erotic Conflict: Condomless Sex

Will consistently maintained his sexual health plan boundaries after 6 months in group. He was now preparing to disclose his HIV status with friends and family. He took a "sabbatical" from church until he could better understand what was realistic to expect from this community. Although he consistently followed his depression medication prescription, he disclosed to the group that he was inconsistent with HIV medication. He decided that he wanted to be accountable to the group when he did not take his daily prescription for HIV treatment and added HIV medication adherence to his Boundary column. His partnered sexual behavior was with men he met online or through social apps, primarily during off-work hours. He had not crossed his workplace boundary since beginning group.

After a year of group, Will turned his treatment focus to learning more about his range of sexual turn-ons and erotic desires. He liked being sexually versatile, being both the insertive and receptive partner during anal intercourse. Condomless sex continually surfaced as an area of competing motivations and intermittent boundary crossing. A clarity began to emerge for Will that connected pleasurable sex with condomless sex. The meaning of condomless sex is an important narrative to consider in OCSB treatment. Bauermeister, Carballo-Diéguez, Ventuneac, and Dolezal (2009) developed a decisional balance scale to measure motivations for men to bareback (anal sex without a condom, usually ejaculating inside the partner). Their findings suggest that condomless sex is a source of coping with racism, homophobia, and loneliness, as well as a source of intimacy and pleasure. The results of Fernández-Dávila's (2009) research examining motivations for condomless anal sex between men found participants' motivation for safety competed with their sexual and nonsexual motivations. The motivations among the study participants include seeking reaffirmation of personal worth or physical attractiveness, to regulate feelings of loneliness and disconnection, being in love, a conversion of the risky behavior into the pleasure of the forbidden, and a desire to rebel against perceived rules. In certain situations, condoms represent a threat to completing the sexual encounter and fulfilling the outcomes that either consciously or unconsciously motivated the experience. How might a gay men's OCSB group leader facilitate the emotional activating reactions of group members exploring competing motivations between the sexual health principles of pleasure and STI/HIV protection?

WILL: I have been seeing a guy for about a month now. His name is Nicholas. We are both positive and want to have sex without condoms. I want to change my sexual health plan so that having sex without a condom is not a boundary crossing. I'm excited because we are both versatile. Our health is good. He knows I am in this group and he has his own therapist, which helps. We have talked about not using condoms, but I told him I needed to talk with you guys about it because it means changing my plan.

BRENT: Was it hard to wait?

WILL: We really wanted to ditch the condoms this weekend, but I said, "You know, it's important that I do this." I didn't want to come into group and have to talk about a boundary crossing. Frankly, I was surprised that I could regulate myself like that, but I realized that this wasn't a "sex emergency" that I wanted to wait until I talked to you guys. So, that's why I brought it up. It wasn't as hard to wait as I thought it would be.

BRENT: What do you want from us?

WILL: Well, I just wanted to talk about it here, to see what the group thought.

DOUG: Will, a way to think about Brent's question is to see whether you are seeking the group's approval. Or perhaps you want a dialogue to explore what this change means to you? Sex without condoms has meaning well beyond your sexual health plan boundary. I assume other men in the group have thoughts and feelings about what condomless sex means for them.

WILL: I don't want the group's approval. It's more like I needed a place to talk about it privately, where I can think about the decision without having to immediately get concerned about what Nicholas thinks. I think the group can help me think about what this decision is about for me.

DOUG: Is there someone in the group you would like to ask?

WILL: Well, Brent, you're positive. What does it mean to you when you have sex without a condom?

BRENT: I wish I had thought about it as much as you think I have. Just listening to you has made me wonder if I even know for myself. I know what I liked the most. But, I am primarily a bottom, so for me it is all mixed up with crystal meth, HIV, and being a bottom. It has taken me a while to have sex without thinking about crystal or fantasizing about using when I masturbate. To think about what barebacking means, well, it will take me a while to think about that.

GIL: I have a different take. I've never liked using condoms. They interrupt the flow. I have to stop what I'm doing, open the wrapper, which is hard to do when my hands have lube on them. It is not always easy to put it on without losing my erection. And when I have it on, it doesn't feel right and I lose my erection. So, there have been times where a guy is so hot and he doesn't care about the condom. I think, "if he doesn't care, I don't care." I'd rather have sex being hard than risk ruining the moment fumbling with a condom.

ELLIOT: I get why you want to stop using condoms with Nicholas. I have the same goal when I'm in a committed relationship. Besides not wanting to have to deal with condoms

DOUG: in the moment, like Gil said, I feel closer to my boyfriend when I have sex without condoms. There's something about skin to skin that feels more intimate than skin to latex to skin. Plus, I don't want to have to think about HIV when I'm trying to be intimate. I just want to enjoy the moment.

DOUG: Will, what are you hearing from the group that resonates with you?

WILL: This might sound strange, but I am thinking about church. I was remembering a sermon I heard in 2008 during the Prop 8 campaign against gay marriage. The preacher was railing against the gay community. I looked over at my Mom and saw the face she gets when she is feeling really connected. It was like Jesus was speaking through my preacher and my Mom was listening. I felt so alone; like I belonged somewhere else and yet this was home. Listening to you guys makes it so clear about what I've been missing at church and in my family. It's a place to feel connected and not be judged. Like we are in this together. So I get it. I liked hearing how both Gil and Elliot took time to understand their sexual behavior without automatically thinking it was wrong or sick. It's so hard to not to hear that preacher's voice in my head. I think there is still a part of me that believes HIV is a punishment. The condom is like a symbol of being immoral, to cover my sin. That's why I want to change my boundary, just see what it is like to give myself permission to not wear a condom and be honest about living with HIV. That's my new sexual health plan boundary.

Will continued to explore his erotic interests in the ensuing months. He discussed his attraction to White men and realized he judged himself about this erotic preference in much the way he judged White men who were into Black guys. Will practiced revealing his diverse sexual interests with the group, which led to unraveling the political, racial, and religious narratives contained in the use of a condom and processing the internalized shame that inhibited his sexual intimacy with his boyfriend. Each time he disclosed details of his erotic orientation, he found new ways to decouple his shame from his sexual and erotic desires. Much to his delight, Will's primary focus during sex ceased to be "just get through it."

Will attended group for approximately 3 years and continued individual therapy with Michael for another year.

REFERENCES

Bauermeister, J. A., Carballo-Diéguez, A., Ventuneac, A., & Dolezal, C. (2009). Assessing motivations to engage in intentional condomless anal intercourse in HIV-risk contexts ("bareback sex") among men who have sex with men. *AIDS Education and Prevention: Official Publication of The International Society for AIDS Education, 21*(2), 156.

Fernández-Dávila, P. (2009). The non-sexual needs of men that motivate them to engage in high-risk sexual practices with other men. Forum: Qualitative Social Research, *10*(2), Art. 21. Available at http://nbn-resolving.de/urn:nbn:de:0114-fqs0902219.

Koukounas, E., & McCabe, M. (1997). Sexual and emotional variables influencing sexual response to erotica. *Behavior Research and Therapy, 35*, 221–231.

Lamb, S. (1996). *The trouble with blame: Victims, perpetrators & responsibility.* Cambridge, MA: Harvard University Press.

Le, T., Wright, E. J., Smith, D. M., He, W., Catano, G., Okulicz, J. F., … Ahuja, S. K. (2013). Enhanced CD4+ T-cell recovery with earlier HIV-1 antiretroviral therapy. *New England Journal of Medicine, 368*(3), 218–230.

Loewenstein, G., & O'Donoghue, T. (2007). *The heat of the moment: Modeling interactions between affect and deliberation.* Unpublished manuscript. Retrieved from https://odonoghue.economics.cornell.edu/heat.pdf

McNulty, J. K., & Widman, L. (2013). The implications of sexual narcissism for sexual and marital satisfaction. *Archives of Sexual Behavior, 42*(6), 1021–1032.

Morin, J. (2010). *Anal pleasure & health: A guide for men, women, and couples.* Burlingame, CA: Down There Press.

Torres-Harding, S., & Turner, T. (2014). Assessing racial microaggression distress in a diverse sample. *Evaluation & the Health Professions,* pp. 1–27. Advance online publication. Available at http://ehp.sagepub.com/content/early/2014/09/16/0163278714550860

Tybur, J. M., Lieberman, D., & Griskevicus, V. (2009). Microbes, mating, and morality: Individual differences in three functional domains of disgust. *Journal of Personality and Social Psychology, 97*(1), 103–122.

Vonderheide, S. G., & Mosher, D. L. (1988). Should I put in my diaphragm? Sex-guilt and turn-offs. *Journal of Psychology and Human Sexuality, 1*, 97–111.

Sexual Health Group Therapy for Men*

GROUP THERAPY COMMITMENTS AND GUIDELINES

Welcome to Sexual Health Group Therapy for Men. This form provides a brief description of the commitments and guidelines of group membership, which were developed to maintain group therapeutic value and integrity and serve the needs of every member. Consequently, these commitments and guidelines support both individuals and the whole group. We hope that all group members will feel free to discuss these expectations within the group itself. We also welcome any ideas and suggestions that will help the group work together more productively.

Attendance Commitment
- Group members are expected to be present each week, arrive on time, and remain throughout the entire session.
- Group members are expected to announce planned absences during a group prior to the absence.
- Group members are expected to leave a voicemail with a group leader on the day of an unplanned absence from group.

Financial Commitment
- Group members are fully responsible for their bills. Payment is due monthly, at the first group session of the month. Monthly payment includes all group sessions for the upcoming month.
- The fee for group participation is $50.00 per session.

---

*The guidelines for both the heterosexual and gay men's group are the same; we have not included orientation in these guideline titles.

- Group members are charged for their place in the group and are required to pay for any missed sessions. Two uncharged absences are allowed for each 6 months of group participation.

Group Participation Commitment

- Group members are expected to create goals for group treatment during their assessments.
- Group members are expected, as agreed upon during their assessment, to share their treatment goals and sexual health plan with the group.
- Group members are expected to create and follow a written sexual health plan. Members are expected to disclose when they cross the boundaries listed in their sexual health plan during the next group session.
- Upon entering the group, members are expected to remain in the group for a minimum of 6 months. At the end of the first 6 months, group members may remain in the group until their treatment goals are achieved.
- Group members are expected to receive concurrent individual psychotherapy with a psychotherapist of their choice (one session per month at minimum) during the entirety of their group participation.
- Group members are expected to discuss with the group any changes in their treatment plan or sexual health plan prior to acting on them.
- Group members are expected to not eat, drink, or smoke during group sessions.
- Group members are expected to be as honest as possible during group discussions.
- Group members are expected to express feelings, ideas, and opinions in a manner that maintains the physical and personal safety of all members.
- Group members are expected to discuss within the group any contact among group members outside of the group sessions.
- Group members are expected not to engage in sexual, dating, or business relationships with other group members.
- Group members are expected to give the group a minimum three (3) sessions notice prior to ending their group participation.

Confidentiality Commitment

- Group members are expected to protect the names and identities of fellow group members. Please be advised, confidentiality in group therapy cannot be guaranteed because the members are not held to the same legal and ethical expectation as the group leaders. However, prior to entering the group, each group member is informed of the importance of confidentiality and has agreed to the confidentiality expectation.

- The law protects the privacy of the majority of the communication between group members and leaders. In most situations, the group leaders can only release information about a member's participation to others if the member signs a written authorization form that meets certain legal requirements imposed by state law and/or Health Insurance Portability and Accountability Act (HIPAA) guidelines. There are, however, important exceptions in which the leaders are required or permitted to disclose information about a member without either his consent or authorization. The following list provides an overview of the relevant exceptions:
  1. A group leader must notify the intended victim and the appropriate law enforcement agencies if he judges that a group member has an intention to cause grave harm or death to another individual.
  2. If a group member's mental or emotional condition is assessed as dangerous to the member or the property of others, the group leader may disclose confidential information if it's determined disclosure is necessary to prevent the threatened danger.
  3. A group leader must report any suspicion of child abuse or sexual abuse to protect the child/children involved.
  4. A group leader must report the witnessing of domestic violence by minor children, even if the children themselves are not physically harmed.
  5. A group leader must report any suspected abuse, neglect, or sexual abuse of an elderly person or dependent adult to protect the elderly person or dependent adult involved.
  6. In cases of alleged criminal or civil liability, a group leader may be court ordered to release treatment information and/or records. If a group member files a complaint or lawsuit against one or both of the leaders, relevant information regarding that member may be disclosed in the defense of the leader(s).
  7. A group leader may determine it clinically necessary to discuss some aspects of your psychotherapy with another qualified professional in order to further treatment goals. If a leader seeks such a consultation, neither the group member's name nor any identifying information will be communicated.
  8. A group leader may release a member's name for collections processing. However, no treatment-related information will accompany the disclosure.

9. If a group member files a worker's compensation claim, a group leader must, on appropriate request, disclose the information relevant to the claimant's condition to the worker's compensation insurer.

General Guidelines for Successful Group Therapy

- Group therapy is most successful when group members encourage participation of everyone during group discussions. However, group members are free to talk or not talk during group sessions.
- Group therapy is most successful when group members discuss major life decision with the group prior to acting on them.
- Group therapy is most successful when group members develop and manage their relationships with other group members in a manner that is therapeutic and supportive of each member's treatment goals.

Consent for Treatment

Before signing this form, make sure that all of your questions and concerns have been addressed. Your signature indicates that you understand the following:

- All of the commitments and expectations described here.
- (Names of group coleaders) agree to follow the group leader commitments and expectations.
- You are voluntarily consenting to and authorizing (names of group coleaders) to provide group psychotherapy services.

Name of Group Member	Signature of Group Member	Date
Name of Group Coleader	Signature of Group Leader	Date
Name of Group Coleader	Signature of Group Leader	Date

INDEX

Printed in the United States
By Bookmasters